MW00826227

A WOMAN'S GUIDE TO HER BODY AND HER TOTAL HEALTH

Barbara Entsuah. MD, MHSc. Fellow GCPS

(Board Certified In Family Medicine USA)

Reviews

"When I was 20 years old about to marry, my mother gave me the *Betty Crocker Cookbook.* It was the "American Bible" for cooking. My copy is so loved that the cover is taped together, the pages scribbled on and many well used pages have lost their binding. *A Woman's Guide to Her Body and Her Total Health* is an International "Bible" for women's health. I looked at this book with my own personal health in mind and found suggestions to alleviate several systemic issues. I viewed it from the eyes of my daughters and I want them to know this information. I scrutinized it as an Executive Director of a nonprofit organization working to educate women in developing nations on health issues often treated as a curse instead of a disease or one that can be prevented. In the end of my examination I found the information presented in this book is relevant to every woman regardless of age, race, or social economic status. I applaud you, Dr. Entsuah, for creating a well needed reference for women's health."

— Ms. Deborah Frock, Founder/Executive Director
Ghanaian Mothers Hope Inc., Florida, USA

"As I read through the pages of this book, *A Woman's Guide to Her Body and Her Total Health,* I knew that it was a book which I would not only keep close by to make reference from time to time, but also a book which I would recommend to many ladies – especially "lay people" (like me). Dr Barbara Entsuah seems to have covered every possible condition, especially those affecting women and to me she has succeeded in her aim to help women have a better understanding of medical conditions they have been diagnosed with or symptoms they may be experiencing. The language used is not complicated and can be easily grasped by a non-medical person.

The World Health Organization (WHO) has defined health as "a state of complete physical, mental and social wellbeing and not merely the absence of disease or infirmity". Dr Entsuah, knowing and recognizing the beneficial effects of a healthy soul and spirit on the body, also prescribes effective remedies for the soul and spirit thereby supporting the WHO definition of health. I found the layout of the book helpful – health from a global view and the types and practices of medicine; understanding medicines and why we take them and the various systems in the body and diseases associated with each system.It is clear that Dr. Entsuah is passionate about the fact that women should take charge of their health and with this informative book, women can appreciate to a greater extent the way their bodies work and become more knowledgeable, for as the old saying goes, "Knowledge is power". I want to congratulate Dr. Entsuah on writing this book and pray that many women may read it, find it useful, and be blessed by it.

— Rachel Baddoo, Esq. (Barrister at Law)
Chair, Board of International Needs Ghana
Board, Great Commission Movement Ghana

TAKE CHARGE OF YOUR HEALTH

By

Keeping a Healthy Body, Soul and Spirit

That is your right and responsibility

This book is not meant to replace Physical examination and diagnosis by a qualified health provider. It is to help you have a better understanding of medical conditions you may have been diagnosed with or symptoms you may be experiencing. It teaches among other things how to treat minor illnesses like common cold, allergies etc. at home for symptom relief; and the need to see a health professional if there is no improvement after a few days. New scientific information is continually emerging and recommended treatments and tests are always changing in medicine. I have tried to provide the most accurate and current information present at time of publication. This is just a guide and neither me, or my publishers are responsible for errors or consequences resulting from application of any part of the book by a reader in your quest to live a healthy life. It is to encourage you to have the necessary information in order to have a meaningful visit when you go to see your health care provider. Regular visits and communications with your health care provider for all your ongoing medical problems cannot be replaced by anything else.

Books are available at special discounts when purchased in bulk for premiums and sales promotions as well as for fund-raising or educational use. For details, contact us at barbara.entsuah@gmail.com.

Author photograph: South Lake Hospital/Orlando Health

Book Cover Design by Amma Aboagye, Founding Curator of The Afropole
Cover Pictures: We acknowledge the following:
1. Women drinking water from DAPA Images
2. Woman stretching on yoga ball in gym from Getty Images Pro
3. Women praying for each other by pixelheadphoto from Getty Images Pro
4. Gym doctor with a patient checking her ankle from Latino Life

Diagrams: Produced by Adotstudio (Fiverr) and others mentioned in text

Typeset in India by Imprint Digital Ltd

Dedication

First and foremost to God my Father and his Son, Christ Jesus, my Lord and Savior, my mentor, advisor, and encourager who provided the grace and wisdom needed to write this book.

In loving memory of my late parents, Isaac Amoo-Lamptey (Esq.) and Mary Amoo-Lamptey, who encouraged me to study Medicine.

To my husband, Jojo Entsuah, who patiently encouraged me to fulfill my dreams and aspirations.

To my Family Medicine Residency Program 'In His Image', where I learnt how to practice whole person medicine – bringing healing to Body, Soul and Spirit.

Her Unique Body

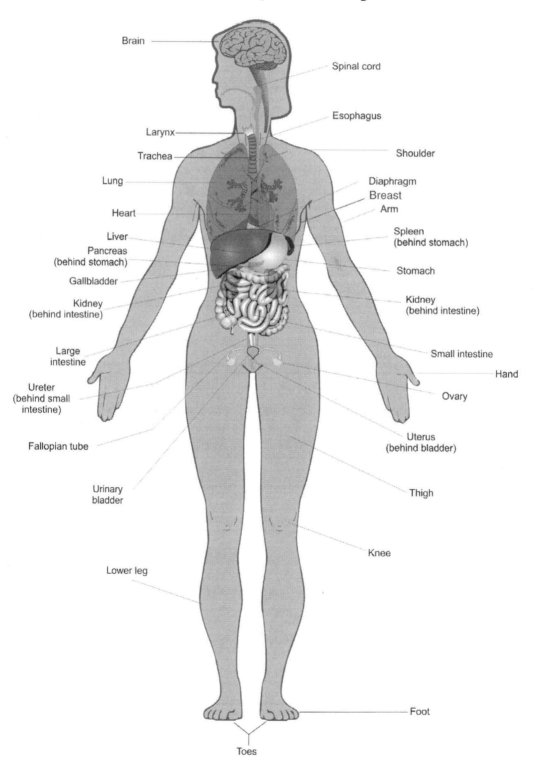

Brain

Spinal cord

Esophagus

Larynx

Trachea

Shoulder

Lung

Diaphragm
Breast
Arm

Heart

Spleen
(behind stomach)

Liver

Pancreas
(behind stomach)

Stomach

Gallbladder

Kidney
(behind intestine)

Kidney
(behind intestine)

Large
intestine

Small intestine

Ureter
(behind small
intestine)

Hand

Ovary

Fallopian tube

Uterus
(behind bladder)

Urinary
bladder

Thigh

Knee

Lower leg

Foot

Toes

Contents

PART FIVE

Foreword

Dr. Barbara Entsuah has written a very comprehensive guide to a woman's body, encompassing physical, spiritual, and mental health. The format is easy to read for the lay person. The advice given is well thought out and thoroughly researched. Although this book provides detailed self-help instructions for various ailments, Dr. Entsuah makes it clear that her intent is to supplement and not replace regular care by your physician.

It has been my privilege to practice in the clinic alongside Dr. Entsuah and to observe her work in other medical settings. I remain impressed at the broad scope of her medical knowledge and the compassion with which she treats each patient. Whether in an office setting in Florida, or on the mission field in Africa, she serves each patient with excellence and commitment. I attribute her excellence as a physician to her extensive training and practice on multiple continents, in several different countries and in a variety of practice settings. Even more than that, I attribute her excellence to the calling and Hand of the Lord on her life. Dr. Entsuah is one of those people whom God called to be a doctor from the foundation of the world. She has embraced this calling with all her heart, mind and soul.

The book that you are about to read is an outpouring of her many years of experience, and of her heartfelt desire to use her calling as a physician to help as many people as possible. You will find it both practical and comprehensive in scope. Although she may have never met you, Dr. Entsuah has written this book with you in mind.

Vivian J Woodard, M.D.
Medical Director, Emmanuel Christian Health Center

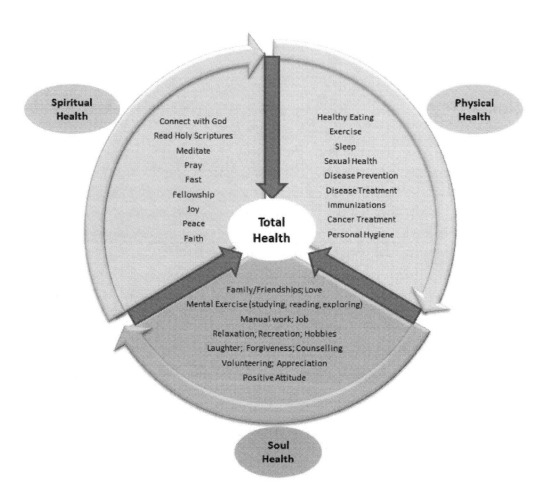

Preface

"Employ your time in improving yourself by other men's writing so that you shall come easily by what others have labored hard for." Socrates

This book is primarily for women everywhere, in developed and developing countries alike. It aims at helping women understand how their bodies work so they can manage their health more effectively. A girl starts becoming a woman through a process called puberty. By sixteen years or thereabout she would have developed into a young woman. Women have unique health challenges and certain medical conditions which are prominent in their lives. Sexuality, fertility, childbirth and menopause are all part of being female. The changes that continue to take place in the body (physiological and anatomical) and what causes these changes must be understood by every woman: young, middle-aged and seniors.

My extensive practice as a Medical Doctor in both Africa (Ghana & Liberia) and North America (Canada & USA) over these three decades have made me realize that "Practice reaps valuable observations." Some of my most fascinating medical experiences have been my involvement in medical missions with Gateway of Hope, a non-profit founded by my husband and I. We partner with women's groups, churches, medical personnel, non-governmental organizations, along with donations from friends, family, colleagues, and church members to provide free medical clinics in poor urban centers and rural areas in Ghana.

Since 2000, I have undertaken medical missions to over 36 different communities in Ghana. Making a difference depends on one's perspective. Free medical clinics meet a present need, whether acute or chronic and do contribute to addressing health challenges, however temporary. Education about chronic diseases and referrals to clinics are made for continuity of care. We do clinical breast exams and teach breast self-examinations, and have lately added cervical cancer screening to our medical mission work.

In the span of three weeks, our team sees hundreds of patients with medical conditions of all levels of severity. We also do a lot of health education for women in churches and communities. For adolescents, we focus on interactive sexual health education presentations in high schools (especially all-girls' high schools) teaching students that they can achieve their dreams and aspirations through education, and so they can postpone sexually active until later.

My extensive work with high school students brought me face to face with the stark reality: the extent of sexual abuse and the challenges, coupled with increased vulnerability these young people face. My response was to equip them with information that will help them avoid or manage these challenges, which I have carefully elaborated in three books I have written on sexual abuse: *The Dawning of a New Day*, *A Parental Guide on Teaching Children How to Avoid Abuse* and *Young People's Guide to Personal Safety*.

The first book helps victims of sexual abuse to recover and move on with their lives; the second book equips guardians and parents to teach their children to avoid sexual abuse, and the third book, targeting elementary and middle school students teaches safety at home, at school, and in one's neighborhood. In addition, I have written several newspaper articles in news print and on line for readership on chronic medical conditions, child sexual abuse and cancer prevention.

In my community in Florida where I live and practice medicine, I have organized health fairs in conjunction with church and nonprofit organizations. I also give presentations at my local church on the importance of screening for breast cancer and offer free medical care to low income families.

If medical practice were an experiment one would wonder why there doesn't seem to be a major significant rise in patient knowledge while the count goes up? Why do I say this? Because of the blank stare and awkward moments I encounter when a patient is unable to name medications they have been taking for years or to adequately communicate a health condition they have been battling for a while. This scenario is of course more prevalent in developing countries. However, there are also many women in North America, both average and well educated with the same attitude because they cannot be bothered, underestimate their own abilities or just lazy.

But patients are not to blame alone. Some doctors create the impression that our bodies and medical terms are so complex the lay person may not be able to understand it, even though there are simplified explanations about various medical conditions. Rethinking and addressing this challenge to help women manage their health is also the subject of this book.

What are the global trends in women's health that every woman should be aware of? Which diseases have been identified to affect women in the future? How do you navigate the vast field of different practices of medicine in the world? Where should you go and who should you consult? Part 1 addresses these questions.

Your physical body is important because it is the instrument by which you carry out your passion, pursuit and purpose. You cannot accomplish anything without your physical body. That is why it is important to acquire the necessary information and skills to listen to its needs and respond by improving the functions of its systems and organs with appropriate food, exercise, and medication regimen supported by a good healthcare provider. Understanding how your body works and the underlying physiological (body) changes, common diseases, and treatment requires committing to some basic science education, which is covered in Part 2.

Learn how to take simple steps to avoid problems with your medicines and supplements and the important role of pharmacists and health systems in preventing medication errors in Part 3.

What good is a great car without a driver? How beneficial is a great body without a sound mind? Your body thrives when your mind is sound and peaceful. Mental health and spiritual health work together to make you happy and fulfilled. So Part 4 is devoted to mental and spiritual health.

This book is for you if you

Want to know more about the physiology of a woman's body and its relation to mental and spiritual health to help you create balance in your life

Need a quick reference about common diseases which affect women and how to treat them

Want to know how to diagnose and improve your mental health as a woman

Acquire basic understanding of your medication (prescription or countertop or supplements), interactions and side effects

Want to improve your relationship with God to boost your spiritual health

Wanting to make a difference in people's lives

This book has been reviewed by other practicing physicians and healthcare providers and it is written in easy and clear to understand language. You can read the book both as a whole and as individual chapters when a situation or need arises. The scientific or medical name of a health condition or disease is always attached so you will know the name and be familiar with it. The benefit of having a readily available information and using it to manage your overall health cannot be overemphasized. However, since not all health conditions can be covered, do well to look up for more information on a condition in the references used, on the internet, or other credible medical books to broaden your knowledge. An informed patient is a more compliant patient.

Studies and References used in this book

....

You will notice that throughout the book, the references and studies or research results associated with various medical conditions will be cited for your reference to give you the opportunity to validate the statements I make here. No one should be intimidated by inclusions of studies and references because they make you more confident about the information. I present what is based on valid scientific research. In this age of "fake news", there are many health related information being circulated which are not true, but one can have more assurance in those facts coming from scientific reviewed articles or from reputable sources.

Acknowledgements

This book has been over five years in the making. The world of medicine like other fields is ever changing and so over the last few years, I have been constantly updating with the latest research and information available. It has been many hours of researching, corrections and typing and I want to thank my Lord and Savior Jesus Christ who gave me the idea and the grace to write this book. My husband Jojo has been very supportive and read through the earlier manuscripts. I thank you for your patience as I took over the bed to write. I love you. I thank all my children for encouraging and praying with and for me on this journey and helping with some diagrams.

I thank the following physicians in the USA who reviewed the topics which dealt with their specialties: Dr. Anthony Gyang – Gynecology; Dr. Ahmed Al-Hazzouri and Dr. Isaac Odame (Canada) – Hematology/Oncology, Dr. Ken Sampong – Cardiology, Dr. Ernest Asamoah – Endocrinology, and Dr. Eric Boye (UK) who read the medical part of the manuscript and offered useful suggestions. I am grateful to you. My thanks to Mrs. Ohui A. Allotey and Mr. Eli Tetteh for reading through parts of the manuscript, I appreciate your help as always. Thanks to Mrs. Nicole Asher (medical student) who read through the whole manuscript offering helpful suggestions, Nicole you are a gem. Thanks to Mrs. Flora Adjaye who edited and contributed to the first part of the book. My Thanks also to the Late Dr. Vivian Woodard, my colleague, sister in Christ and friend who wrote the foreword. Unfortunately, she transitioned from this world in August 2019. Over the last 15 years we have worked together and prayed together. My Thanks also to my dear friends and prayer partners in my church who supported and prayed for me during this task. Profound thanks also to my friends Rachel Badoe and Debi Frock for writing the reviews for the book, and to Ms. Amma Aboagye for the cover design. Amma, Thanks for your patience.

Layout, editing and typesetting was done by Paul Walker and his team at Imprint Press UK, you guys were great.

May God richly bless all of you for contributing to this book.

Barbara Entsuah MD.

This book promises to provide you with adequate education to help identify the common diseases that affect women, established interventions, nutritional changes, supplement/herbal support, exercises, mental and spiritual practices that can help you optimize your health. Read it so you may be filled with hope.

A life of balance will help you reduce the risk of most diseases; including heart disease, stroke and diabetes, joint and muscular conditions. It will also reduce the symptoms of stress, anxiety and depression, and improve your sense of wellness and mood. Others include improvement in self-esteem, self-confidence, sharpness and clarity of mind, memory, and ability to recover from illness speedily. It will also boost your immune system, and all of these will lead to increase in longevity.

Women are naturally good communicators of information: users and sharers. Therefore equipping a woman with adequate information to help her manage her health has practical benefits for her immediate family, as well as her extended family and social circles.

Every woman can strive towards TOTAL HEALTH by taking charge of her own health by acquiring knowledge, improving self-knowledge and taking actions that will help her achieve this goal.

Killer Diseases in Countries with Limited and Rich Resources

Diseases causing most deaths in middle income (limited resources) countries

....

In limited resource countries, the maximum number of deaths is caused by infectious diseases, like Malaria, Diarrhea, and HIV/AIDS, on the contrary, developed countries are battling with deaths caused by chronic diseases, like Coronary heart disease, Cancers, and Cardiovascular diseases (affecting the heart and vessels). According to WHO (World Health Organization) report published in 2011, the top 20 causes of death in Ghana (a middle income country) are as follows:

1.	Diarrhea
2.	Stroke
3.	Coronary Heart Disease
4.	HIV/AIDS
5.	Influenza & Pneumonia
6.	Tuberculosis
7.	Lung Disease
8.	Malaria
9.	Road traffic accidents
10.	Kidney Disease
11.	Diabetes Mellitus
12.	Other Injuries
13.	Hypertension

14.	Violence
15.	Liver Cancer
16.	Liver Diseases
17.	Breast Cancer
18.	Low Birth Weight
19.	Skin Disease
20.	Asthma

*Source: www.world life expectancy.com; and WHO – 2011 data

In these limited resource countries, it is being noticed that even chronic diseases which are not caused by infections from bacteria or viruses are also prevalent and the cases of these diseases are gradually increasing. This is caused by the changes in society and in the lifestyle of people who are adopting a western world or developed countries cultures.

There is less walking and more riding in cars, less consumption of fresh fruits, vegetables, or natural produce and more stress with less leisure time. People are eating more processed foods, drinking more sugary drinks, smoking tobacco, and using alcoholic beverages. All these contribute to chronic diseases like Heart diseases, Hypertension, Diabetes, Lung diseases, and some Cancers.

Killer diseases causing most deaths in Developed (resource rich) countries

....

According to WHO (World Health Organization) data the top 10 causes of death in high income countries in 2012 are mostly chronic diseases and cancers

| Ischemic heart disease |
| Stroke |
| Cancer of lungs, bronchus, trachea |
| Alzheimer's disease and other dementias |
| Chronic Obstructive Lung Disease |
| Lower Respiratory infections |
| Colon and rectal cancers |
| Diabetes Mellitus |
| Hypertensive heart Disease |
| Breast Cancer |

*(WHO Fact sheet No 310. Updated May 2014)

What is Medicine

"It is the science of healing which involves the practice of the diagnosis, treatment and prevention of disease, and the promotion of health. Treatment and prevention involves using various medications and healing methods."

www.medicalnewstoday.com/info/medicine

I must add that it is also an art, demonstrated by how healthcare providers show compassion, empathy and listen to their patients.

Part One

Healthcare Providers
and
Health Trends

Types of Practice of Medicine in the World

Conventional or Allopathic Medicine

This practice of medicine is based on modern science

A

Complementary and Alternative Medicine (CAM)

This practice of medicine is based on well-organized systems of traditional health care with long traditions dating back thousands of years. This field includes:
Acupuncture, Ayurveda, Homeopathy, Naturopathy, Chinese or Oriental medicine, (body) Chiropractic, Massage, Body movement therapies, Tai chi, Yoga, (diet & herbs) Dietary supplements, Herbal medicine, Nutrition/diet, (external energy) Electromagnetic therapy, Reiki, Qigong, (mind) Meditation, Biofeedback, Hypnosis, (senses) Art, dance, and music, Visualization and guided imagery.

B

Traditional Healers

This system of providing health care is not formalized and dates back thousands of years. They use indigenous theories, beliefs and experiences handed down by elders or experienced traditional healers to treat physical, mental and spiritual illnesses.

C

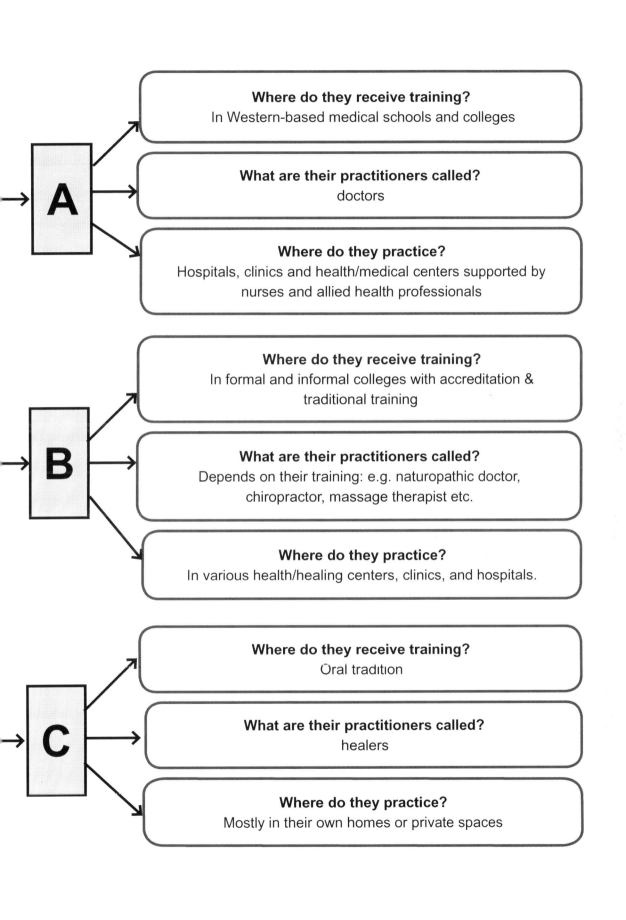

A

Where do they receive training?
In Western-based medical schools and colleges

What are their practitioners called?
doctors

Where do they practice?
Hospitals, clinics and health/medical centers supported by nurses and allied health professionals

B

Where do they receive training?
In formal and informal colleges with accreditation & traditional training

What are their practitioners called?
Depends on their training: e.g. naturopathic doctor, chiropractor, massage therapist etc.

Where do they practice?
In various health/healing centers, clinics, and hospitals.

C

Where do they receive training?
Oral tradition

What are their practitioners called?
healers

Where do they practice?
Mostly in their own homes or private spaces

Let's Pause and Say Thank You to:

All who work in the modern medical field (Allopathic Medicine) to help us manage our health. Included are:

Doctors: They generally examine a patient for signs and symptoms, and sometimes request laboratory and imaging tests to help them arrive at proper diagnosis of a disease. Special doctors like surgeons undertake surgical procedures to remove or replace diseased tissue or organs in patients.

Nurses: The nurse is the link between you and your doctor. They monitor and evaluate patient's overall care. They plan and administer daily treatment. They also offer advice and emotional support to patients and their families and take care of your paperwork.

Medical Assistant: Medical Assistants help doctors and other providers in Ambulatory Clinics, medical offices and they do both administrative and clinical duties. Administratively they may be at the front desk, welcoming patients, answer phones, schedule appointments, pull and store medical records, handle correspondence, and billing, make arrangements for hospital admissions and use computer applications. Clinically, they take patient's history, triage patients take patients' vitals, and prepare patients for exams. They also draw blood and prepare specimens to be sent to the laboratory, and assist physicians in doing office procedures, and relaying instructions to patients about their medications, referrals and treatment procedures. They also administer medications as directed by physicians remove sutures and do dressing changes, as well as perform electrocardiograms in the office. (www.aama-ntl.org/medical-assisting).

Pharmacists: They fill prescriptions, advise other health professionals on the proper dose, provide information about medication side effects, disease prevention, nutrition, addictions, diabetes management, and more.

Allied Health Professionals: They are university-qualified practitioners who work as part of your multidisciplinary healthcare team. They assess, diagnose, treat, discharge and/or refer patients to other services and provide specialist advice. They include dietitians, occupational therapists, physiotherapists, podiatrists, speech pathologists and support staff.

Technicians: Diagnostic Imaging technicians assist doctors by running tests like x-rays, MRIs, CT scans, or ultrasound, to diagnose any medical problems patients may have and medical lab technicians perform tests on tissue, blood and other body fluids.

Hospital Support Staff:
Clinical Assistants – take care of ward housekeeping
Patient Services and dietary Assistants – bring meals and drinks
Porters – take care of patient lifting and transport

Volunteers – help with fundraising, help visitors with ward visits

Ward Clerks – staff the ward reception desks and help with paper work

Healthcare Scientists: The work of a healthcare scientist or clinical scientist as some call them covers a broad area in medical care. Their work covers three areas: life sciences, physiological science, clinical engineering and physical sciences. They generally work in labs investigating diseases, genetic make-up, and the embryo to develop successful treatments and cures. Those working in clinical engineering and physical sciences research develop techniques and technology for medical equipment like radiography, ultrasound and nuclear medicine for diagnosis and monitoring patients. Biomedical engineering is also included.

1

Types of Practice of Medicine

If you are a mother, a grandma, aunt or sister you may be familiar with such inquiries from children: "Ma, I have a bump inside my nose, do you know what it is?" Women tend to possess better nurturing skills. Because of this they are naturally the providers for their families' health and wellbeing and their link to various health care systems. As managers of their own health and that of their families' it is important for every woman to know what types of practice of medicine there are, who their practitioners are, and what advantages or disadvantages each of them has. There are three broad types of practice of medicine in the world (Figure 3). These include Conventional or Allopathic, Complementary and Alternative (CAM), and thirdly Traditional. I will use Conventional and Allopathic interchangeably.

Conventional or Allopathic Medicine

....

Conventional or allopathic medicine is practiced by graduates with degrees in MBChB, M.D. (medical doctor) and D.O. (doctor of osteopathy). These are the ones who successfully graduate from medical schools and are fully licensed to practice medicine. Doctors are also called physicians, however this term is sometimes used for physicians who have been trained to treat adults, also referred to as internist or Physician Specialists.

What do doctors do? A doctor diagnoses and treats diseases and conditions, and provides treatment in the form of medication, procedures, surgery, or therapy. If you go back to Figure 3 you will see that Allopathic medicine involves many other professions apart from doctors. This group is referred to as allied health professionals. They include physical therapists, psychologists, advanced nurse practitioners, registered nurses, midwives physician assistants and dietitians among others who together with doctors, help a person recover from illness, manage a disease, or prevent one.

Preventive Health

And talking about prevention. Our bodies have developed all sorts of mechanisms and techniques to help us avoid being sick. All we have to do is to identify them and optimize them. This is the work of Public Health workers who have been trained to use population-based measures to protect and promote the health of people and their communities and prevent diseases. Most communities have Public Health Centers. To optimize our bodies' mechanisms and techniques to prevent diseases, Public Health workers emphasize lifestyle changes and safe environments, for example: exercise/physical activity, healthy eating, weight loss if obese, smoking cessation, occupational health for workers and safety issues in communities like good drinking water etc.

Immunization

However, at other times, our bodies' immune system isn't quick or strong enough to prevent pathogens from infectious diseases from making us sick. This is where we need immunization or vaccines which is largely carried out by Public Health workers. Some communities in the world are constantly faced with dangerous diseases like Hepatitis B, cholera and polio and we need vaccines to bolster our immune systems to protect us from these diseases. For example children who are eleven and twelve years old in some countries receive Human Papillomavirus (HPV) vaccine to prevent cancers of the cervix, penis, vulva, vagina, anus, back of the throat, base of the tongue and tonsils (oropharynx) in the future. And note, when enough people in a community are vaccinated against dangerous diseases (about 95%), it stops infections from spreading so the lives of those who may have allergies to the vaccine or may have certain conditions that may not allow them to take the vaccine can be protected. This is known as herd protection or herd immunity.

Most countries have scheduled immunizations for children, teenagers and even adults to prevention infections. Some of these have to have booster doses a few years later to keep the immunity in the body up.

Apart from using vaccines to prevent diseases, medication and use of screening tests for early detection of certain diseases are also employed by Public Health workers. For example Aspirin is given to a patient to prevent a first or second heart attack in a specific population. Mammogram or Pap smear are employed to detect breast or cervical cancer respectively.

Sometimes a request from your doctor for a test from a medical lab or a diagnostic center can be distressing for many. Not to talk about the needles and the awkward procedures of undressing and dressing. But the work of the technologists who work in medical labs and Diagnostic Imaging Centers are a very important part of allopathic medicine, both curative and preventive. Diagnostic Imaging Technicians use tests like x-rays, MRIs and CT scans, or ultrasound to scan the body to diagnose any medical problems patients may have. Medical laboratory technicians perform tests on tissue, blood and other body fluids. It is estimated that about 60 to 70% of medical decisions are based on laboratory results.

Another important aspect of allopathic medicine is scientific research. The goal of healthcare scientists is to research the science, technology and practice used in healthcare to innovate and improve services.

Where do doctors and allied health professionals work? They work at public health organizations, teaching facilities, private practices, group practices, community health centers, hospitals, polyclinics, health posts and centers. Some also work in long term residential facilities like nursing homes, and assisted living facilities for seniors who cannot take care of themselves at home and also children or adults who may have physical and mental challenges and so may need care in an institution. There are also hospitals just for women and or children.

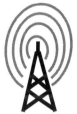

Reminders on Your Radar

"Vaccines prevent an estimated 2–3 million deaths worldwide every year. But, a further 1.5 million lives could be saved annually with better global vaccine coverage."
Source: wellcome.ac.uk/news/why-do-we-need-vaccines

"HPV is a very common virus; nearly 80 million people—about one in four—are currently infected in the United States. About 14 million people, including teens, become infected with HPV each year."
Source: www.cdc.gov/hpv/parents/vaccine.html

A doctor for every major system or condition in your body. Really? Mostly So. Here are some

. . . .

Family Medicine: Family Medicine provide general medical care for the whole family, including children, adults, and the elderly and refer you to a medical specialist when they find it necessary. They can treat up to 90% of diseases, including chronic and acute conditions, treat behavioral/psychiatric problems, do gynecological and surgical procedures and deliver babies.

The Rest

Allergists/Immunologists: experts in asthma, eczema, environmental/food/insect sting allergies, etc.

Anesthesiologists: administer drugs to numb pain and consciousness for various surgical procedures

Cardiologists: experts on the heart and blood vessels

Colon and Rectal Surgeons: experts on colon, rectum and anus (bottom)

Critical Care Medicine Specialists: experts in caring for the critically ill or injured

Dermatologists: experts on skin, hair, nails

Endocrinologists: experts on diabetes, obesity, thyroid problems, adrenal glands, reproductive and sexual maturation, calcium and bone disorders.

Emergency Medicine Specialists: experts on life-or-death decisions for sick and injured people they work in emergency departments

Gastroenterologists: experts on esophagus, stomach, bowels, pancreas, liver, and gallbladder diseases

Geriatric Medicine Specialists: experts in caring for the elderly or seniors

Hematologists: specialists in diseases of the blood, spleen, and lymph glands, e.g. anemia

Hospice and Palliative Medicine Specialists: experts in working with people who are nearing death and their families

Infectious Disease Specialists: experts in diagnosing and treating infections in any part of your body

Internists: experts in treating both common and complex illnesses, usually only in adults.

Medical Geneticists: experts in diagnosing and treating hereditary disorders passed down from parents to children

Nephrologists: experts in treating kidney diseases, high blood pressure and fluid and mineral imbalances linked to kidney disease.

Neurologists: specialists in the nervous system – the brain, spinal cord, and nerves

Obstetricians and Gynecologists: experts on women's health, infertility, pregnancy, and childbirth

Oncologists: experts in cancer treatment.

Ophthalmologists: they treat every kind of eye condition as well as operate on the eyes

Osteopaths: they are trained like other allopathic physicians to diagnose and treat medical conditions, but they also specialize in hands on manipulation of the body's skeletal and Muscular systems so as to use the body's natural ability to heal itself.

Otolaryngologists: experts in treating diseases in the ears, nose, throat, sinuses, larynx, head, neck, and upper respiratory system

Pathologists: They identify the causes of diseases by examining body tissues and fluids under microscopes. They also do post mortems on dead people to find out causes of death

Pediatricians: experts in caring for children from birth to young adulthood

Physiatrists: experts in physical medicine and rehabilitation, treat neck or back pain and sports or spinal cord injuries

Plastic Surgeons: They rebuild or repair your skin, face, hands, breasts, or body. They include cosmetic surgeons

Podiatrists: They care for problems in your ankles and feet. They are not trained medical doctors

Public Health Specialists: They may work in public health or at hospitals

Psychiatrists: They work with people with mental, emotional, eating or addictive disorders.

Pulmonologists: specialists for problems like lung cancer, pneumonia, asthma, emphysema, and trouble sleeping caused by breathing issues. They tend to concentrate on the lower respiratory system

Radiologists: They use X-rays, ultrasound, and other imaging tests to diagnose diseases

Rheumatologists: They specialize in arthritis and other diseases which affect your joints, muscles, bones, and tendons like Lupus, and autoimmune conditions

Sleep Medicine Specialists: They find and treat causes behind your poor sleep

Sports Medicine Specialists: they diagnose, treat, and prevent injuries related to sports and exercise.

General Surgeons: experts in operating on all parts of your body.

Urologists: they are surgeons who care for men and women for problems in the urinary tract, like a leaky bladder and prostate problems in men.

<u>**Caution:**</u> Conventional Medicine has many useful diagnostic techniques unknown to many traditional practitioners. Conventional Medicine works quickly and saves

lives in many situations. Surgery for example can be life-saving in cases of trauma, serious accidents, broken bones, wounds, and certain infections. However:

- Make sure the doctor you are seeing is accredited with a national body
- Seek a second opinion if you are not sure of your doctor's advice to avoid incorrect diagnosis or treatments. In the province Québec, Canada, the Code of ethics of physicians is unequivocal: "A physician must acknowledge the patient's right to consult a colleague, another professional, or any other competent person. He must not, by any means, interfere with the patient's freedom of choice."
- Make sure your pharmacist educates you about your prescriptions from your doctor. All drugs in conventional medicine may have side-effects which can negatively affect one's health. Some patients have been addicted to some drugs while adverse drug reactions have resulted in many deaths.

Complementary and Alternative Medicine (CAM)

....

On the face of it Allopathic Medicine might seem an unlikely ally for ancient medicinal systems. But here it is, CAM. CAM is a type of practice of medicine generally not considered as part of conventional medicine. It is defined as medical products and practices that are not part of standard Allopathic or Conventional Medicine. CAM practices developed in both non-Western cultures and the traditional medicinal system of Europe. They are referred to as 'Whole Medicinal Systems.' Why are they called Whole Medicinal Systems? Because they are complete systems of healthcare built upon philosophy, practices, diagnosis and treatment that have evolved and predate the conventional medical approach.

The interface between Whole Medicinal Systems and Allopathic Medicine has been particularly susceptible to great stumbles until recent years. CAM has been welcomed along Allopathic Medicine mostly because of the many scientific investigations in recent years that have partly supported their medical efficacy through preclinical and clinical experiments. However, there are other practices of CAM that are yet to be subjected to standard scientific inquiry. The four major whole medicinal systems are Ayurveda, Homeopathy, Naturopathy, and Traditional Chinese medicine. A detailed description of each of these systems is discussed below under the topic Whole Medicinal Systems.

People often use Complementary and Alternative interchangeably and it has caused a lot of confusion, until in the US they were defined more clearly, because strictly speaking they are not the same. Let's take an exploratory expedition into CAM practices.

Complementary or Integrative Medicine

These days some doctors may use Conventional medicine (medication) in addition to a non-allopathic practice like acupuncture to treat a patient for pain. Yoga and massage have been used to help some cancer patients who have pain, anxiety and fatigue. This is called Complementary medicine because the doctor added another approach to Conventional medicine to treat the patient.

Probably this is no news to you especially if you live in Africa or Asia because they have been combining these two approaches for a while now, using both modern medicine and traditional medical practices (herbs and manipulative body practices). Interesting enough, it's catching on in developed countries. In the USA, about 30% of adults and 12% of children use health care methods which are outside conventional medicine and so the general public has been doing this for a while, and it is only recently that some allopathic physicians are incorporating non-western or alternative methods into their practices.

A new field of medical training or specialization has emerged where Allopathic trained doctors are specializing in Integrative Medicine. Integrative Medicine combines both conventional practice and aspects of whole medicinal systems in a coordinated way to treat the whole person. A 'whole-person' approach to meeting health needs addresses the mind and body, lifestyle and nutrition, inflammation, infections, immune system, toxic burden, allergies, hormone balancing and the gut. It's about time and there is a lot of ground to be covered.

Alternative Medicine

So where does the Alternative Medicine come in? Alternative medicine refers to the use of only CAM or aspects of Whole Medicinal Systems in place of Conventional Medicine. For example using Acupuncture for arthritic pain. Products and manipulations which may come under Alternative (non-main stream) Medicine include acupuncture, massage, chiropractic manipulations, dietary supplements and herbs.

Note: Most use of CAM by the Western world is complementary, however in developing countries (especially in rural areas) due to lack of western trained health workers and or resources, some individuals will mainly use Alternative medicine as the means to take care of their health needs.

CAM Practices

....

Alternative medicines practiced in CAM are divided into two main groups: Botanicals/Natural products and Mind and Body practices. The latter can be further divided into sub groups as shown in Figures 4 & 5.

Examples of Botanicals/natural products: Dietary supplements, Herbal medicine, Nutrition/diet

Examples of body therapies: Chiropractic and Osteopathic medicine manipulations, Massage, Body movement therapies, Tai chi, and Yoga

Examples of external energy therapy: Electromagnetic therapy, Reiki, and Qigong. This form of therapy is based on the belief that external energies from objects or other sources directly affect a person's health

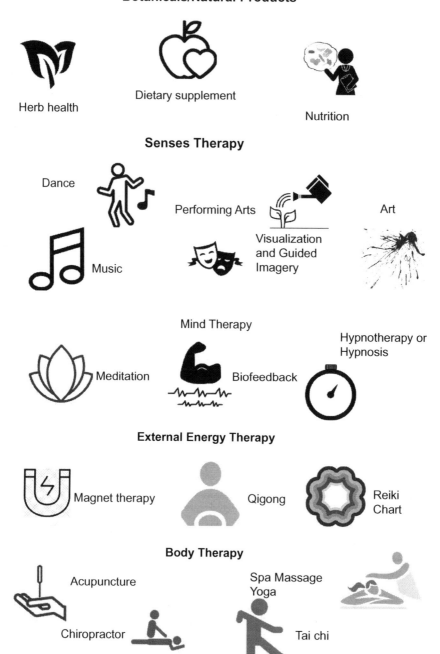

Botanicals/Natural Products

Herb health

Dietary supplement

Nutrition

Senses Therapy

Dance

Music

Performing Arts

Visualization and Guided Imagery

Art

Mind Therapy

Meditation

Biofeedback

Hypnotherapy or Hypnosis

External Energy Therapy

Magnet therapy

Qigong

Reiki Chart

Body Therapy

Acupuncture

Chiropractor

Tai chi

Spa Massage Yoga

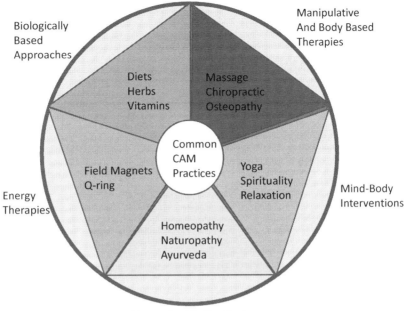

Alternative Medical Systems

Examples of Mind therapies: Meditation, Christian meditation, Biofeedback, and Hypnosis. Even standard or conventional medicine recognizes the power of the connection between mind and body.

Whole Medicinal Systems

··············

It's rather normal that herbs have been the natural choice for treating various health conditions since ancient times in all cultures. So naturally it has remained in most cultures to date. The underlying principle that underpins whole medical systems is to treat the whole person and not just the symptoms to obtain optimal emotional and physical health.

Homeopathy and Naturopathy medicinal systems have developed in Western culture while Traditional Chinese Medicine (TCM) and Ayurvedic Medicinal systems developed in non-Western cultures.

Traditional Chinese Medicine (TCM)

TCM practitioners use herbal medicines and various mind and body techniques to treat or prevent health problems. TCM is based on the concept of restoring balance. Included is the notion that each individual is made up of five essential substances, wood, fire, earth, metal, and water and imbalance among these elements can result in mental and physical health problems, and this is what their approach aims at balancing. Secondly, there is the concept of vital life force known as Qi that makes up and binds together all things in the universe. The push and pull factors, yin and yang, are the two aspects of Qi. One enjoys good health, wellbeing and contentment when all of the yin and yang aspects of Qi are in harmony with one another. Too much or too little of yin or yang relative to another results in illness, pain and suffering. The approach of TCM is to restore harmony or balance when these two forces go out of Kilter (out of sync).

Acupuncture is one of the major practices of TCM. Another practice is moxibustion commonly used around the abdomen and feet. Others are cupping, a therapeutic procedure, Chinese herbal medicine, and tui na, which is a Chinese therapeutic massage. Then there is dietary therapy, and tai chi and qi gong which are forms of martial arts. Let's discuss the dominant practices within TCM: Chinese herbal medicine, acupuncture, and tai chi.

Chinese Herbal Medicine

Chinese herbal medicine primarily consists of parts of plants, such as the leaves, roots, stems, flowers, and seeds formulated as teas, capsules, liquid extracts, granules, or powders to treat or prevent diseases.

Caution: There are many benefits of using Chinese herbal medicine but as with all drugs we all need to exercise caution. Here are a few to consider.
- Be careful as sometimes herbal medicines are marketed as dietary supplements
- Some herbal products have been reported as being "contaminated with drugs, toxins, or heavy metals or not containing the listed ingredients."
- Some Chinese herb formulations have been known to interact with drugs resulting in serious side effects. And some have been reported to be unsafe for people with various medical conditions. For example, "the Chinese herb ephedra (ma huang) has been linked to serious health complications, including heart attack and stroke." nccih.nih.gov/health/whatiscam/chinesemed.htm
- Make your doctor aware of any herbal medicines you may be taking so he or she can coordinate your health properly

Acupuncture

This technique uses special needles to penetrate the skin and stimulate various points on the body (acupuncture points) to balance the flow of energy through pathways between different organ systems in the body. However, western practitioners view the acupuncture points as places which stimulate nerves, muscles and connective tissue, and boost the activity of a person's body's natural painkillers and increase blood flow to the area. Acupuncture is used to treat chronic pain, chemotherapy-induced nausea and vomiting, fibromyalgia, headaches, labor pain, low back pain, menstrual cramps, migraines, osteoarthritis, dental pain, and elbow pain.

Caution: Use of acupuncture have been mostly safe. However, should you need this intervention, make sure to use a qualified practitioner who follows the standard practice of proper sterilization of needles and the use of nontoxic needles labeled for single use.

Tai chi

Tai chi is a martial art which involves gentle physical movements, stretching, relaxation and breathing which must all be done with mental focus. In some studies, it has been found to strengthen the lower extremities and helps prevent falls in seniors and those with Parkinson's disease. It helps with pain, posture and balance. Some people with painful osteoarthritis (from wear and tear of joints) have had less pain when they practice Tai Chi.

Caution: Tai chi and qi gong are generally safe.

Other TCM Practices

Moxibustion: This technique uses the herb mugwort or Ai Ya, which involves burning it above the skin to apply heat to acupuncture points. It is believed to help increase blood circulation and energy, stimulate the digestive system and boost the immune.

Caution: There have been reports of allergic reactions, burns and infections.

Cupping: Cupping involves "applying a heated cup to the skin to create a slight suction." How is the vacuum created? "By means of heat from a burning alcohol cotton ball inside the cup or by pump." Though cupping can be used alone it is generally combined with acupuncture.

Caution: Skin may be marked temporarily from applying heated cup. Make sure to let your healthcare provider know about it so it is not mistaken for a symptom of a disease or physical abuse.

Ayurveda Medicinal System

Ayurveda is the traditional Hindu system of medicine from India. The word is derived from two roots, namely 'Ayus' and 'Veda,' meaning life and knowledge, respectively. It is based on the idea of balance in the body, mind and spirit. Ayurveda treatment consists of the use of herbal preparations and emphasizes the practice of yoga and meditation as well as massage, special diets, and cleansing techniques.

Ayurveda uses five approaches in treating diseases: internal, external, surgical, mental and spiritual therapies and herbs. Included in the internal approach is the use of Shodhana (detoxification) and Shamana to improve quality of life. Included in the external approach is the use of Snehana (oil treatments), Svedana (steam therapy using herbal steam), and herbal pastes. Included in the surgical approach is removal of tissues, organs, and harmful growths. Mental and spiritual therapies are called Daivya Chikitsa. And lastly the herbal approach includes rasa shastra, that is, the use of various herbal and trace metal formulations.

Caution: Some Ayurvedic products have been reported to contain metals, minerals, or other materials that may be harmful. And just as in Chinese herbal medicine do your research as sometimes herbal medicines are marketed as dietary supplements.

Homeopathy Medicinal System

This medicinal system was developed in Germany over 200 years ago. It treats diseases by minute doses of natural substances that in large amounts in a healthy person would produce symptoms of disease. It is based on the theory that "like cures like." The diluted substance is believed to help with the symptoms and work with the body to heal it.

So what do homeopathic products contain and look like? Homeopathic products come in the form of sugar pellets, ointments, gels, drops, creams, and tablets consisting of plants (such as red onion, arnica [mountain herb], poison ivy, belladonna [deadly nightshade], and stinging nettle), minerals (such as white arsenic), or animals (such as crushed whole bees).

Caution:
- Let your physician know of any homeopathic products you may be using. Some homeopathic teething tablets have been reported to contain amounts of the toxic substance belladonna. Should you want to use homeopathy consult doctors who have acquired the necessary training
- Homeopathy is CAM so make sure to use conventional care as your first choice for any medical problems you may encounter.

Naturopathy Medicinal System

This medicinal system developed in Europe in the 19th century by combining various strands of traditional medicine and health care practices. Naturopathic practitioners use dietary and lifestyle changes, stress reduction, herbs and other dietary supplements, homeopathy, manipulative therapies, exercise therapy, practitioner-guided detoxification, psychotherapy and counseling as treatment and prevention of diseases in their patients.

Naturopathic physicians are graduates from naturopathic medical schools accredited by the Council on Naturopathic Medical Education. However, there are also traditional naturopath practitioners who are not licensed because they receive their training from training programs that have no accreditation.

Caution: Should you want to use a naturopathic practitioner do your homework and consult one that is licensed with accreditation.

Traditional Healers

These are found in most cultures and they use indigenous theories, beliefs and experiences handed down by elders or experienced traditional healers to treat physical, mental and spiritual illnesses. They may use herbs and botanicals and some incorporate some spiritual ceremony to the physical or mental healing process.

Caution: Because there is no standardization of their practices and training methods, many lives are endangered by wrongful doses of herbs, herb formulations, and ritual practices that have no bearing on the disease being treated. Inform your primary healthcare provider of any consultation with traditional healers and the form of treatment you may receive.

Christian Meditation

Christian meditation offers a complete lifestyle approach to health and it has been used as a means of healing for many centuries. In Christian meditation, Bible reading and reflection (including listening to soft Christian music) and prayers are used to draw one closer to God and bring healing to the body, soul and spirit.

Christian meditation has been known to heal broken relationship with God and to draw one closer to Him, overcome negative thoughts and restore peace of mind, uncover past pains and releasing them to God for inner healing. It also eliminates daily stress and does away with frustrations, anger, and ugly dispositions. Christian mediation also include taking nature walks to appreciate God's creation. There are various videos and music on Christian Guided Meditation and Imagery for healing on YouTube as well as various resources online you can use.

Caution: If Christ is not the only center and only focus of the meditation then beware it is not Christian meditation.

Reminders on Your Radar

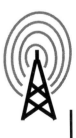

Despite the ancient beliefs upon which Whole Medicinal Systems are based, their techniques adopted in CAM are solely based on the science of the effects on the body and how helpful the practices help in managing symptoms.

2

Trends in Women's Health

"Being a man or a woman has a significant impact on health, as a result of both biological and gender-related differences. The health of women and girls is of particular concern because, in many societies, they are disadvantaged by discrimination rooted in sociocultural factors."

(WHO-Women's Health)

What's making women sick and which regions of the world are more prone to certain diseases, and what outbreaks may be headed your way? A decent predictability of diseases goes a long way to help health systems undertake appropriate research and improve services. And individuals are alerted to take the necessary precautions needed to safeguard themselves and reduce the rate of incidence.

Globally, there are differences in the health challenges which women and men face, and for women, there are also differences depending on age group and whether they live in high-income (developed) or low-income (developing) countries. Take a look.

Low-Middle Income Countries – Women (15-44)

Communicable diseases (primarily acquired immunodeficiency syndrome [AIDS]), maternal causes of death, unsafe sex, breast cancer, cervical cancer, tuberculosis, depression, iron-deficiency anemia, increases the risk of hemorrhage and sepsis during childbirth, chronic obstructive pulmonary disease (COPD) and deaths mostly due to "exposure to indoor smoke from cooking with open fires or inefficient stoves"; unsafe abortions, and fire-related injuries.

Women Over 50 – Everywhere in the world

Cardiovascular diseases – 45%, cancers – 15% (mainly of the lung, breast, colon and stomach), chronic obstructive pulmonary disease – 10%, disability

Low-Income Countries – Female Adolescents

Anemia, pregnancy, unsafe abortions, sex abuse, and HIV infections

Americas – Female Adolescents

Substance use (tobacco & alcohol)

Female Adolescents – Everywhere in the world

Self-inflicted injuries, road traffic injuries, drowning, depressive disorders, schizophrenia

WHO is projecting that maternal mortality rates will keep declining rapidly in both low and middle income countries and "as a result, mortality patterns in all countries will increasingly resemble those currently seen in high-income countries. In other words, deaths will be increasingly delayed to older ages and cancers will cause a larger proportion of deaths in people between the ages of 20 and 75 years."

This is also true with other chronic diseases, which are not caused by infections from bacteria or viruses. These are slowly increasing in developing countries as their societies adopt Western and modern lifestyles. There is less walking and more riding in cars, less consumption of fresh fruits and vegetables coupled with increased stress and shrinking leisure time. They are also eating more processed foods, drinking more sugary drinks, smoking tobacco and there is a marked increase in the use alcoholic beverages. All these contribute to chronic diseases like heart diseases, hypertension, diabetes, lung diseases, and some cancers.

These trends call for not just "adapting health systems to better meet the changing health-care needs of women in low- and middle-income countries primarily by improving the capacity to prevent and manage non-communicable diseases" but also equipping women everywhere with readily available information about how to manage their health, which this book is attempting to provide.

It is also apparent that diseases affect the totality of the person. It is therefore imperative that women take a proactive and holistic approach to managing their health which should address not just their physical body and mental health but also their spiritual health and this is the approach this book is adopting.

Part Two

Medications

MEDICINES

Medicines play an important part in treating diseases and conditions and in Allopathic medicine, most medicines are produced by pharmaceutical companies using chemical synthesis. We shall discuss various aspects of medicines which all users should be aware of.

Know your medicines and why you take them
Side effects of medicines
Drug allergies
Classification of medicines
Prescription medicines
Over the counter medicines (OTC)
Polypharmacy
Medicines and expiry dates
Vitamins and Minerals
Antioxidants
Do anti-oxidants prevent cancer?
Probiotics and Prebiotics
Medical Foods
Classes of Pharmaceutical medicines for treating illnesses
Complementary or Alternative medicines (CAM)

3

Be in Charge of Your Medicines: Know Why You Take Them

Introduction

....

When I began practicing medicine in North America (Canada and USA), I was surprised at how knowledgeable most of my patients were of their medical conditions and the names of their medicines. As a result, when they come to see a doctor, there is a meaningful exchange and understanding of how the doctor is treating and managing their disease or condition. Now, not every North American patient is informed about their medical condition or knows the names of their medicines, however, even among the uninformed I find that some keep a list of their medications, the dosage, and the number of times they take it written on a piece of

"Drugs are of priceless value when needed, but they are at best emergency measures of most temporary utility. . . . The more effective they are in the right place, the more harmful in the wrong one".

—Woods Hutchinson,
A.M., M.D. Civilization and Health, 1914

paper or stored on their cell phones. This makes the work of a health professional so much easier in managing your condition and prevents dangerous duplication of medications and serious side effects which may arise. Informed patients also know what medicine they take for what condition, if they have several medical problems.

For simplicity, we will be using medicines, medications or drugs interchangeably in the book. In many places where I have worked, I met educated individuals who would tell me "I take a small, white pill".

First of all, there are so many small white pills available, so I will have no clue as to what medicine is being referred to.

Secondly, because the same medication may be produced by different pharmaceutical companies, there are chances that one may receive a medicine with one shape at one time and at another time may get the same medicine but with a different shape or color.

Thirdly, all medications have adverse or side effects (including CAM supplements). So, it is important to know the names of medicines one is taking, in case an adverse reaction occurs.

In most advanced countries, if you have a medicine prescribed, you can easily identify a particular pill by its color and any inscription written on it. In the USA, websites like, www.drugs.com and www.webmd.com contain "pill identification" content which I sometimes refer to when a patient comes with a pill she is not sure of.

Know Which Medicine is for What Condition or Disease

If you are aware of what medicine is used to treat which medical condition that is very useful and keeps you safe. Many individuals are on several different medicines for managing a variety of diseases. It is important that you learn which medication is being used for which disease or medical condition. Be familiar with your medicines. Another important reason to be familiar with your medicines is that if you suddenly develop a possible side effect, then supplying this information can help your health provider quickly recognize the link and cause of the problem or side effect. Your knowledge about medicines can be used as a great help for both, you and your health care providers. It is possible that the same medicine may be used to treat many different medical conditions and there is possibility that a new doctor treating you may make a wrong assumption a particular medicine you are taking is for a certain condition which may not be the case. For example, a common medicine called METOPROLOL is used to treat hypertension (high blood pressure or BP), heart disease, migraine, and rapid or irregular heartbeat. A doctor meeting a patient for the first time may think he/she is using it for BP, but in actual fact it may be for correcting or regulating an irregular heartbeat.

You can list your medicines as shown in example below:

Examples:

Medicine	Dosage	Indication
Lisinopril 10 mg	once a day	High Blood Pressure
Atorvastatin 20 mg	once at bedtime	High Cholesterol

Tips to Remembering What Medicines You Take

So, it is important YOU know the names of your medicines and the conditions you are taking them for. Writing them on a piece of paper or keeping the names on your cell or mobile phone is a good idea. I even have patients who take pictures of their labeled pill container or packet and keep them on their phones to show to me when I ask them what medicines they are on. One other important reason for keeping your medication list on your phone is that the person who is assisting you will be able to quickly access them in cause of an emergency when you end up in a hospital or emergency room. That medication list can let the doctors know what medicines you are taking and for what conditions.

Side Effects of Medications

A side effect or adverse effect of a medicine is an unintended effect of a medicine on the patient who is taking it. All medicines have some side effects and these tend to be predictable and can be minor or severe. Minor ones may include stomach pain, diarrhea, constipation or dry mouth.

For example:

1. Aspirin may cause stomach pain or irritation. However, if taken with food or use of an enteric coated one (has a coating which protects the stomach lining) may prevent this

2. Taking higher doses of Amlodipine or Nifedipine (blood pressure pills) may cause swelling of the legs in some people. However, lower doses may not cause this problem

3. Certain medicines may affect or decrease levels of minerals and vitamins in your body, and these include some in the categories of blood pressure or cholesterol lowering medications and antibiotics

4. For example, Diuretics used for treating high blood pressure, heart failure, liver, and kidney diseases may lower levels of potassium, magnesium, and zinc. If you take a diuretic, occasional blood work checking the levels of potassium or magnesium, or taking OTC supplements with your health provider's knowledge may be helpful

5. Statins (cholesterol lowering medicines) may decrease level of Coenzyme Q10 (CoQ 10) in the blood. This is an antioxidant and it also helps to protect the heart and skeletal muscles, however; low levels may cause muscle pain for those taking Statins

6. CoQ 10 lowers blood sugar level of those on Diabetes medicines and may also cause low blood pressure. Therefore, a health care provider has to be aware of all supplements one is taking

7. Antibiotics may also lower B Vitamins (B1, B2, B6, folic acid, and B12) level if taken for a long time. They may also affect the "normal" bacteria levels in the intestines or gut because they kill both bad and good bacterial colonies in the gut. The two types (bad and good bacteria) have a good balance which gets upset after taking antibiotics, leading to many problems including diarrhea,

overgrowth of clostridium difficile which is a bad bacteria, and vaginal yeast infections. That is why it is important to TAKE ANTIBIOTICS and other medicines as specified (amount and duration) by a qualified health care provider. Taking Probiotics with antibiotics may help prevent these adverse effects

Drug Allergies
What are They?

Drug allergies involve the body's immune system reacting to the drug as a harmful substance and producing cells to fight it. In the process, chemicals are released which cause the symptoms.

Minor allergies include: Cough, itching, or hives (itchy skin wheals or raised rash).

Serious reactions include: Angioedema when there is swelling beneath the skin leading to swelling of face, tongues, hands, legs, and belly. Some breathing problems may occur if neck, mouth, and tongue are involved.

Most severe reaction is called Anaphylaxis: This is life threatening and may include difficulty in breathing, shortness of breath, severe rash, dizziness, chest pain, rapid heartbeat (palpitations), low blood pressure, and death.

Examples of drugs causing any of the reactions mentioned above are antibiotics like Penicillin, and Sulfa drugs, Aspirin, Ibuprofen, and other Non-Steroidal Anti-Inflammatory Drugs (NSAIDs), Radiological contrasts, and some Cancer medicines.

How to Prevent A Severe Reaction Or A Recurrence

1. If someone has such a severe reaction he/she will have to always carry an injectable drug called EPINEPHERINE PEN (EPI PEN) with him/her all the times to self-administer when needed
2. Reaction to one drug in a class means you may be allergic to all those in that class. So, a reaction to PENICILLIN V means any of the others in the class like PENICILLIN G, AMOXICILLIN, DICLOXACILLIN, or AMOXICILLIN/ CLAVUNALATE may also cause similar allergic reaction in the person, and so they all need to be avoided
3. For example, if you have a rash or get any of the other above mentioned reactions to Penicillin, then you are aware that PENICILLIN type medications give you an ALLERGIC REACTION. So, if your doctor prescribes you Penicillin antibiotic, you can confidently tell her or him that you are allergic to Penicillin
4. In fact, all doctors and healthcare providers should be in the habit of asking patients whether they are allergic to any medicine or not, and if they are, then document that medicine before starting the consultation. However, if you are knowledgeable about any allergy or intolerance that you have had to any med-

icine, you should volunteer or mention that information to your doctor so that it could be recorded in your medical records. THIS IS BEING PROACTIVE

Drug Intolerance
What is This?

A reaction to a drug that does not involve activation of the immune system.

There are some medicines to which people are INTOLERANT which means they may have a minor reaction to them, but these reactions are not regarded as allergic in nature. For example, a class of medicine called narcotics (such as codeine, hydrocodone, morphine, oxycodone, and pethidine) is used for treating severe pain. They can, however, cause nausea, vomiting or constipation in many individuals. These symptoms are more of INTOLERANCE and once such a medicine is given and you get symptoms like nausea, for example, you will be often given anti-nausea (against nausea) medication to counteract the nausea.

In the course of the book, I will mention some side effects of the common medicines that are used to treat the different medical conditions. Due to possible side effects, it is important that you know the names of medicines you are taking.

Reminders on Your Radar

Make your doctor visits meaningful by knowing the names of what medicines you take, and for which medical conditions. Have the names and doses written on paper or save on your cell phone so that you can make it available when needed. All medicines have some type of adverse effects, some more serious than others. Discuss side effects with your health provider in case they appear.

4

Classification of Medications

The above discussions on side effects refer to drugs or formulated chemicals produced by pharmaceutical companies that are used to treat medical illnesses. Worldwide, there are two broad classifications of medicines used by doctors who practice western or conventional medicine. These are:

1. PRESCRIPTION MEDICINES (Prescription only medications – POM) and
2. OVER THE COUNTER MEDICINES (OTC) or NON PRESCRIPTION MEDICATIONS

Prescription Medications

....

Prescription Medication are usually prescribed by a qualified and licensed health provider and the production and purity of these are regulated by a government body, like the Food and Drug Administration, of the particular country. These medicines have to be prescribed by a medical professional only and obtained at a pharmacy, chemist or drug shop because misuse or abuse may lead to serious complications. These are not supposed to be sold over the counter without a prescription and always should be kept BEHIND THE COUNTER next to where the pharmacist stands in the shop. These medicines should never be available for a patient just to take and pay for without a valid prescription.

Misuse and Adulteration of Prescription Medications

....

However, it is being observed that unfortunately in many developing or low resource countries, one can easily buy some of them without a valid medical prescription.

Secondly, some are being sold unregulated in markets, shops, or retail outlets etc. by unqualified medical or non-medical individuals. Examples of these medicines include anti-malaria or antibiotics medicines which are used to treat serious conditions like malaria and infections, respectively. In many developing countries, antibiotics sold in the marketplace or street corners may be substandard or adulterated with other products. For example, yam flour, wheat flour, or cassava powder is mixed with a small amount of the proper antibiotics and then are sold in capsules without a medical prescription. Due to lack of rules and regulations, these may be produced in other countries and brought into a country illegally. For example in Nigeria, fake antimalarial medicines have led to the deaths of many innocent children who were being treated for malaria with those medicines. In developing countries at many places, Licensed Chemical retail shops are only supposed to sell over the counter medicines and not prescription medications; however, some do get away with doing that because there is no monitoring or enforcement. Any shop selling prescription medicines should have a licensed pharmacist working in the shop, unless it is a clinic with a dispensary for dispensing medicines for its patients.

How to Avoid Buying Fake Medicines

Everyone has to be aware about fake medicines especially in developing countries. The solution is simple; always buy from the reputable pharmacies even if it is a little more expensive or from the Government pharmacies in the hospitals. Don't buy from the markets, questionable retailers, road side hawkers, or over the internet. It is also important to read the label carefully to make sure you have the correct medicine and as well as the expiration date of the medicine, since some pharmacy shops may carry expired medicines, have wrong labelling, give you another medicine with a similar name or someone else's prescription medicine. Always check your medicines when you pick them up from the pharmacy.

Over the Counter Medicines

There are some medical conditions you can self-treat with "Over the Counter" (OTC) medications or be told by a doctor to get and use. These medications you can buy without a prescription written by a medical professional. In the history of pharmaceuticals, these medicines have been deemed safe enough for individuals to buy without a written prescription from a medical professional. They are known as OTC drugs because they are kept in front of the drug store or pharmacy counter and one can just take them and pay for them without a prescription. Just like the prescription medicines, these OTC medicines may also have adverse effects if not used as directed on the medicine box or container. They are also known as NON PRESCRIPTION medicines because one does not need a prescription from a health care professional to buy them.

Examples of OTC Medicines

These medications include Aspirin, Paracetamol (Acetaminophen), Brufen (Ibu-profen), cough syrup, medicines for flu, cough, catarrhs, or head colds etc. One should be aware that just because it's an OTC medicine does not mean that it cannot cause adverse effects if there is excessive use, overdose or not using it as directed. All medicines have adverse or side effects if not used as prescribed. Most medications from reliable sources would have instructions on how to take them and may have instructions in case of overdose on the box or container.

For example, the maximum dose of Acetaminophen (Tylenol) also known as paracetamol should not exceed 3000 mg in a 24 hour period. Regular use of excessive amounts can lead to poisoning and acute liver failure (the liver stops working and chemicals that need to be broken down by the liver into harmless chemicals or byproducts accumulate in the body). These OTC medicines are sold in pharmacies, markets, grocery shops, and licensed chemical shops etc. and to be sure they are authentic and safe, it is best to buy them at reputable shops and pharmacies.

Polypharmacy

This is a term used when one is taking more than five different medications on a daily basis. Some seniors take up to 10 medications on a daily basis. While most may be necessary, still there may be some that should have been stopped but they continuously take them. Sometimes, when a person is admitted to the hospital they may be put on certain medications like: stool softeners for constipa-tion e.g. – Docusate, (Colace) sleep aids like Benzodiazepines e.g. Temazepam (Restoril), for sleep, or peptic/stress ulcer prevention medicine like Omeprazole. However, upon discharge from the hospital, they continue taking these, thinking they are still necessary for them. To prevent this one should visit your home primary care provider soon after discharge and let him/her know about all the medicines one was discharged home with. There are also several medicines that may cause side effects and are not very effective for long term treatment for the condition these were given for. For example, Benzodiazepines given for short term sleep problems, could in the elderly cause falls and confusion at times.

Medications and Expiry Dates

In examining research that has been done on stability of long expired prescription medications, I found that groups like the American Medical Association (AMA) had questioned the validity of expiration dates and in a review of the procedures used for setting expiration dates, they concluded that the actual shelf lives of some prod-ucts are longer than the set expiry dates. The FDA of the USA has administered for over 20 years a program for the US Department of Defense with regards to shelf lives of drugs. This program is called the Shelf Life Extension Program (SLEP) and a review of 122 different drug products tested showed that many drugs if stored properly can be extended past the expiration date. Another study had shown that for four products studied, when stored at room temperature, maintained at least 98% potency for 18–170 months past the labeled expiration dates (Lyon R, Taylor J et al. Stability profiles of drug products extended beyond labeled expiration dates. www.interscience.wiley.com March 2006). So, the bottom line is most drugs can be taken without any bad consequences even if past the expiration date so far as they have been well stored and have been produced by a reputable company. Of course, if it has changed it's color or if it has turned powdery in the case of pills or if it has absorbed moisture then it's best to dispose them.

Reminders on Your Radar

Reading directions about how much and how often a medication should be taken is very important in order to avoid overdose or adverse effects. If you are on any medicines and are not sure why you take them, let your doctor know about them and ask if they still need to be taken. Substandard medicines exist depending on where they were produced and some countries are notorious for producing substandard medicines which do not work.

5

Vitamins, Minerals, Antioxidants, Probiotics and Medical Foods

Vitamins and Minerals

. . . .

What are These?

Many patients want to know whether they should take vitamins like, Vitamin A, C, E, B12, beta carotene and some minerals like, iron, calcium, potassium, zinc, and selenium etc.

Vitamins are chemicals needed in small amount to help in various chemical reactions and metabolic activities in the body. Vitamins mixed with trace minerals are very important for many reactions at the cellular level.

What are the effects of Vitamin Supplementation?

Excessive amount of some of these can lead to problems. The fat soluble vitamins are A, D, E, and K and if used in excessive amount, can accumulate in the fat cells and are not easily eliminated from the body; so, this can cause adverse effects. Not getting enough of vitamins from ones diet or being deficient as seen in blood work results; means one would require supplements. Some people also need certain supplements due to insufficient absorption from the intestines, intestinal problems, or surgery. Women who have undergone gastric bypass surgery for obesity, for example, may be low in Vitamin B12 and may need this supplement for life. Black women or veiled women (Muslims) who cover themselves and those with dark skin are not able to produce adequate Vitamin D from the Sun (sun interacts with skin to produce Vitamin D) and tend to be low in Vitamin D; which has been found to be very important for many body functions apart from preventing bone loss problems. Individuals with heavy monthly menses may need Iron supplements to make up for excessive blood losses. Some vitamins are also important as they act as antioxidants.

What are Antioxidants?

Antioxidants neutralize chemicals known as "free radicals" which occur naturally in the body when molecules in our cells undergo a process called Oxidation. The free radicles damage DNA or genetic material.

Antioxidants are produced by the body and also found in several foods. The free radicals are unstable and if present in large amounts in cells can destroy them by damaging DNA, Proteins and other components. The body also produces high amount of free radicals from exposure to ionizing radiation, cigarette smoking, and high oxygen environments. The antioxidants react with them making them harmless and also prevent and slow down cellular damage. If there are low levels of antioxidants in the cells, the cells go through oxidative stress and get damaged or die. Examples of antioxidants are Vitamin C, A, E, glutathione, (an Amino acid), and those found in plants like beta carotene, lycopene, and lutein.

Dietary Sources of Antioxidants

Fruits with deep pigments, vegetables, and grains are high in antioxidants and specific foods high in antioxidants include red grapes, red bell peppers, blueberries, cranberries, strawberries, guava, coffee, tea (black and green), oranges, mango, whole grains, kidney beans, dark chocolate, pecans, walnuts, hazelnuts, apples, and red wine.

Studies About Effects of Supplementary Antioxidants

Studies have shown that taking certain antioxidant supplements like Vitamin A or Vitamin E in high doses do not prevent cell damage but rather can be harmful. Several studies show that high levels of Vitamin E, beta carotene, and Vitamin A caused increased death in people. Vitamin E and selenium have been found to increase risk of prostate cancer; and Vitamin E and beta-carotene increase risk of lung cancer or make it worse. It is believed this may be because they repair damaged DNA in abnormal cells and prevent the body's own cancer defense system from attacking the damaged cells and so those cancer cells multiple rapidly. On the other hand, Vitamin C which is a water soluble does not increase the number of deaths because perhaps excessive amount can be quickly removed from the body. Interestingly enough, this is not the case with antioxidants found in foods. It is believed that when antioxidants are in combination with foods, then they collectively hinder the free radicals and prevent oxidative stress. So, it's important to eat foods which are high in antioxidants and use them to replenish the body's supply of antioxidants rather than supplements.

Do Supplementary Antioxidants Prevent Cancer?

According to the US National Cancer Institute, which is a US government entity, several studies have been done to find out if supplementary antioxidants can help prevent or lower risk of cancer in humans. The results have been mixed, however, most of the high powered studies conducted did not show benefit and few surprisingly showed increased cancer incidences. The explanation given above about food derived antioxidants acting differently (positively) may be the reason for the discrepancy. Now, for those who already have cancer, some studies have been done to find out whether they will benefit from taking supplementary antioxidants or not. The results are mixed; but, most of them showed cancer patients did worse. So, cancer patients need to be careful about taking supplementary antioxidants. As usual, your doctor should know about any medications or supplements that you are taking.

Probiotics

Probiotics are made up of live bacteria and some types of yeast and they are "good" organisms which may help with digestion and improve the health of the intestinal tract, protecting you from "bad" bacteria present in your gut. These bacteria include *Lactobacillus acidophilus*, *bifidus*, and *Bifidobacterium bifidum* to name a few. Probiotics are found in fermented dairy and soy products; for example, foods like certain yogurt, Kefir, Miso, Tempeh (from soy), fermented cheese like Gouda, cheddar, and Swiss cheese as well as those which are aged or made from raw, unpasteurized milk. Other foods include fermented cabbage (sauerkraut), and ginger beer. They also can be bought as supplements and the refrigerated ones are said to be better.

Research on Probiotics

Apart from gut health, emerging research shows that probiotics may help in diarrhea, antibiotic associated diarrhea, irritable bowel syndrome, allergic disorders, decrease recurrent vaginal yeast, and Bacterial Vaginosis infections. Some pilot research indicate they may help with symptoms of depression, stress, and memory because it is emerging that gut bacteria may have effects on brain and mental health.

Prebiotics

Prebiotics are complex carbohydrates, like insoluble fiber that are consumed by probiotics, and therefore they can increase probiotic levels. They are found in foods high in fiber like soybeans, artichoke, garlic, wheat bran, onion, and banana. There are also commercial prebiotic supplements available.

Medical Foods

....

According to the US Food and Drug Administration (FDA), a Medical Food is "a food which is formulated to be consumed or administered enterally under the supervision of a physician and which is intended for the specific dietary management of a disease or condition for which distinctive nutritional requirements, based on recognized scientific principles, are established by medical evaluation" (section 5(b) of the Orphan Drug Act (21 U.S.C. 360ee (b) (3)) They are specially produced to meet nutritional requirements and are associated with certain medical conditions. They do not require extensive studies and testing which regular pharmaceutical produced medicines require before approval by FDA. Examples of a few of these include the following:

NAME	MEDICAL CONDITION
Metanx	Depression
Foltanx	Depression
Vayarin	ADHD
Deplin	Depression
PoDiaPN	Diabetic peripheral neuropathy
Axona	Mild to Moderate Alzheimer's

For example, Axona is made from median chain triglycerides called Caprylic acid produced from coconut oil or palm kernel oil. Caprylic acid is broken down into ketone bodies which is believed to be an alternate energy source for brain cells affected by Alzheimer's disease. It seems such brain cells are not able to utilize glucose which is the brain's energy source. The Alzheimer's Association has stated that there is not enough evidence to assess the benefits of Medical foods for the treatment of Alzheimer's disease. However, some caregivers of Alzheimer patients have been using Axona or cheaper supermarket Coconut Oil for their loved ones and some have claimed anecdotally that it has been helpful.

Different Classes of Pharmaceutical Medicines

....

There are many categories of medicines used for treating different symptoms and diseases and below are examples of some classes and their uses. It is not by any means an all-encompassing list and a particular medicine that you may be taking for one of the conditions listed below may not be included but do not be disturbed or worried.

Condition	Class of Medicine	Examples of Medications
Inflammation	Anti-Inflammatory	Naproxen, Ibuprofen, Diclofenac
Inflammation	Anti-inflammatory	Steroids – hydrocortisone, Betamethasone
Pain	Analgesics	Ibuprofen, Acetaminophen, Brufen, Paracetamol, Diclofenac, Naproxen
Infection	Antibacterial	Penicillin, Gentamicin, Azithromycin
Infection	Antifungal	Miconazole, Fluconazole, Terbinafine
HIV	Antiretroviral	Zidovudine, Kaletra, Ritonavir, Tenofovir
Malaria	Antimalarial	Quinine, Artemether-lumefantrine, Doxycycline
Worms	Anti parasitic	Albendazole, Mintezol, Pyrantel pamoate
Viral infections	Antiherpes virus	Acyclovir, Valacyclovir, Famciclovir
Hypertension	Blood pressure (several classes)	Amlodipine, Nifedepine, Atenolol, Metoprolol, Lisinopril, Ramipril, Losartan, Cardizem, Verapamil, Hydrochlorothiazide lasix, Bendrofluothiazide, Clonidine
Anticholesterol	Cholesterol (several classes)	Atorvastatin, Simvastatin, Pravastatin Niacin, Fenofibrate, Ezetimibe
Anti dysrhythmics	Correct abnormal heart beat	Digoxin, Cordarone, Sotaolol
Heart failure	Several classes	Lisinopril, Spironolactone, Furosemide, Carvedilol
Antiplatelet	Blood thinners	Aspirin, Clopidogrel
Anti-coagulants	Inhibit clot formation	Warfarin, Dabigatran, Rivaroxaban, Apixaban
Diabetes Mellitus (DM)	Sugar lowering injections	Insulin, Liraglutide, Exenatide
Diabetes Mellitus	Sugar lowering Oral	Glipizide, Metformin, Pioglitazone, Glimepiride, Repaglinide, Sitagliptin
Antidepressant	Treat depression and Anxiety	Paroxetine, Fluoxetine, Bupropion, Amitriptyline

Condition	Class of Medicine	Examples of Medications
Hypothyroid	Thyroid Replacement medicines	Levothyroxine, Synthroid, Armour thyroid, Cytomel
Acid Reflux	Acid reducer	Cimetidine, Zantac, Ranitidine, Famotidine
Acid Reflux	Acid reducer	Omeprazole, Pantoprazole, Esomeprazole

Note: These are just a few examples of the groups of the different classes of medicines available. Most examples given are the generic names, but a few are brand names.

Complementary and Alternative Medicines (CAM)

....

What are These?

"Decisions about your health care are important—including decisions about whether or not to use complementary health products and practices. ------ Find out and consider what scientific studies have been done on the safety and effectiveness of the product or practice that interests you"

(https://nccih.nih.gov/health/decisions).

According to the USA government body called National Center for Complementary and Integrative Health – NCCIH (formally called National Center for Complementary and Alternative Medicine – NCCAM), Complementary and Alternative Medicines (CAM) are drugs made from a varieties of Herbal and Botanicals, Vitamins, Minerals, and other "Natural Products". These have been used in the world for many centuries by many cultures and we are familiar with CAM practices by Herbalists, Naturopaths, or some who do so with some elements of Spiritualism or Religion as well.

Dietary Supplements

....

What are These?

Many CAM products are sold over the counter (OTC) under a broad group known as DIETARY SUPPLEMENTS. The dietary supplements, according to the National Center or Complementary and Integrative Health (NCCIH), are a variety of products, including Herbs, Vitamins and Minerals, and Probiotics, which are taken by mouth and used to supplement the diet. Some of them are beneficial to health but with others there is no good scientific evidence to back their claims.

Can They Cure Diseases?

In the USA, these are not supposed to be used to treat or diagnose medical conditions and most of them will have that disclaimer on the bottle or package. Some have been well studied by rigorous scientific research and found to perform as specified, however, some according to the NCCIH have gained their popularity due to tradition. For some, scientific research done to ascertain their effectiveness in treating the said condition they are supposed to treat have proved to be disappointing and they have fared no better than placebo or a pill filled with sugar.

Below, we will discuss the whole aspect of medicine practiced using plant medicines or supplements and also their interaction with drugs. Examples of such common herbal medications are MORINGA, GINGKO BILOBA, GINGER, TURMERIC, and GINSENG etc.

Natural Products

These include herbal medicines/botanicals, animal products, vitamins, and minerals. Examples are Black Cohosh, Soybean products, Gingko Biloba, fish oil, and glucosamine. Taking dietary supplements like calcium to meet needed dietary recommendations because one is not getting enough from one's diet is not considered as using it as a dietary supplement. That is like treating a deficiency.

Regulation of CAM products

Most CAMs are sold "over the counter" but the sad thing is that they are not regulated by a government body. These complementary medicines are used by people as a treatment for an illness or specific symptoms or to try and improve their overall health and prevent illness. In fact some manufacturers of supplements, in order not to get into trouble with the USA Food and Drug Administration (FDA), put on their bottle label that the product and its claims are "not intended to diagnose, treat, cure or prevent any disease". They may also have stated "these statements have not been evaluated by the FDA". Most lay people believe anything natural is safe and effective; however, this is not always the case, since there is lack of regulation of these supplements by government agencies. For example, to help men who are sexually impotent or having problems with erectile dysfunction (not able to maintain an erection) many products have been put out as being natural and effective. However, over 330 dietary supplements containing undeclared active ingredients have been identified by the FDA over the past five years. These products claim to be "all natural" alternatives to prescription drugs; however, they may contain substances like "Viagra" or "Cialis" which are prescription allopathic medicines used to treat erectile problems.

Safety and effectiveness of Herbal Products

Most consumers believe anything "natural" is safe and effective. However, as mentioned above even in most developed countries they are not regulated and so their safety and effectiveness are not guaranteed. There is lack of regulatory oversight during production of these supplements in most countries including the USA. It is estimated that there are over 30,000 different CAM products on the market produced by several different companies in the USA alone. The purity or effectiveness of the herbal products is also a problem. Interaction with some common drugs may also be an issue (herb/drug interaction). Contaminations with heavy metals like Lead and Mercury, adulteration with real pharmaceuticals like Ibuprofen, Hormones, and Antibiotics occur regularly. For example, a product called Red Yeast Rice, which is used to treat high cholesterol, is often adulterated with a pharmaceutical product called lovastatin by some Chinese drug manufacturers. Most countries may also have traditional herbs prepared as teas, potions, powders, liquids, etc. which herbalists or naturopaths may sell for various ailments. Caution needs to be taken with these since their production may be by questionable means and are not regulated by any agency. Most supplements when taken in amounts specified may not cause any harm, however, it is always important to check with your health care provider. According to recent research (2015) by the CDC (Center for Disease Control) and FDA of the USA, side effects from dietary supplements send about 23,000 people to emergency rooms each year. The majority was from those used for energy and weight loss and the most serious side effects were heart related. (Geller, A. et al. N Engl J Med 2015; 373:1531–1540).

The National Center for Complementary and Integrative Health (https://nccih. nih.gov) is a good website to check the health claims made for different supplements, so keep this website handy. Remember not all internet sites are reliable or carry accurate information.

Herbal Dietary Supplements and Drug Interactions

There are some dietary supplements which have high risk of interactions while others have low risk, and that is why you should always inform your doctor/provider about what medicines you are taking whether they are OTC or herbal supplements. Those with high risk of interactions with pharmaceutical drugs include, St. John's Wort and Goldenseal and need to be avoided with other OTC or prescription drugs. A good site to check drug and herbal interactions is www.drugs.com/drug_interactions.html.

Examples of Dietary Supplements

....

Below are a few of the popular supplements which are used as dietary supplements. References are from the NCCIH website and Medscape.com. We will discuss some of the complementary medicines that are also typically used to treat various medical diseases and conditions, and what medical experts think about their use.

Ginkgo Biloba

One of the oldest type of trees in the world whose leaf extract has been used to prevent Alzheimer's Disease and other dementias, to decrease leg cramps in those with blocked blood vessels in their legs, and to treat sexual dysfunction, multiple sclerosis, and ringing in the ears (tinnitus).

Scientific evidence: shows that after a 6 year study following over 6000 subjects it was found to be ineffective in lowering Blood Pressure, decreasing memory loss, or prevent Alzheimer's disease (dementia).

Side Effects

The side effects include headache, dizziness, stomach problems, and allergic skin reactions in some people. There is increased bleeding risk for people on Warfarin (a drug that is used to thin the blood) or those with bleeding disorders. Caution is needed for those scheduled for surgery or dental procedures, since it may result in excessive bleeding.

Glucosamine Sulphate

Glucosamine sulphate/sulfate is produced from shellfish and is used for treating OSTEOARTHRITIS. Osteoarthritis is the most common type of arthritis and it is due to inflammation of the joints with degeneration and loss of the cartilage between the joints, which increases with age. It is found mostly in adults above 40 years; however, younger people who get an injury to a joint may end up getting arthritis in that joint at a much earlier age than most people will. This supplement comes mostly combined with Chondroitin (obtained from shark/cow cartilage).

Scientific evidence: A study done in 2001 suggested it improved symptoms and preserved joint space in moderate and severe arthritis compared to placebo or a sugar pill.

Side Effects

There are no significant side effects from taking this medication. The usual dosage is 1500 mg a day and it needs to be taken for at least 8–12 weeks to be effective. A note of caution is that it should be avoided in patients allergic to shellfish.

Asian Ginseng Root

The Asian Ginseng root source comes from Japan, Korea or China, and is used for a variety of conditions. It is believed that it is used to improve well-being and recovery from illness, help stimulate the immune system, control blood pressure, diabetes, mellitus, menopausal symptoms, erectile dysfunction, treat hepatitis C, and improve physical and mental performance.

Scientific evidence: Has denied most of the above, however it seems to suggest that Asian Ginseng may lower blood sugar and may benefit boosting the immune system. This is different from Siberian Ginseng.

Side Effects

Short term use at recommended doses appears to be safe. Most common side effects are headache, insomnia, stomach problems, and allergic reactions. It may decrease the actions of many drugs including chemotherapy, HIV drugs, Statins, certain Blood Pressure medicines, and some antidepressants. It is best to avoid this if one is on any of the above drugs.

Omega 3 Fatty Acids (Fish Oil)

Omega 3 fatty acids also known as Fish oil are found in fatty fish like sardines, salmon, mackerel, and oysters, as well as in nuts and seeds. Main fatty acid components in fish oil are called EPA and DHA. There is also a type called ALA found in vegetable oils like soy and canola. Many health claims have been made about Omega 3 fatty acids but according to the NCCIH some of the science results are not conclusive. Fish oil, because of its antioxidant properties increase levels of antioxidants which mop up chemicals known as free radicals.

USES: They have been used for many conditions that may involve inflammation. These include:

- Increased cholesterol and triglycerides
- Coronary Heart Disease and Hypertension
- Dysmenorrhea (painful periods)
- Brain health
- Depression and bipolar disorder if the content of EPA is high
- Psoriasis (skin disease)
- Raynaud's Syndrome (constriction of arteries in the extremities causing pain, cold and discolored toes, and fingers especially in cold weather)
- Breast cancer prevention and recurrence in high risk women
- Numbness and tingling (neuropathy) caused by chemotherapy

Scientific evidence: It helps in development of the eye and brain of babies and infants, and been found to decrease pain in Rheumatoid Arthritis (type of arthritis in which the body turns against itself, attacking joints, and causing swelling – autoimmune type). In Cardiology, research has shown that fish oil may decrease the tendency for blood clot formation and inflammation in people who may have coronary heart disease. However more research is needed.

There is Insufficient evidence that Omega 3 supplements (compared to dietary sources) help prevent or treat strokes, eye problems like macular degeneration, depression, mental problems, or dementia. A prescription fish oil does reduce risk of CVD and Coronary Artery Diseases (CAD) in some populations. A study analyzing several studies done on Marine Omega 3 supplementation found it lowered risk for MI, CAD, and deaths from cardiovascular diseases with exception of strokes. (Hu,Y et al. Jr of American Heart Association Vol 8, No 19, sept. 2019).

What About Fish itself?

Dietary fish itself has been reported to decrease risk of prostate cancer and help to increase antidepressant medication effects in the treatment of depression. Eating fish but not the supplements (capsules) have been associated with reduction of heart diseases like Heart Attack as well as Strokes.

Watch Out for Cod Liver Oil

It is important to know that fish oil is not the same as Cod liver oil, because Cod liver oil contains Omega 3 as well as Vitamin A and Vitamin D, and excess intake of these can cause serious problems.

Side Effects of Omega 3

This is a fairly safe supplement but it may cause some abdominal symptoms like gassy feeling, belching, bloating, and fishy smell on one's breath. It may also thin the blood causing bruising (slight bleeding or discoloration under skin when it is rubbed or hit) especially for those taking blood thinners like Aspirin, Warfarin, or even the group of drugs called NSAIDS (non – steroidal anti-inflammatory drugs like Ibuprofen, Diclofenac, Advil, Motrin etc.). Freezing the capsules or putting them in the fridge is said to take away some of the fishy smell when swallowing it.

Ginger

This is used to relieve nausea and vomiting in pregnant women, nausea after surgery, and also nausea and vomiting during Chemotherapy treatment for Cancer. Other uses are for migraine headaches, motion sickness, vertigo (type of dizziness), and painful periods in young girls (Dysmenorrhea). It is believed to have anti-inflammatory effects and so is used for Osteoarthritis of joints.

Scientific evidence: It may help with nausea related to pregnancy and chemotherapy, but not for osteoarthritis or rheumatoid arthritis.

Side Effects

These may include diarrhea, heartburn, stomach pain, throat irritation, skin irritation, or rash if used for skin problems, irregular heart beat, and bleeding tendencies.

Like any medicine, excess amount taken may lead to these side effects, however, some people will not experience any of these.

Garlic

Used for treating high cholesterol, heart disease, and hypertension. It is also thought to be able to prevent Stomach and Colon Cancer.

Scientific evidence: Its effect in lowering both blood pressure and cholesterol are small, however, it does not seem to lower the "bad" cholesterol called LDL. It has not been found to reduce risk of above cancers, but may have potential anti-cancer ability according to the National Cancer Institute. Many forms of garlic are available as raw, cooked, and powdered in capsule or tablet forms.

Side Effects

These include allergic reaction resulting in swelling of face and skin rash. Others include tendency to bleed, asthma, diarrhea, gassy feeling, bad breath, heartburn, and upset stomach. It may decrease concentration of drugs like Verapamil, Digoxin, Rosuvastatin, and Tacrolimus and so it is best to avoid if on any of these.

MSM: (Methylsulfonylmethane)

This is a supplement used to treat Osteoarthritis (degeneration of joints).

Scientific evidence: has not been able to confirm that it helps with Osteoarthritis, however, some people think it does and it is either used alone or combined with Glucosamine or Ginger. It is taken orally or used topically. For example, a topical lotion is made from MSM granules and ginger powder mixed with two teaspoons of water and added to 16 oz. of a moisturizing lotion. This is applied to painful back or joints.

Side Effects

Allergic reaction, skin rashes, stomach upset, or diarrhea.

Black Cohosh

Black Cohosh has been used for many years by women for hot flashes and night sweats associated with menopause and in some European countries it has been prescribed by doctors for treating hot flashes.

Scientific evidence: Studies show it is not better than a placebo (dummy or sugar pill) in preventing or treating hot flashes and night sweats.

Side Effects

It has been found to cause liver damage, rash, stomach ache, and headache in some women. Make sure your liver function is tested before trying this if you chose to use it. It may also interact with drugs like Fexofenadine (Allegra), Glyburide, and Statins and so one must avoid it, if on any of these drugs.

Melatonin

This is produced naturally in the brain and helps in maintaining a normal sleep cycle, by causing more to be released at night and less during daytime or in light environs at night. This supplement is used to help with sleep disorders.

Scientific studies: Studies show it may help with inability to fall asleep, jet lag, and night shift work sleep problems. It has also been used for headache and tinnitus (ringing in the ears), but research on these is scanty. It has to be taken close to one's bedtime. Research showed it helps to improve sleep and fatigue in people who are taking beta blockers like Metoprolol and Atenolol for Hypertension or heart disease. It is believed these drugs may decrease melatonin levels leading to the problems.

Side Effects

It is fairly safe and possible side effects include drowsiness, nausea, and dizziness.

Coenzyme Q10 (CoQ10)

This fairly expensive supplement is used by people for heart conditions. It is an antioxidant and is involved in energy production in the cells. It is also used to treat muscle ache/pain in patients taking Statins for high cholesterol (about 5–10% of patients taking these may have muscle problems).

Scientific evidence: Studies show it may help the heart in people with heart failure and those who are recovering from heart bypass surgery. Some few studies suggest it may help individuals who suffer from muscle pain after taking the cholesterol medicines known as "Statins" (e.g. Atorvastatin-Lipitor), but most good ones refute that (Beth Taylor, Am J Cardiovasc Drugs 2018; 18(2): 75–82). More good research are needed. However, many cardiologists may prescribe it.

Side Effects

It is fairly safe, however, may cause dizziness, stomach upset, nausea, and increased liver enzymes in some individuals. Increased liver enzymes are seen in the blood when there is liver cell damage or inflammation.

Evening Primrose Oil

This oil is extracted from the seeds of the Primrose plant. This contains fatty acids (gamma-linolenic acid – GLA) and is believed to have anti-inflammatory effects. Women use evening primrose oil for premenstrual syndrome (PMS), breast pain, endometriosis, and symptoms of menopause such as hot flashes. It is also used for eczema, acne and rheumatoid arthritis.

Scientific evidence: Results are mixed regarding its use for rheumatoid arthritis and breast pain and no convincing effect was found for its use for PMS or eczema. It is usually sold in capsules.

Side Effects

Upset stomach, nausea, soft stools, or headache may occur. If any of these effects persist or worsen, stop medicine and contact your doctor or pharmacist promptly. A very serious allergic reaction to this product is rare. However, seek immediate medical attention if you notice any of the following symptoms of a serious allergic reaction: rash, itching/swelling (especially of the face/tongue/throat), severe dizziness, and trouble breathing.

Reminders on Your Radar

There are different types of Medicines: Prescription, OTC, Complementary/Alternative Supplements, Vitamins, Minerals, and Medical Foods. There may be different classes of medicines used to treat a particular condition and a choice may depend on other medical conditions that you have. Make sure your health care provider is aware of all medicines you are taking, because there may be interactions between some which may cancel the effect of others.

Therapeutic Lifestyle Changes (TLC)

. . . .

What Are These?

Through out this book you will read about Therapeutic Lifestyle Changes (TLC) that is a part of treatment and prevention of many chronic medical conditions. These are lifestyle changes one has to make in order to treat a particular disease or medical condition. They are part of the "therapy" together with medications or whatever is needed to control a disease and make you feel better. They include: healthy eating, increased regular exercise, quit smoking, and weight

> **"The secret of change is to focus all your energy, not on fighting the old, but on building the new"**
>
> —Socrates
> (Ancient Greek philosopher).

management. Everyone should try and incorporate this into their treatment proto-col and sometimes they may let one get off certain medicines or decrease the number of medicines being used for a medical condition.

Food or Dietary Preferences

"Let food be thy medicine and med-icine be thy food."

— Hippocrates.
Ancient Greek physician.

Healthy eating which includes eating more fruits, vegetables, and whole grains like whole wheat bread, brown rice, whole rye, buckwheat, bulgur, etc. has to be the norm for all of us. Try to avoid what I term "the white stuff". These include: white flour, white sugar, white bread, regular pasta, and white rice. Minimize cooking methods which involve a lot of frying, especially deep frying, instead try baking, grilling, broiling, or boiling which do not use as much oil or fats. Use of an "Air Fryer" can brown foods which are lightly sprayed with cooking spray products and therefore reduce the use of oils and fats for cooking.

The Mediterranean Diet

This has been found to help lower cholesterol, prevent heart attacks and strokes, decrease Alzheimer's disease (dementia), and Parkinson's disease among other things. The Mediterranean diet can be considered as a food pyramid which has 4 levels. More of the lower level foods are to be eaten. It is made up of a wide base consisting of lots of fruits, vegetables, nuts, olive oil, grains, beans, and seeds; fol-lowed by moderate amounts of fish and sea food (level 2), minimal eggs, cheese and yogurt (level 3), and less amounts of meats and sweets (level 4) at the top of the pyramid.

A glass of red wine or pure grape juice is included in the Mediterranean diet.

Decreasing red meat and making sure that fat around chicken, pork, or beef is trimmed before cooking, all helps cut down on cholesterol and saturated fats.

Weight Loss

Losing weight has been found to lower high cholesterol, blood sugar, and blood pressure. From discussions in the book, you will find out that these risk factors are for many other health problems. Extensive discussion on this is discussed else-where in the book.

Exercise

Do what you enjoy, whether walking, dancing, Zumba, salsa, going to the gym to use exercise equipment, gardening, swimming, jogging, or movement exercises like Yoga or Tai Chi etc. Do anything that will get you moving and get your heart rate up. You may wear a tracker or watch that tracks how many steps you walk in a day. It is good to aim at 10,000 steps a day. This is equivalent to 5 miles, and it takes about 20 minutes to complete one mile.

Use Alcohol in Moderation

Decrease excessive alcohol use (this is more than 2 drinks by women and 3 drinks by men per day). Moderate alcohol intake is one drink a day for women and two drinks a day for men. If you are wondering what one drink constitutes of, it is either:

- Beer: 12 fluid ounces (355 milliliters)
- Wine: 5 fluid ounces (148 milliliters)
- Distilled spirits (80 proof alcohol): 1.5 fluid ounces (44 milliliters)

Quit Smoking Tobacco

Smoking increases one's risk of heart disease, stroke, lung problems, and different Cancers just to name a few. To stop smoking some do it "cold turkey" – that is without any help. However, smoking cessation is possible with medication, tobacco substitute products like nicotine patch or gum, laser therapy, acupuncture, hypnosis, and e-cigarettes. E-cigarettes may, however, not be as harmless as people think it is and so one has to be careful about its prolonged use. Recently there have been incidents of serious lung diseases especially in young people who are using it.

Reminders on Your Radar

TLC examples like healthy eating, exercise, weight loss, smoking cessation, and cutting back on alcohol consumption are all ways which help one either reduce risks for certain chronic diseases or are part of treating chronic diseases. These are the things which YOU personally undertake. Scientific evidence support their very important role in being healthy.

Part Three

Physical Health

6

Physical Health

Introduction

....

The third part of the book deals with the physical, and aims to empower you to know about what common diseases can affect you, and how you can develop the ability to prevent certain chronic diseases in your body. It will also equip you with knowledge about the various life transitions a woman goes through and how to deal with health issues that may arise with changes that your body goes through due to age.

"Physical fitness is not only one of the most important keys to a healthy body, it is the basis of dynamic and creative intellectual activity."

John F Kennedy. American President
May 29, 1917—Nov. 22, 1963.

Each chapter deals with a different organ system and the common diseases that may occur within that organ system. We do not discuss all medical conditions, however, I hope this will encourage the reader to look up from other sources, any conditions that are not addressed here. To make for easy reading and reference we will discuss the various conditions and diseases that affect us starting from the head region and moving down to the neck, chest, abdomen, and so on. Some of the systems may have diagrams to help better understand the problems that can affect them.

Remember, the internet is a great source of information and you can use it to find out more about conditions we discuss in this book. However, look up from credible sources like those referenced in this book. Use this book as a reference or look up book to know more about a certain medical condition or any disease you are diagnosed with.

Importance of Knowing About Your Body and Staying Healthy

1. One has to be physically healthy in order to live long and fulfill your God given dreams and purpose in life
2. Knowledge of how your body functions and the reason why certain symptoms or ailments occur empowers you to take quick action to preempt any serious condition which may result
3. Knowledge will help you recognize and be reassured when certain symptoms occur as a result of normal changes in your body as you go through the female transitions
4. As an EDUCATED person you should know the names of your medical conditions and as previously mentioned the names of your medicines
5. Don't underestimate your ability to know about how the body works and diseases affecting the body. The information is NOT ABOVE your head. Don't buy into the idea that only medical doctors or other health providers are entitled to medical information
6. Once you know about your medical condition, you are in a better position to know what will make you feel better or make it worse, and prevent its progression
7. Armed with this knowledge, you have the ability to control your health outlook as far as it is humanly possible and you are not totally clueless about your disease(s)
8. Knowledge makes YOU know and feel in control of the future direction of your health
9. Many doctors including myself get very excited when patients ask me serious questions about their disease/illness or have taken the initiative to do something to improve their condition or health in general. This is being PROACTIVE and many doctors are impressed with proactive patients, although some doctors get intimidated by that.

Second Medical Opinions

As a patient, you are entitled to seek a second medical opinion or switch doctors when you are faced with a new medical condition, life threatening disease, or improper care of an established health issue. Other situations include: If your present doctor is not communicating well with you, does not take time to explain things relating to your health concerns, displays a poor attitude or rudeness toward you, or you are not satisfied with your care. You can go to consult another doctor or health care provider if that will give you peace of mind because one has to be comfortable with and trust their health care provider.

The Human Body

"I will praise You, for I am fear-
fully and wonderfully made;"

Psalms 139:14 NKJV.

The human body is a remarkable one
and is programed to work in a beautiful
way with every part being in sync with
the others. However, disease and the
normal process of aging bring about certain changes including results of normal
wear and tear e.g. joint degeneration. When a change is just due to the "normal"
lifecycle process it is known as physiological change. For example at puberty, boys
or girls experience differences in their bodies. The boys have deeper voices and
grow hairs in the pubic (genital area) and underarms (axillae); the girls start developing breasts, pubic and axillae hairs, and start having their monthly periods or
menses/menstruations. Some physiological changes later in life may bring issues
which may bother women e.g. menopause; and we will discuss some of these in
later chapters of the book.

Before discussing diseases by systems, it is important to mention two group of
diseases known as hereditary and congenital diseases which may affect either one
system or several organs in the body.

Hereditary and Congenital Diseases
Hereditary diseases

These are diseases that ran in families and are inherited from either or both parents' genes. Each person is made up of cells and each cell has a nucleus which
carries genetic material in a chromosome. This genetic material is called DNA
(Deoxyribonucleic acid) and it is from this genetic material that instructions are
received to cause growth, multiplication, repair, metabolic processes, and reproduction in all living beings. When there is a defect in the genetic material and it is
handed down to an offspring then we get hereditary diseases. Examples are sickle
cell anemia, cystic fibrosis, polycystic kidney disease, some clotting diseases, and
familiar hypercholesterolemia. However, not all genetic disorders in new born are
inherited genetic disorders and some babies are born with genetic disorders from
mutations (changes in DNA) which were not passed down from families – meaning
there is no family history of that disease, and the babies developed the mutation
during development. Sickle cell disease, which is inherited and is therefore passed
down, is discussed under blood or hematological conditions; and familiar hyper-
cholesteremia is discussed under cardiovascular diseases. In some resource rich
countries, newborns are screened for many genetic diseases. For example, in
some states in America, 34 core conditions are recommended for newborn screening with some states screening even more conditions.

Congenital diseases

These are diseases that exist before or are present at birth and may be due to genetic, infectious, trauma, or environmental causes. The most common ones are cerebral palsy (disorder in the brain resulting in a movement disorder), heart defects like septal defects (hole in the heart), neural tube defects as in spinal bifida (there is incomplete development of the spinal cord and its coverings or membranes), and Down's syndrome (this is a genetic disorder present at birth and presents with developmental and intellectual delay, but it's not hereditary). Others are club foot (inward twisting of the foot or feet) and cleft palate and lips (openings in the roof of the mouth and lips).

7

Eyes, Ears and Nose

We will discuss common conditions affecting the eyes. Ears and nose in the next chapters.

Common Conditions Affecting the Eyes

....

Introduction

"The eye is the window of the human body through which it feels its way and enjoys the beauty of the world".

—Leonardo da Vincian Italian polymath of the Renaissance, who was also a great painter/artist.

The eyes are a very important part of the body providing sight which is one of the five senses we use to contact or appreciate our environment, whether it is other individuals or innate things. The eyes enable us to read, watch TV or movies, and protect ourselves from danger, etc.; they are the window to our outside world and so we have to protect them as best as we can.

How Vision Occurs

In order for vision to occur light from an object is focused by the cornea and then the clear crystal LENS; with the object registering as an image at the back of the eye on a tissue known as the RETINA. This is the light sensitive part of the eye which sends the image by nerve impulses to the brain that creates the visual image. The center of the retina is the area of sharpest vision and is called the macula.

Causes of Impaired Vision or Blindness

Vision can be affected in many ways from mild impaired vision to more serious permanent blindness. The common conditions leading to blindness include Trachoma, Diabetes Mellitus, Cataract, Glaucoma, and Injury. Impaired vision and blindness can also result from tumor and cancers of the eye or brain, and in the elderly a condition called macular degeneration is also common. We will discuss just a few here. As part of your eye health care, it is important to have an eye exam every 1 to 2 years by an optometrist or ophthalmologist.

Eye Health Professionals

An optometrist is a primary care provider who exams eyes, checks vision, and provides treatment for normal vision problems, and also does yearly eye checkups for individuals.

The Ophthalmologist is a medical doctor who is highly qualified to diagnose and treat more serious eye diseases, does what the optometrist does, and also performs eye surgeries. Some ophathalmologists have specialized in pediatric care and particular areas of the eye like the eye lids, retina, and cornea.

An optician is an eye technician who fits and dispenses corrective lenses ordered by either an ophthalmologist or optometrist.

Vision Testing

When you visit an eye care provider, you will first have a "Visual Acuity" test. This is when you either stand about 20 feet away from a board and read letters or numbers or do it sitting down in the chair with a special gadget in front of your eyes. Perfect or sharp normal vision is 20/20. This means you can see clearly at 20 feet what should normally be seen at that distance. If your visual acuity is 20/100, then it means you can see at 20 feet what a person with unimpaired vision can see at 100 feet. In countries which use the metric system, normal vision is 6/6 in meters. The eye professionals normally use a chart called a "Snellen Eye Chart" to do this test. Your primary care provider may also have one in her office to do eye screening test.

Complete Eye Exam

During a complete eye exam, you will first have a Visual Acuity test, and this will be followed by testing of the muscles that move the eyes, and how your pupils respond to light shown through them. Next is inspection of the eye lids and lashes, followed by the various eye chambers; after which the eye pressure is measured by a special instrument. The pupil of the eye may be dilated with eye drops, so that the retina can be thoroughly examined.

We will now discuss some of the common eye conditions or diseases and how they are treated.

Cataract (Ca-ta-rat)

What is it?

This is the most common cause of blindness in the world and it is due to the clouding of the lenses in the eye. Cataracts tend to occur with age, and 60% of those over 60 years have cataracts; however prior injury, diabetes, prior infections, chronic steroid use, or being born with congenital cataract from an infection called Rubella (German Measles) can all lead to cataracts.

Signs and Symptoms

Signs of cataract include fuzzy or clouded vision, blindness and sensitivity to light or glare. When it is severe, an individual's central part of the eye appears white or cloudy.

Diagnosis

Your vision will be checked (visual acuity), followed by a complete exam. The examiner will usually observe that the lens is clouded in one or both eyes.

Treatment

Treatment initially may include: use of stronger corrective glasses, brighter lighting, anti-glare sunglasses, or magnifying lenses, however advance cases are treated by surgery to remove the lens, followed by implantation with an artificial lens, or use of corrective spectacles (glasses) with high powered lens to enable one to see clearly.

Prevention

To prevent or delay cataract the use of broad brim hats and sun glasses to reduce ultraviolet light from the sun has been suggested.

Glaucoma (Gla-co-ma)

What is it?

It is the second most common cause of blindness in the world, the first being cataracts. Glaucoma is mostly caused by increased pressure in the eye leading to damage of the optic nerve, which is the nerve involved with vision. The eye contains special fluids which help with its function and contribute to maintain the pressure in the eye and keeping the shape of the eye ball. There is a normal pressure which is maintained by a system which circulates the fluids, however; sometimes the pressure increases as a result of blockage of the fluid drainage system in the eye, and this is called increased Intra Ocular Pressure.

Signs and Symptoms

Vision decreases gradually or suddenly depending on the type of glaucoma. Most people will have elevated internal pressure of the eye (Intra Ocular Pressure), although there are some individuals with glaucoma who have normal eye pressure. Normal pressure in the eye is less than 14 mm Hg, but this may increase in Glaucoma.

Diagnosis

Your vision will be checked by making you read the letters on a chart and the various eye chambers inspected after which the eye pressure is measured. The eye may be dilated so that the retina can be thoroughly examined.

Treatment

Treatment of glaucoma is either by surgery, special eye drops (e.g. Timolol, Betaxolol), and or oral medications (Methazolamide and Acetazolamide) to lower the pressure and prevent damage to the optic nerve. Your eye doctor or ophthalmologist will let you know which treatment is best for you.

Prevention

It is important to have regular eyes examinations about every one to two years after the age of 40 years or earlier if you have a family history of glaucoma.

Red Eye
What is it?

Red eye is inflammation or infection of the eye, causing increased blood flow to the surface of the eye which results in the redness seen on the front of the eyeball. The most common causes are viral or bacterial infections involving the thin, transparent membrane that covers the surface of the eye ball (CONJUNCTIVA), allergies from dust and pollen from plants, or foreign body in the eye like an eye lash. Other causes of redness include glaucoma (see above), and infections or inflammation involving the deeper tissues of the eye, for example the sclera or white tissue covering the eye ball. Below are explanations of some of them.

Conjunctivitis

Inflammation or infection of the conjunctiva can be caused by infection due to viruses, bacteria and fungi, allergy to an environmental agent like pollen and grass, irritants like smoke, chlorine in swimming pools, or foreign body in the eyes like a piece of hair.

Signs and Symptoms
Viral conjunctivitis

Caused by many viruses and it is commonly called "pink eye". They don't usually present with much pus, but watery eye, slightly swollen eyelid, and one may have a swollen lump (lymph node) right in front of the ear on the affected side. Frequently, the individual may have had a recent cold or upper respiratory infection. It is very contagious and can be spread to others when one touches the eye and touches door handles, bed sheets, or someone's hands or face.

Bacterial conjunctivitis

Can be caused by several organisms or germs but the serious ones are those caused by gonorrhea and chlamydia, both of which are sexually transmitted bacteria. An individual with the bacterial type will have a lot of pus looking creamy discharge from the eyes, the eyelids are difficult to open in the morning (matted together), and there may be swelling of the eyelids with discomfort or pain.

Allergic conjunctivitis

This may present with itchy, watery eyes, with no pus but may have a stringy discharge. It may be accompanied by itchy, watery nose, throat or ears, and a lot of sneezing and throat clearing.

Treatment

It is important that you see a doctor to make the right diagnosis and get the right treatment.

1. Bacterial Conjunctivitis is treated with antibiotic eye drops, and if severe, or caused by gonorrhea or chlamydia, oral, or intravenous antibiotics are used. In resource poor countries, Povidone-iodine 1.25% ophthalmic solution is used if antibiotic drops are expensive. If not treated some can lead to complications of blindness and cataract formation
2. Allergic conjunctivitis is treated with allergy eye drops and sometimes oral or nasal allergy medicines if needed. Sometimes steroid eye drops are used if the symptoms are severe
3. Viral conjunctivitis is usually allowed to take its own course since it is self limiting, with the body's own immune system fighting the infection. Sometimes lubricating eye drops or eye drops for red eye are used to sooth the burning. However, sometimes antibiotic eye drops are prescribed as a precaution

against a resulting secondary bacterial infection. If the infection is deemed to be caused by HERPES SIMPLEX virus, then specific anti-herpes eye drops are used

Prevention

Hands have to be washed well (good hand hygiene) and avoid touching the eyes to prevent transmitting the infection to other people if infection is the cause. For those with a history of allergies, make sure you take your allergy medicines and do the other things discussed under Allergic Rhinitis in Diseases affecting the Nose. In many countries to prevent bacterial infection with gonorrhea or chlamydia of a newborn baby as it passes through the birth canal, prophylactic (preventive medication) antibiotic called Erythromycin antibiotic is put in the eyes after delivery.

Trachoma

What is it?

Trachoma is caused by a bacterial infection of the clear tissue which covers the front surface of the eye ball – conjunctiva and the cornea. This is the leading cause of blindness in most developing or resource poor countries and it is spread from human to human as a result of poor sanitation and contaminated water. It has largely been eliminated from developed countries, however worldwide about 80 million people suffer from it. It is caused by spread from contact with an infected person's eyes or nose, or throat secretions, or through indirect means from surfaces, clothes, bedsheets, and even flies that have been contaminated by an infected person.

Signs and Symptoms

May be asymptomatic initially, but may present with time, as redness and a granular surface under upper eyelid, as well as scarring of the conjunctiva and dry eyes due to destruction of glands producing eye lubricating fluids. Eye lashes may grow inward, scarring the cornea and conjunctiva and leading to loss of vision and blindness.

Treatment

The WHO recommends use of surgery, antibiotics, facial washing, and environmental cleanliness, in all endemic countries. The two mostly prescribed antibiotics for trachoma treatment in the early stages are combined oral Azithromycin tablets and Tetracycline, or Azithromycin eye drops. Both oral and eye drops have to be used. Facial cleanliness by washing is stressed, as well as environmental cleanliness, and good water supply. There is sometimes need for surgery to correct deformed eyelids, which if not corrected will lead to injury of the cornea and subsequent blindness.

Prevention

Ways to prevent the spread is through washing of face with soap and water, widespread treatment with antibiotics of communities where it is present in large numbers (endemic), and improving environmental sanitation to prevent transmission or spread.

Decreased Vision Associated With Age (PRESBYOPIA)
What is it?

Most individuals over the age of 40 years realize it is hard to read words that are close up or at normal reading distance. This decreased vision associated with age, is known as PRESBYOPIA (pres-bye-o-pia). The crystalline lens in the eye loses its ability to focus or change its shape because it loses its flexibility and images are not well focused on the retina.

Signs and Symptoms

Vision becomes blurred at arm's length, making the eyes tired through straining in order to focus, although seeing far away is fine.

Treatment

READING GLASSES: To correct this, an individual has to get Reading Glasses or Reading Spectacles, after seeing an eye professional who will examine your vision and prescribe appropriate reading glasses for you. For those who already wear glasses for near vision or long vision, they will need bifocal lenses, which have the bottom part of the lenses for reading and the top part for distant vision. One may also obtain LINELESS or PROGRESSIVE BIFOCAL lenses. These do not show the typical line separating the two types of lenses

SURGERY: There is also a surgical procedure which can correct this vision problem. In a surgery called LASIK surgery, one eye is corrected for distant vision and the other eye is made nearsighted and so the need for reading glasses is eliminated

Myopia and Hyperopia (Hypermetropia)
What are These?

The two other types of vision defects known as refractive errors:

1. MYOPIA (nearsightedness, short sightedness) in which one can see near objects close to the eye clearly, but far objects appear blurred

2. HYPEROPIA (farsightedness), one can see far or distant objects well, but close objects do not come into proper focus or are blurred. In this state the eye ball is smaller or the lens and cornea don't have the correct shape preventing images from focusing on the retina

Signs and Symptoms

Both cause blurred vision as mentioned above. If straining to see occurs, then people may even end up with eye fatigue or headaches. In younger students who cannot see well at school their performance in school may be affected, resulting in bad grades.

Treatment

Both are treated with eye glasses, contact lenses, or laser procedures after an examination by an eye professional.

Dry Eyes Syndrome – "Strange-But My Eyes are Watery"??
What is it?

Dry Eye Syndrome (DES) also known as keratitis sicca is a condition caused by a problem with any one of several parts of the eye involved with tears. These include: the tear film on the surface of the eye, the tear ducts and production apparatus, the eye lids, the nerves supplying the eye, or the tear gland. Abnormalities in any of these may result in DES. Tears usually lubricate and provide moisture to the eye; however, in DES there is abnormality of the quality or quantity of the tears produced. The tears produced are not the usual type and tend to be more watery and have less of the oily component, and the excessive tearing often seen is due to a reflex reaction called reflex tearing. In reflex tearing, the dryness causes the nerves to send a message for more tears to be produced. Factors that may contribute to dry eyes include:

Causes of Dry Eyes Syndrome

1. Medications: For example, BP medicines, antihistamine, psychiatric medicines, and preservatives in certain eye drops
2. Age: Dry eyes increase with age as the glands quality and quantity of tears decrease
3. Medical conditions: Diabetes Mellitus, Rheumatoid arthritis, and Sjogrens' syndome which are autoimmune related
4. Abnormal eyelid position: This can result in increased evaporation of tears such as in Trachoma, Bell's Palsy (there is damage to nerve which normally causes eyelids to shut, so eyelid stays open), blockage of the glands called Meibomian glands which produce the oily layer of tears

5. Eye conditions: Conditions like conjunctivitis, contact lens wearers, Vitamin A deficiency, and cornea problems which all cause dry eyes

Signs and Symptoms

There is excessive tearing and runny nose, and other symptoms include foreign body sensation (gritty sensation on eye surface), blurred vision, red eye, sensitivity to light, and mucus like discharge. If not treated early, the excessive dryness results in damage or scarring of the eye layers.

Treatment

Tests the eye doctor may do include vision testing, staining of the surface of the eye to check for abrasions/scratches, and checking the quality and quantity of the tears produced.

Treatment is related to treating underlying specific cause if that is reversible, and it is also based on severity of DES.

1. Medications: Alternatives have to be used, e.g. change antihistamines for allergic rhinitis from oral to steroid nasal drops
2. Medical or eye conditions: Treat underlying condition. e.g. eye lids may be repaired or reposition if that is the cause
3. Infections: If infection is present as in blepharitis, antibiotic eye drops may be used
4. Increasing tear production: Cyclosporine (Restasis brand) prescription eye drops increases tear production
5. Conserving tears: Plugs are put into the tear duct holes so the tears stay longer on surface of eye and do not drain out quickly
6. Improving the quality of tears: Omega 3 fatty acid or flax seed oil have been found to increase the oily part of the tears. Oily eye drops such as Liposomal eye sprays can be sprayed on the edges of eyelids to replace oily part of tears. Warm compresses and sometimes antibiotics are used if there is infection of the oil producing glands (Meibomian glands) so they can produce enough of the oily layer of the tears
7. Replacement of tears or lubrication: If mild, one uses mild lubricants called artificial tears which are obtained over the counter. If moderate to severe, immuno-suppressive eye drops e.g. Cyclosporine (Restasis) have been found to stimulate tear production
8. Antibiotics, anti-inflammatory, and steroids may be used to treat infections or inflammation of the meibomian glands or the eye lids. Sometimes, oral tetracyclines are given for a few weeks on a daily basis to reduce inflammation

9. Surgery is used to treat DES if it is very severe. This includes the punctate plugs or occlusion of the tear ducts using heat (cauterization). In very severe cases if all else fails salivary glands are transplanted to area around the eyes and then saliva acts like tears and lubricates the eye(s)

Prevention

If the cause is reversible, then as soon as it is noted, changes should be made, e.g. change of medications with resolution of the dry eyes. In other cases treatment of dry eyes sooner than later prevents further damage to eyes.

Age Related Macular Degeneration (Maa-cue-lar) – AMD
What is this?

This is the leading cause of severe vision loss and blindness in adults aged 65 years and above in most of the developed world and Asia. Factors that put one at increased risk include family history (genetics), diet, smoking, and hardening of the arteries also called arteriosclerosis or atherosclerosis. Atherosclerosis is a condition where there is blockage of arteries caused by cholesterol and other substances, and this can lead to diseases like heart attacks or strokes when vessels in the heart or brain are affected.

This occurs with age and genetics (inherited characteristics), with lifestyle and environmental conditions contributing to its development.

Signs and Symptoms

There is central vision loss due to new tiny blood vessels forming in the part of the eye called the Macula of the Retina, where sharp central vision occurs. A sufferer will see the periphery of an object but the central part will be blurred or dark, progressing to severe vision loss and blindness with time.

Treatment

It is treated by vitamins, medications injected into the eye, eye drops, laser treatment, or individuals may use vision aids like magnifying glasses to see or read. A study by the US National Eye Institute (age related eye disease study-AREDS) found that taking high levels of antioxidants and zinc can reduce risk of developing ADVANCED AMD by about 25% (https://nei.nih.gov/research/clinical-trials/age-related-eye-disease-study-areds).

STUDY SUMMARY: It did not show that it prevented development of AMD, just slowed progression to an advance form. The formula used for the study contained VIT C 500mg, VIT E 400 IU, VIT A 25,000 IU or Beta Carotene 15mg, Zinc Oxide

80mg, Cupric oxide 2mg (copper). A regular daily multivitamin does not provide the formulation used in the study. A second study AREDS 2 completed in 2011, tested omega 3 fatty acid and 2 other beta carotenoids (Lutein and Zeaxanthin) with exclusion of beta carotene itself. They found study participants benefited from the formulas with the two beta carotenoids, but omega 3 did not seem to decrease progression to Advance AMD. These results were important since high doses of beta carotene has been associated with lung cancer in smokers, but not lutein and zeaxanthin.

Prevention

To prevent PROGRESSION the two beta carotenoids which are antioxidants, are being used in supplements. These two are also found in leafy green plants. Many companies are selling supplements based on the combination of vitamins minerals and antioxidants of the AREDS2 Study to prevent progression to advanced AMD.

Diabetic Retinopathy (ray-ti-no-pattie)
What is this?

This is the most serious eye/vision complication related to diabetes mellitus. It affects about 9 million diabetics and is the most common cause of blindness in adults in the USA. It affects the blood vessels in the retina or the light sensitive part at the back of the eye and uncontrolled diabetes may hasten its development.

Signs and Symptoms

Initial retinopathy may be asymptomatic, with no change in vision, however, with time fuzziness, blurred vision, floaters, and distortion of images may occur. Advanced cases have swelling of tissues, leakage of blood vessels, and new abnormal ones forming on the retina, leading to vision loss and blindness.

Treatment

The various treatments will delay or prevent further vision loss and do not cure it. These include medications like injection of steroids which decreases swelling of macula and injections of "anti-VEGF" medication which reduces the formation of abnormal blood vessels and bleeding as well as scar tissue formation. All of these – swelling, abnormal vessels, and bleeding lead to vision loss if not treated. Additionally, Laser surgery is used to seal off leaky blood vessels and shrink them as well. Surgery called Vitrectomy removes the gel in front of the retina and any blood that has leaked into it causing one to have better vision.

Prevention

Individuals with diabetes need to have a complete diabetic eye screening exam every year, which involves dilation of the pupil so that trained doctors can look at the state of the retina. Careful control of blood sugar and any accompanying high blood pressure and cholesterol is needed to delay or prevent this condition. If you notice change in your vision, see an eye doctor as soon as possible for an eye exam.

Reminders on Your Radar

There are many diseases affecting the eyes and some of the chronic ones can be detected early if as an adult you have regular eye exams every one to two years. Certain medical conditions require yearly eye exams and screening, and the most important one is Diabetes Mellitus. Common causes of blindness include Diabetes Retinal disease, Age related Macular degeneration, cataract, glaucoma, and trachoma. Save your eyes: have regular eye check ups.

8

Common Conditions Affecting the Ears

Structure of the Ear

....

The ear has the pinna or outside portion we see and an inner part divided into 3 chambers. The pinna protects the part inside the skull and directs sound waves through a canal or passage known as the EXTERNAL CANAL. The ear drum is a thin sheet which separates the external canal from the middle canal or space. This space has tiny bones which help transmit sound into the INNER EAR which converts sound waves to electrical impulses which are transmitted to the brain by the ear nerve called the Auditory nerve. The inner ear has another organ that controls balance. An earache can be due to infection or inflammation of the external canal, middle, or inner ear.

> "So then, my beloved brethren, let every man be swift to hear, slow to speak, slow to wrath;"
>
> —James 1v 19 (NKJV)

Otitis Externa

What is it?

This is also known as swimmer's ear and occurs when the external canal which connects the outside of the ear to the middle ear becomes infected or inflamed, causing the passage way to become painful and narrow as the tissues swell. The external canal can be affected by infection involving the ear drum, or infection occurs when one uses Q tips and bobby pins to relieve itching in the external canal. The scratching of the canal can cause breaks in the lining, causing bacteria to penetrate it. Infection may also start from the middle ear or fungal infection may affect the external canal of those exposed to aquatic sports and during summer time or in hot climate. It may also occur when the canal is dry due to excess removal of cerumen (wax). Skin conditions like eczema (a skin condition related to allergy), rash due to sensitivity to jewelry or hair products, or psoriasis also cause scaly, red, itchy skin of the ear lobe or canal.

Signs and Symptoms

This results in pain and or ulceration around the opening of the affected ear, causing the external canal and ear lobe to be crusty, scaly, itchy, or red. The canal may be very swollen and hearing may be decreased. Sometimes when an otoscope (instrument used to view the ear canal and drum) is used to try and examine the ear, it cannot be placed into it due to pain.

Treatment

Antibiotic pills and or topical drops and pain medication are used to treat the infection and pain. Anti-fungal drops are used if fungus is suspected. If allergy or psoriasis is involved, steroid drops or creams may be prescribed. If a lot of debris is present, a healthcare provider may need to clear the canal and then prescribe the steroid or antibiotic drops.

Prevention

1. Avoid putting foreign objects in the ears. I do not recommend the use of objects to clean the external canal of the ears because the lining of the canal is thin and can be easily damaged causing bacteria to cause infection of the external canal, ear drum, and middle ear
2. Cerumen or wax has its function as it can trap bacteria and protect the ear and also keeps it clean. If you have excess wax and cannot hear, the best thing is to let a health professional clean it out, or you can purchase a small OTC ear suction device which operates by battery or suction and can remove excess wax without the problems inserted objects cause. One can also put a few drops of any type of oil, like baby oil, mineral oil etc. into the external canal an hour or so before bedtime and plug it with cotton ball. When you sleep, lie down with that side on the pillow, it will soften the wax and may help it fall out of the canal
3. Prevention of infection in those who do aquatic sports is by using "swimmer's ear" solution as soon as one comes out of the water after swimming or scuba diving or use of ear plugs while swimming. This dries up water in the canal. You can make your own solution by mixing equal amounts Acetic acid (white vinegar) and Isopropyl alcohol and putting a few drops in the canal after being in water

Middle Ear Infection

....

Otitis Media

What is it?

Infection of the middle ear chamber is called OTITIS MEDIA or middle ear infection. Ear infection is caused by bacteria or viruses and to a lesser extent fungi. This often occurs in children but can affect adults as well. The infection may also start from the external canal and then involve the middle ear.

Signs and Symptoms

An individual may have sore throat, runny nose, cough, and pain in one or both ears. There may be muffled or hearing loss, pressure in the ears or ears may feel clogged. Pulling on the ear may be painful. There may be a smelly discharge coming from the affected ear if drum is perforated or punctured and this actually causes reduced pressure and pain when it occurs. In children they may have a mild fever and even diarrhea. Examination by a health worker using an Otoscope will reveal the ear drum to be red and swollen or it may be perforated. If the external canal is involved then it will be swollen, narrow, and may have pus in it.

Treatment

Oral antibiotics and pain medicines may be given for the infection. If it is not severe then antibiotic ear drops may be prescribed.

Prevention

1. Immediately treat an upper respiratory infection with OTC medications like decongestants and anti-inflammatory medicines like Ibuprofen, and these may help minimize swelling and redness, and may decrease the progression to a middle ear infection
2. Avoid use of Q tips or bobby pins in the external canal since these can lead to infection of the middle ear
3. Good hand washing and use of hand sanitizers may minimize one's tendency to catch a cold, which is usually caused by a virus

Ringing in the Ears Tinnitus (Tin-ni-tus)

What is it?

Ringing in the ears is known as TINNITUS and it can be very annoying. The sound may be ringing, humming, or roaring. It is a symptom (meaning something you feel) and so it may signify an underlying disease or condition. Most of the time, it is heard in both ears although it may be in just one ear. It may be due to conditions within the ear itself or outside of the ear.

Causes

AGE: Advanced age or normal aging may cause ringing and most times it is a result of hearing loss associated with age

EARS: Several problems within the ears themselves can cause tinnitus. These include

  Excessive wax in the external ear canal

  Collection of fluid in the middle ear (behind the ear drum)

  Allergies and colds

HEARING LOSS from any condition: Examples include:

Exposure to loud noise for a prolong time (includes young people listening to loud music with ear phones or plugs), calcium build-up in the tiny bones present in the middle part of the ears, tumors, and Meniere's disease (see below)

MEDICATIONS: May result from use of several medicines over a long period of time. Common ones include Aspirin, Antibiotics like Gentamycin, Doxycycline, and Tetracycline; Ibuprofen (Brufen, Motrin), Furosemide (Lasix), and Atorvastatin (Lipitor) to name just a few

EAR INFECTIONS: Those caused by bacteria, viruses, and fungi of the middle and inner ear

MUSCLE AND BONY STRUCTURES: Structures near the ears, e.g. Temporomandibular Joint TMJ (joint of the upper jaw near the ear) problems, and even neck injuries like whiplash (muscle spasm)

DENTAL: Some dental or jaw problems

CIRCULATION PROBLEMS: Sound may be like a "wuss" or "heart beat" in your ears (pulsation). This may be due to veins or arteries in the head and neck area which may be partially blocked or kinked, arteriosclerosis or blockage of carotid vessels at the sides of the neck, and hypertension. Neck vessel malformations with irregular blood flow may also be a cause

MEDICAL CONDITIONS: Hypertension, hypothyroid and hyperthyroid

Treatment of Tinnitus

Depending on the history of the patient and the examination results, a health care provider may order some imaging studies, Ultrasound of neck vessels and a hearing test.

Treatment depends on the cause.

1. If due to a specific medication, stopping it will decrease or stop the tinnitus
2. If due to wax in the ears, the wax can be removed by irrigating the ears
3. If circulation problems are suspected, your health care provider may order imaging studies to find out more about your circulation in the head and neck areas. If there is blockage that can be treated by medication or surgery
4. If due to hearing loss associated with old age, some coping skills can be learnt, or use of hearing aid if hearing loss is the cause.
5. Avoidance of caffeinated drinks e.g. colas, salty foods, and beverages may also help
6. MEDICATIONS:
    Several prescription types have been tried with varying success. These include ANTIDEPRESSANT medicines called NORTRIPTYLINE and PAROXETINE. Certain medications called BENZODIAZEPAMS used to treat anxiety and stress may be useful, but these can lead to addiction and so are best avoided, and will not be the first choice medicines to use
7. HEARING AIDS:
    For those with hearing loss, the use of a hearing aid helps with tinnitus and can mask or decrease the sound
8. MASKING THE NOISE:
    These include drowning out the ringing (masking) with music; sounds e.g. ocean sounds or forest sounds, or use of "white noise". This is the sound between 2 FM radio stations or frequencies, which will mask the tinnitus or ringing
9. DIETARY SUPPLEMENTS:
    Over the counter (OTC) supplements like Niacin, Lycopodium, Melatonin, CoQ10, Ginkgo biloba have been found to be helpful at times by some patients, however, with Ginkgo biloba there are some studies which show it may somewhat improve tinnitus. However, inform your doctor if you decide to use any of these

Meniere's Disease
What is it?

Meniere's disease is a condition affecting the inner ears and consists of a combination of fluctuating hearing loss, tinnitus, and pressure or fullness in ears and occasional vertigo. It may be a result of high inner ear pressure due to increase in the fluid normally present in the inner ears which affects sound, balance, and pressure. Meniere's disease is usually idiopathic (unknown cause) but Meniere's syndrome which has the same symptoms and signs also occurs but it has identified causes which are believed to increase the inner ear fluid production or removal. The symptoms may be episodic (come and then go away, only to return later).

Causes of Meniere's Syndrome

These include:

1. Inner ear tumors
2. Medications e.g. Stimulants like Ritalin
3. Autoimmune diseases (diseases where your body's immune system is fighting against its tissues) like Hashimoto's Thyroiditis, Lupus, and Rheumatoid arthritis
4. Head and brain injury
5. High cholesterol and other fats
6. Infections like parasitic infections and syphilis
7. Food allergies

Signs and Symptoms

Sudden attacks of vertigo with episodes lasting from 20 minutes to four hours may occur. Vertigo is perceived spinning of the room especially with change of position of the body or the head. There may be feeling of pressure or pain in affected ear with hearing being decreased. Tinnitus has been discussed above as buzzing, humming, whistling sounds in the ears. There may be nausea and vomiting associated with the vertigo. If it is due to an underlying condition, then there will be symptoms of that disease present e.g. Rheumatoid Arthritis will present with severe joint pain, swelling, and deformity.

Treatment

You need to see your doctor who will examine your ears and do some hearing tests, positional tests – lying down and getting up etc., eye movement, and balance testing. They may require blood work and brain imaging to make sure you don't have a tumor in the brain or inner ears, etc.

Treatment of Meniere's Syndrome

If the cause is found, then treating it will get rid of the symptoms. For example, if it is due to thyroid problems, treating this will get rid of the symptoms. If it is due to a medication e.g. Methylphenidate (Brand – Ritalin which is a stimulant used to treat attention deficit), it can be replaced with a non-stimulant and the symptoms will go away. Meanwhile, the symptoms in the initial stages can be treated with the medicines mentioned below.

Treatment of Meniere's Disease

As mentioned above, for Meniere's disease there is no cure, but the following can help:

Medicines: There are medicines to treat acute episodes when they come on. These may include anti-motion medicines like Meclizine and Diazepam for vertigo, and anti-nausea drugs like Promethazine for nausea associated with vertigo. Others which decrease body fluids called diuretics, e.g. triamterene (Dyazide, Maxzide) may be used

Diet: Eating foods which are low in salt may reduce fluid retention

Exercise: Balance and vertigo exercises may be prescribed to help these two symptoms

Hearing Aids: For those with hearing problems or tinnitus, hearing aids may be helpful

Injections: Severe cases may have steroid injections into middle ear as a last resort

Surgery: If no other treatment brings relief, surgery is done to either remove excess fluid from the inner ear or sever the nerve supply to the inner ear which controls balance and motion. Sometimes, in order to help with fluid exchange a device called a Meniett pulse generator is used to apply pulses of pressure through an inserted ear tube and the individual has to use it several times a day at home. It has been found to improve all three main symptoms

Hearing Loss

This is when hearing in one or both ears is diminished and there is inability to hear sound. In America, over 48 million individuals suffer from some form of hearing loss. It can be acute or short term or chronic or long term.

Acute hearing loss: This is due to a temporary condition which if treated resolves. These include ear infections of external or middle ears, wax or cerumen, fluid in the middle ear, some medications like furosemide and erectile dysfunction drugs.

Chronic hearing loss: This is more permanent and some of the causes are:

Old age – this is treated below

Hereditary – some genetic abnormalities

Recurrent ear Infections

Medications: Aspirin, Chemotherapy, some antibiotics

Exposure to loud noise for a prolong time from working with machines, factories, mining etc

Young people listening to constant loud music with ear buds or plugs

Musicians exposed to noise

Cholesteatomas (a cyst in middle ear made up of skin tissue which can erode
    into inner ear)

Tumors of the inner ear

Injury to the ear drum or skull

Meniere's disease

Hearing loss can also be classified as conductive, sensorineural or mixed when
both are present.

In conductive hearing loss sound cannot travel from outer to middle ear.
Causes include wax, tumors in the outer or middle ear, foreign body in outer ear,
infections or fluid in the ears. Others are congenital defect of outer ear, or bones
in the middle ear and even simple hole or perforation of ear drum. Treatment is by
medications or surgery.

In sensorineural hearing loss there is damage to the inner ear or to the path
between the inner ear and the brain where sounds are processed. This is mostly
treated by hearing aids.

Symptoms

It may start slowly and may not be obvious initially. The individual may feel people are mumbling when talking, ends up turning the TV or radio volume up, asks
people to repeat what they say or seems to always talk loud, and cannot hear well
while talking on the phone.

Treatment

A history and physical exam would be done by a doctor. Hearing tests by a primary
care doctor, ear doctor, or audiologist will show objective hearing loss recorded as
a graph. It will also tell if the hearing loss is conductive, sensorineural, or mixed.

Treatment depends on the cause.

For example:

1. Advance age – see below for solution
2. Medication – withdrawal of some of the offending medications will resolve the
    issue, e.g. Furosemide, however some medicines cause permanent hearing
    loss due to damage of delicate hair cells in the inner ear, for example Che-
    motherapy like Cisplatin and Bleomycin, and Aminoglycoside antibiotics like
    Neomycin, Gentamicin, and Tobramycin
3. Wax – irrigation of the ear improves hearing
4. Tumor – surgery
5. Perforated ear drum – surgery

Prevention

This is key especially in cases like work place associated noise where wearing ear plugs or muffs should be the rule, musicians wearing hearing plugs, and young people turning music down when using ear buds in their ears.

Hearing Loss Associated With Old Age (PRESBYCUSIS)

What is it?

This is also called PRESBYCUSIS (presbi-cosis), and hearing loss associated with advanced age is the most common cause of hearing loss. About 30% of individuals between the ages of 65–74 years have some degree of hearing loss and the numbers increase after 75 years of age. Exact cause of hearing loss with advanced age is not known, however, factors like long exposure to loud occupation noise e.g. airport workers, factory workers etc. and genetics may play a part.

> *"Old age may have its limitations and challenges, but in spite of them, our latter years can be some of the most rewarding and fulfilling of our lives".*
>
> —Billy Graham, American evangelist (Nov. 7 1918 – Feb. 21, 2018).

Aggravating factors for Presbycusis

The hearing loss may be aggravated by other situations like previous ear infections, excess wax in the ears, certain medications used in the past or present e.g. cancer drugs, certain anti-malaria drugs, drugs used by men for erectile dysfunction, certain water pills or diuretics, antibiotics and aspirin.

Signs and Symptoms

Older people with progressive hearing problems, may turn the TV or radio volume on high, speak loudly when talking, ask people to repeat what they say, or find it difficult following a conversation when several people are involved.

Treatment

An examination and tests by an Ear Nose and Throat (ENT) or OTOLARYNGOLOGY doctor, or AUDIOLOGIST can determine what type of hearing loss is present. It can be corrected by:

1. Some simple devices called sound amplifiers which can amplify sounds
2. A device like a hearing aid. Some newer hearing aids are small and discretely placed inside the ear so they are not noticed

Reminders on Your Radar

There are many diseases affecting the ears including infections, balance, and motion problems. Hearing loss can occur with aging, however, age is not the only cause. Being in close proximity to loud noise for a long time as in work environment or listening to loud music may also result in hearing loss. Both Vertigo (spinning) and Tinnitus also increase with age, and they cannot be cured but can be controlled.

9

Conditions Affecting The Nostrils

Allergic Rhinitis (Hayfever)

. . . .

What Is It?

This is an allergy related condition affecting mainly the nose, but often the ears, eyes, and throat are also affected. This may be seasonal (seasonal allergies) or year round (perennial) condition when one's body reacts to an allergen or several different ones. An ALLERGEN is a substance that produces severe symptoms only in certain individuals when they come into contact with it, because it causes the immune system to work vigorously to neutralize it, as it sees the allergen as a threat. Environmental allergens (those found outside) include pollen, dust, animal dander, feathers, certain trees, plants or grass. Some people may also get reactions to certain foods (food allergens) e.g. milk, soy, wheat, shrimps (seafood); and others to medicines or chemicals.

"A big nose does not necessarily mean a sharper sense of smell."
—Nana Awere Damoah (chemical engineer and author)

Signs and Symptoms

After exposure to an allergen, the person may react by: Sneezing, itchy nose, eyes, ears, throat or skin, thin clear watery runny nose, stuffy nose, watery eyes, coughing, postnasal drainage (dripping of fluid down the back of the throat), throat clearing, discomfort in the face, coughing, change in smell and taste. It may also cause wheezing sound when it causes the airways in the lungs to react and become narrower. There is usually no fever, however, if not treated or controlled, it can lead to sinus infections or congestion, flare up of asthma in asthmatics, development of nasal polyps, and headaches. When secretions stay in the sinuses and do not flow out, it can lead to sinus pain and infections.

Treatment

See your health care provider to make the diagnosis and to treat you. There are some simple things you can do to decrease the frequency and or intensity of attacks.

1. Removal of allergens or the triggers by regular dusting, removal of carpets and use of a dehumidifier may dry out mold, mildew and dustmites. One may need to give pets away
2. Using saline nasal solution or salt water (instructions for making your own is below) copiously irrigate the nostrils several times a day, especially at night time to remove any allergen – pollen, dust etc. that may have accumulated in the nostrils during the daytime. It also loosens any mucus which may block the sinuses and prevent them from draining
3. Sometimes instead of salt water, one may use other store bought irrigation fluids containing natural substances like Eucalyptus oil and Menthol, e.g. Alkalol nasal rinse
4. Using an antihistamine helps decrease the symptoms by halting the actions of the allergens. Non drowsy ones include loratidine, desloratidine, fexofenadine, cetirizine, and levocetirizine. The ones which tend to cause more drowsiness include diphenhydramine, (Benadryl), chlorpheniramine, and clemastine and are best used at night
5. When allergic rhinitis is not well controlled by these, steroid nasal drops (e.g fluticasone, or budesonide) and antihistamine nasal drops (e.g. azelastine) may be added
6. Other oral medicines that can be added are Montelukast (Singular) or Zifirlukast (Accolate) which act to prevent the release of chemicals other than histamines and also cause associated allergy symptoms

How to Make Saline (Salt Water) Solution

TAKE 1 TEASPOON OF SALT (you can add 1/2 teaspoon of baking soda – optional) and add it to 500–750 ml of boiled cooled water or bottled sterile water. This can be used with a bottle or put a small amount in a disposable cup and instill it in your nostrils using a medicine dropper. There are saline rinse kits e.g."Netti Pot" and those that come with a bottle and the salt packages making it easier to use. They are available in pharmacies or chemist shops.

Since the nostrils are part of the respiratory system, other conditions affecting them like the common cold and sinusitis are discussed in that chapter.

Reminders on Your Radar

One common nasal problem associated with allergies is Allergic rhinitis and it may involve the throat, ears, and eyes. Use of oral or nasal antihistamines and removal of allergens may help decrease symptoms. Use of salt water or saline solution to rinse the nostrils at bedtime will wash out any allergens you may have picked up during the day.

10

Skin and Hair Problems

Introduction

....

S kin and hairs are connected because hairs usually protrude from the skin. Diseases may affect both and before we go into specifics we will look at the structure of skin and how it relates to its function.

What is The Skin?

"Be good to your skin. You'll wear it every day for the rest of your life"

—Renée Rouleau (celebrity esthetician, skin care specialist).

The skin is the largest organ of the body and has a surface area of about 20 square feet or 2.2 square yards. It is made up of three layers as described below. There are different skin colors and the basis of the variation is due to the presence of more or less melanin in the skin.

It has many functions including:

1. Protecting our internal organs from the outside elements, ultraviolet radiation, chemicals, bacteria, and viruses
2. Regulates body temperature because we sweat to keep cool when it is hot
3. Produces Vitamin D needed to make our bones strong
4. Glands in the skin secrete sebum which is a water repellent, plus other substances to keep our skin moist and not dry out
5. It excretes waste materials (e.g. urea and ammonia) through sweating
6. It absorbs substances like oxygen and medications (topical and transdermal)
7. It has nerve endings sensitive to pain, touch, heat, pressure etc. which make us respond to these sensations and keeps us safe

Composition of Skin

The three main layers from the outside are: outer layer or epidermis, middle layer or dermis, and lastly the inner layer or hypodermis also called subcutaneous (fat) deeper layer.

OUTER LAYER: The epidermis prevents our body from drying out, produces melanin (gives skin color), and its bottom layer produces cells which move up and form dead cells on the surface. It is constantly shed about every thirty days

MIDDLE LAYER: The dermis is thicker and contains collagen and connective tissue giving the skin support. It also contains sweat glands, sebum producing glands, some blood vessels, and hair roots

INNER LAYER: The subcutaneous layer or hypodermis is mostly fat with some blood vessels, muscles, and nerves which connect with the rest of the body

Classification of Skin

Below is a short description of skin classification based on a system called the Fitzpatrick classification, which is dependent upon on how skin reacts when exposed to ultraviolet rays or sunlight. Some skin types sunburn easily, while others don't and this is a result of the melanin content.

Fitzpatrick Classification of Skin

This ranges from a Type 1 through Type VI based on whether the skin burns easily or its tanning ability when exposed to ultraviolet radiation. In this system, lightly pigmented skin color ("white") is classified as Types I, II and III, while darkly pigmented skin color is classified as ranging from Types IV, V and VI. For example, Type 1 – Burns easily and never tans, and Type VI hardly burns and tans deeply.

Racial and Ethnic Classification

In the USA, a racial or ethnic classification based on skin color exists; with those referred to as "brown people" usually being Hispanics, those of African heritage or African American are referred to as "black people", and Caucasians as "white people". This is more or less used in other parts of the world to describe people.

Skin Color

"The only color we must be cynical about is never skin color but, the color of character for what character can do, skin color may never be able to do."

— Ernest Agyemang Yeboah,
Ghanaian Teacher and Writer

Skin color ranges from white or Caucasian skin seen in people with European ancestry to variations of brown and black which are collectively known as "Skin of Color". Those with darker skin tones are seen in different parts of the world;

and include south east and southern Asia, India, South and Central America, (Hispanic), Native Americans, and those of African descent. The evolution of dark skin is believed to be due to adaptation in order to protect against UVR (Ultraviolet Radiation) exposure.

Skin Diagram

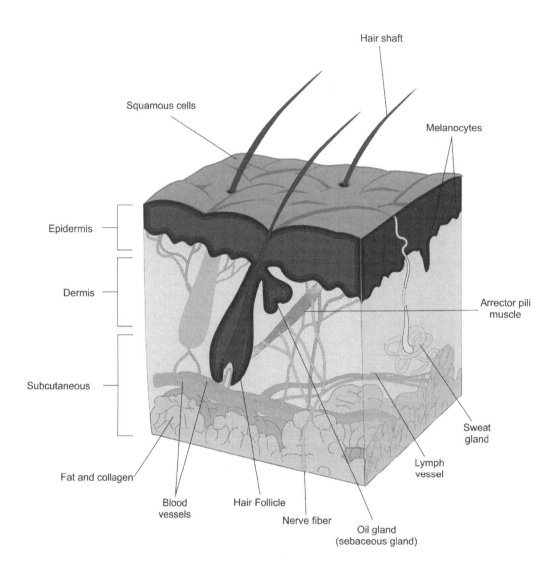

What Produces Skin Color?

How does skin derive its color? In humans melanin determines the color or tone of skin and it is produced by specialized cells called Melanocytes found in the outer layer or epidermis of the skin. Melanin is found in skin, hair, inner ear, the iris and retina of the eye, and even brain tissue. Dark skin or people of color produce more melanin and the tone of darkness varies depending on amount of melanin deposited. Whites produce very little melanin resulting in their skin appearing white. When melanin production slows down as in older people of color the skin may become lighter, or people may have patches of white skin where melanin production is slower than in the rest of the body.

Functions of Melanin

1. Melanin protects the skin from harmful UV (ultraviolet) light from the sun which can damage your DNA, the building blocks of your cells. UV light is regarded as a carcinogen (cancer causing) because it causes skin damage leading to cancer. Melanin containing cells absorb these rays and prevent skin damage from sunburn or development of skin cancer

2. Tanning results as a protection mechanism. As the light rays shine on the skin, the upper layer gets more melanin containing cells sent to it so as to protect the skin from damage

3. Sunburn results, when melanin cannot block all the harmful UV rays, so they penetrate the skin causing damage

4. Melanin protects skin from the sun, so Melanin rich skin is prone to less skin damage from the sun as seen in premature signs of aging, age spots, rough texture, and skin cancer

5. Melanin rich skin produces less wrinkles in people of color (BLACK DON'T CRACK – is a common funny saying in the USA)

6. Melanin present in the inner ear may be the reason blacks have less hearing loss compared to whites

7. Melanin is thought to absorb and destroy reactive oxygen which plays a role in development of macular degeneration of the eyes which was discussed under eye conditions. It is the leading cause of blindness in adults over the age of 60 years in most developed countries

8. Increased melanin may cause increased presence of folic acid in skin of people of color who generally are found to have more folic acid. It may be due to less degradation of this vitamin by UV light due to the excess melanin present. Folic Acid, is a B vitamin necessary for fetal development, prevention of anemia, as well as DNA production

Negative Effects of Melanin

1. Increased melanin makes the skin sensitive because the melanocytes are more reactive; and so in people of color there is tendency for HYPERPIGMENTATION or dark marks following inflammation or injury as would occur in a cut, ear piercing, wound, acne, or mechanical damage from cosmetic procedures. In the healing process the skin becomes darker in color than the rest of the body

2. Increased melanin may decrease production of Vitamin D in the skin from sunlight exposure

3. Folic acid is degraded by UV light in skin; and so more melanin, means less penetration by UV light and therefore more folic acid (stabilizes DNA), and less skin cancer. Alternatively, less melanin, and more UV light, leads to more degradation of folic acid which may in theory increase development of skin cancer. Some researchers believe that topical folate in the skin may protect against skin cancer (Williamson JD, Jacobson EL et al. Folate in Skin cancer Prevention. Subcell Biochem 2012; 56: 181–187)

Albinism

You may have noticed people in all races who have been born with white or pale skin even for those whose ancestry is skin of color, and it is because they have an inherited genetic abnormality – ALBINISM, causing their melanocytes to produce very little melanin. They are known as albinos and are found in all races and even animal species. This condition affects skin, eyes and hair all of which are devoid of pigmentation. They may have vision problems, like sensitivity to light and amblyopia (called lazy eye – with the brain and eye not working together, leading to vision loss); and due to the minimal amount of melanin, they are more prone to skin cancer and sun burn. They have to avoid the sun, use sunscreen, wear long sleeve shirts, and wear sun glasses and hats to protect their eyes.

Skin Color and Disease Presentation

There are structural and functional differences between skin of people of color (Fitzpatrick Types IV through VI) and those with Caucasian skin tones (Types I through III). As a result, there are differences in presentation as well as treatment of diseases and skin conditions in these different skin tones. Hair genetic makeup also differs and so presentations will vary.

Below are examples of presentations found in people who have African ethnicity:

1. Skin may end up as hyperpigmented following inflammation or scratch, acne, wound etc

2. If there is inflammation of the skin as may be seen in acne (pimples), and it is treated, the skin may end up with a milky color known as hypopigmentation, however; it is less common than hyperpigmentation. It often follows procedures with laser, steroids, and chemicals like hydroquinone and Tretinoin (Retin A) which will be discussed later

3. Eczema in people of color may leave excessive scarring and hyperpigmentation resulting from inflammation, scratching, and wound healing

4. In the disease called Lupus which is an autoimmune disease (body's own immune cells are fighting and destroying the body's cells), the skin lesion may present as a butterfly shaped red area on either side of the nose in Caucasians. However, in people of color it may appear as a dark, black, or brown color in the same area

Skin Types Based on Oil Content

There are different skin types and for our purposes there is a simple classification based on oil content of the skin. It is important to know what skin type one has, since it helps one know what skin moisturizer formulation to use; whether cream, gel, or lotion, since each of these is suitable for specific skin types.

There are 4 major types of skin: dry, normal, oily, and combination of dry and oily types. There are simple tests one can do to determine your skin type if it is not too obvious.

DRY SKIN: After washing your face, gently pat it dry, then after about an hour you use tissue paper to blot your face. If there is no sign of oil and your skin appears tight or firm then you probably have dry skin

OILY SKIN: Same actions as above, however, after blotting with tissue paper, oil will appear on the tissue

NORMAL SKIN: Same actions as above, but there is no oil on the tissue and skin does not feel tight or there is no flakiness. Skin feels supple

COMBINATION SKIN: This is a mix of dry and oily skin at different parts of the body. The oily part is usually seen on the forehead, nose, and chin areas (forms like a T)

Some people also have SENSITIVE SKIN, which means they easily develop a rash, may have very dry skin or skin may get red or flush easily. It may also present as burning and stinging when certain chemicals, house products, or fragrances are used on the skin.

Skin Type and Kind of Skin Preparation to Use

Once you know the type of skin you have, then you can know what type of skin preparation to use. Below are some tips.

1. OILY SKIN: May be prone to acne or pimples and the pores are enlarged. Pores are the openings around the hair follicles and help the sebum and oils produced below, move up to the surface of the skin. They get large when they are plugged with bacteria, dead skin, oils, or sebum. Choose skin care preparations which are made of gel or lotion. Wash face two times daily with a gentle

cleanser. Use one that will not clog the pores, and do not squeeze any acne spots, but treat pimples or acne as outlined below. Retinoid gels OTC or pre-scription will shrink and tighten the pores and prevent excessive oil secretions from oil producing glands under the skin

2. DRY SKIN: Skin may be prone to itching. Choose skin care preparations which are creams or ointments. Apply to skin right after shower while skin is still damp. One may need to reapply again as skin dries up quickly. Use of pure SHEA BUTTER moisturizer either alone or mixed with other moisturizers like Vaseline intensive care for dry skin, Lubriderm, aquaphor, petroleum jelly, may keep the skin moisturized for a longer time. Drinking lots of water and use of a humidifier in the bedroom will also help one retain moisture in your skin

3. COMBINATION SKIN: May have different type depending on part of face. Use different products, for appropriate areas of the face. So, treat oily skin areas and normal or dry areas as described above

4. SENSITIVE SKIN: This tends to be present in individuals who have allergies, eczema, or even asthma. You have to avoid chemicals etc. which trigger the reaction. Use soaps, body washes, or creams that are fragrance free or are labeled "for sensitive skin" or "hypoallergenic". Any brand soap labeled for "sensitive skin or hypoallergenic" should be suitable to use or use fragrance free baby soap. Avoid use of excess soap or scrubbing or skin

Skin Conditions of the Face

A woman's face is what reflects her outward beauty (but please remember beauty is more than skin deep) and is the first place most people will observe or look at when they meet her. It is important a woman adopts certain basic facial cleansing methods to maintain supple, blemish free, facial skin. We will address some of the skin issues that affect a woman's face.

Acne Or Pimples
What is it?

These are spots/bumps which appear on the face, chest or upper back, shoulders during adolescence; however some adult women may have them later on in life or during the time of their menses/periods. During adolescence it is more common in males than in females. It affects the base or shaft of the hair follicles which become blocked by the usual secretions produced to lubricate the skin (sebum); and this coupled with inflammation from the presence of bacteria mixed with dead skin cells results in raised white or black spots we call Comedones. Serious ones may involve redness, pustules (filled with pus), papules, (raised bumps on top of skin), and nodules (raised bump under the skin). Adult acne is caused in the same way as teenage acne – excess sebum production, dead skin, and bacteria in blocked pores. When clogged pores are closed they form a bump called a comedone which is also known as a white head; if they open then the contents turn dark when exposed to the air and arc called blackheads.

Signs and Symptoms

Mild ones may have black or white heads, and may be worse close to one's period or menses. Moderate ones will have the above as well as a red base. Serious ones may be large raised bumps called nodules or cysts which are deep seated and can be very disfiguring and make a person feel self-conscious or embarrassed. It can later lead to darkening of the skin and sometimes after healing, scarring may occur if not treated early and effectively. It is also important not to consider acne which is persistent or moderate to severe in adolescents as "part of growing up" and so is not treated. It can lead to poor self – image and affect their self-esteem, leading to withdrawal from friends and social isolation. Acne involving the forehead and sides of the head can be aggravated by use of hair pomade or oily hair products on the scalp in people prone to acne/pimples (POMADE ACNE). These block the pores making acne worse, and are common in African American women and girls.

Aggravating Factors

1. Made worse by stress (probably makes a person with acne produce more sebum)
2. Hormonal changes like during one's menses and pregnancy
3. Excessive scrubbing of the skin and picking and squeezing the spots. The latter may lead to scarring
4. It tends to run in families and so has some genetic elements
5. It is more common in smokers

It is a myth that acne is caused by eating too much chocolate, sugary or fatty foods, and dirt or sex.

Treatment of Acne

Some everyday tips before we consider medicines are important.

1. Keep your hands off your face since that can stimulate oil production and also spread bacteria on the face
2. Wash your face twice a day with a mild facial cleanser or acne wash, using your finger tips or face brush and not an abrasive face towel or scrubbing your face. They will make acne worse
3. Gentle facial brushes that are battery operated are available, and can help remove dead skin and sebum, and unplug the pores, however, avoid harsh ones with hard bristles
4. Avoid oily hair products close to face and neck to prevent pomade acne

Medications

Acne spots can be effectively controlled by OTC (over the counter) or prescription medications which are either topical or oral depending on the severity of the acne. There are ACNE CLEANSERS and ACNE SPECIFIC MEDICATIONS.

> CLEANSERS: A cleanser should be alcohol free and not too abrasive, it works by gently unplugging pores of excess oil and dirt. It should be appropriate for your skin type (dry, oily, or combination). There are many brand name cleansers and most of them contain one of three main medicated ingredients which are: salicyclic acid, benzoyl peroxide, and sodium sulfacetamide in different strengths

Medications

Benzoyl Peroxide: kills bacteria, exfoliates by removing sebum and dead skin, dry and peels the skin, and helps control oil

Salicyclic acid: unplugs the pores, reduces pore size, causing the sebum to drain so it does not plug the pores. It also exfoliates and reduces the inflammation

Sodium Sulfacetamide: slows bacterial growth

These three are usually combined with some hydrators, antioxidants and others that keep the skin hydrated, as well as other exfoliators like alpha hydroxy acids. After washing face, the cleanser is applied with the fingers and washed off. It is good to do this twice a day. However, for more moderate to severe acne, cleansers with higher strengths of the medicines are used and other forms of treatment may be needed.

Moisturizers

After the cleanser, a moisturizer may be applied and that may be sufficient for mild acne. Moisturizers are important because they keep face moist and prevent build up of sebum and clogging of pores. If you have oily skin, you have to use a gel moisturizer. A good moisturizer for acne prone skin should not be oil based or should be light oil based and be non comedogenic (meaning it does not cause comedones to develop). Oil absorbing moisturizers are also good and usually contain dimethicone. Avoid mineral oil or petrolatum-based moisturizers.

OTC Medications

These do not require a doctor's prescription and these are SALICYLIC ACID, BENZOYL PEROXIDE, any low strength RETINOIDS (e.g. Adapalene 0.1% – Differin) which are available as lotions, creams, pads, and face washing soaps. Retinoids are derivatives of Vitamin A and work by decreasing inflammation and swelling. They also unclog the pores making them look smaller. A combination of a retinoid and benzoyl peroxide can be used to treat acne initially and seems to work better than either alone, for example, Adapalene 0.1% and Benzoyl Peroxide 5%.

Prescription Medications

It is important to see a doctor and be treated if one's acne does not improve with OTC medicines, otherwise, scarring and discoloration of skin occur, and they affect the tone and smoothness of one's face, chest or upper back. Prescription medications can be topical or oral.

Topical Medications

These include antibiotic or retinoid gels and cream, alone or in combination with benzoyl peroxide or salicylic acid. Benzoyl peroxide's antibiotic effect adds to that of other topical antibiotics like Erythromycin and Clindamycin and it also helps prevent bacterial resistance to the oral ones. Example of a retinoid is Tretinoin which has several brands like Renova, Retin A, Retin A micro, and Stieva A. Retinoids are also combined with Benzoyl Peroxide (BP) for topical use as mentioned under OTC medicines or with other antibiotics. They penetrates deep into skin to absorb excess oil, and the BP or antibiotics limit bacterial growth. Example is combined Adapalene and Clindamycin cream. Sometimes, acne may get worse with redness of face and dryness before it gets better when using retinoid products.

Oral Medications

For moderate to severe acne, oral medications are used along with acne cleansers. These include oral antibiotics (e.g. Doxycycline, Minocycline), birth control pills, retinoid pills, and androgen blockers. Those with acne related to hormones may be treated with a drug called Spironolactone since it increases removal of testosterone and increases estrogen production. To prevent bacterial antibiotic resistance both topical Benzoyl Peroxide and oral antibiotics should be used together. It is important to know that Benzoyl Peroxide can cause bleaching of dark fabrics and so if being used, care must be taken not to brush it on dark clothes. Wearing white T shirts under clothes may help prevent this.

Make Up for Acne Prone Face

One has to use foundation or powder products that are water based or oil free. The label on such cosmetics may read "NON COMEDOGENIC" – meaning they do not cause pimples/acne. Oil or cream based cosmetics and foundations will clog the pores and cause more acne spots. Before going to bed it is important to remove all facial make up. Ono can use a mild soap with water or better to use a makeup removal cream/solution with a cotton pad or make up removal pad, and then rinse with water. If acne is present then a medicated acne cleanser is used.

Keratosis Pilaris (Goose bumps or chicken bumps skin)
What is it?

This is a disorder of KERATIN which is a protein present in hair, nails, etc. giving them structure or form. This condition is mostly inherited and affects the skin, appearing on upper arms and upper thighs as are horny-like rough structures which present as white or red bumps.

Signs and Symptoms

They give the skin a chicken or goose bump appearance. The condition is seen in children and young people and is commonly seen in people who have eczema, asthma, dry skin, or allergies. A few adults may suffer from it. It is worse during the dry season and in the winter time and it tends to improve with age. It is not itchy and is usually harmless, however; some who have it do not like the way their skin look or the roughness to touch.

TREATMENT: It usually clears by itself with time or the following can be used;

1. Use of soapless cleanser or mild soap which does not dry the skin
2. Skin has to be well moisturized with any cream or lotion moisturizer
3. ALPHA HYDROXY ACID like Lactic acid and Glycolic acid which remove the top layer of the skin and the keratin present
4. UREA BASED CREAMS: remove the horny layer making skin soft
5. RETINOID ACID BASED CREAMS: remove
6. MILD STEROIDS: Like hydrocortisone or Triamcinolone creams
7. Other OTC skin medicines which are used to remove the keratin (called keratolytics) and make the skin soft include: salicylic acid, trichloroacetic acid, Beta hydroxy Acid and coal tar

Dark Mark(s) on Skin (Hyperpigmentation)
What is it?

Excessive production of melanin occurs when there is triggering of the cells (melanocytes) by several conditions. The triggers include:

Medications
Acne, Eczema, Inflammation
Harsh Creams and Skin lightening Creams

Infections, Injury
Laser Treatments, and Surgery

The general term used to describe this condition is POSTINFLAMMATORY HYPERPIGMENTATION. It tends to occur in people of color because in caucasians post inflammatory changes will appear as red.

Signs and Symptoms

Individuals will have darkening of the skin in patches or in certain areas of the skin. Some women have them on their cheeks while others on their foreheads. The color may appear as brown, black or even blue depending on the depth of the inflammation. Dermatologists are able to determine the depth of the hyperpigmentation when they shine a special light on the skin.

1. If the depth is minimal and affects just the superficial skin, the color tends to be brown or light black
2. If it is in the deeper layers, especially on the skin of the face then the color will be blue-black, black, or blue

Treatment

If depth of hyperpigmentation is minimal, then treatment tends to be successful, and doctors give creams called depigmenting agents which remove the dark pigment. Examples are: Hydroquinone, Glycolic Acid, Azelaic Acid, Kojic Acid, Niacinamide (Vitamin B3). We will discuss a few of them in details since they are used for other conditions that affect the skin.

Medicines For Treating Hyperpigmentation

....

Hydroquinone
What it does

This lightens age spots (senile lentigines or sun spots), inflammatory hyperpigmentation, other dark spots, freckles, and dark skin associated with female hormones (melasma).

Types available include

Lustra, Milquin, Alphaquin, Claripel, Clarite, Eldopaque, Eldoquin, Epiquin Micro, Esoterica, Melanex, Ambi, Melpaque, Nuquin HP Cream, Nuquin HP Gel, and Solaquin. There are over the counter (OTC) ones that are of mild strengths (2%) and prescription ones which have higher strengths like 4% and 8%.

Length of use

Usually if no effect is seen after 2 months discontinuation is advised. If used for long periods, this medication can cause darkening of the skin. If using OTC products, always make sure you first test the medication on a little part of your forearm (called patch testing) and check within 24 hours for severe skin reaction. A little redness or pink color is acceptable. This gives you an idea of what reaction you will get when it is applied to a larger area like your face or other affected areas. Excessive use may lead to darkening of face especially in black people, a condition called Exogenous Ochronosis. This gives a black bluish coloration and it has to be discontinued if darkening starts.

Adverse effects

Hydroquinone may cause irritation of the skin e.g. stinging, drying, burning, and cracking of the skin of the face, or allergic reaction to the medicine which may manifest as a red itchy rash or raised itchy spots. Hydroquinone also contains sulfites and so may cause allergic reaction in some who are allergic to sulfa. Talk to your doctor before using any of them.

Glycolic Acid (Alpha Hydroxy Acids)
What is it?

This belongs to the group of products called Alpha Hydroxy Acids (AHA). There are five AHAs found naturally, however Glycolic acid (derived originally from sugar cane) is the one commonly used in skin care products. These remove dead surface cells (exfoliate), firm the skin, and may smooth the appearance of skin. Higher strengths are used as chemical peelers and are used to peel the surface layer of the skin and in the process remove the dark marks along with it. There are OTC ones (5–10%) and higher prescription strengths. A cleanser form may be used to wash the skin followed by a cream, gel, or lotion which does the peeling. Which type one uses depends on whether the skin tends to be oily or dry. Oily skin will need a gel and dry skin will require a cream. It may come as a cleanser, serum, facial peel, or moisturizer. It is important to read the label and make sure an OTC product has a milder concentration.

Kojic Acid

This is a natural substance found in fungus, mushrooms, or malted rice which is used to make rice wine. Among other uses, it works as a skin lightener by decreasing melanin in the epidermis. It is also used in anti-aging creams, age spots, freckles, and to treat Melasma (chloasma) which is dark skin coloration of face associated with hormonal changes like in pregnancy, use of oral contraceptives, and hormone replacement therapy in postmenopausal women.

Azelaic Acid

This is also used for many skin conditions including skin lightening in post inflammatory hyperpigmentation, melasma, acne, and rosacea. It decreases melanin, bacteria, keratin, and inflammation of the skin.

Natural Skin Lightening Creams

Some natural skin lightening creams may contain a combination of Alpha Arbutin (a hydroquinone from the bearberry plant), Kojic acid, Extrapone Nutgrass (inhibits melanin production). To these may be added sun screen and also antioxidants like Vitamin C.

Skin Brightening Products

1. This has nothing to do with lightening but more to do with turning dull skin into youthful glowing skin. It is a result of dead skin cells piling up and so to get skin to be brighter, exfoliants are used to remove dead cells and stimulant growth of new cells. To do so, these products include AHAs, e.g. Glycolic acid or lactic acid and BHAs e.g. Salicylic acid as well as Retinoids can be used. Fruit enzymes are also used as chemical exfoliants and are found in fruits like Papaya (pawpaw), Pumpkin, and Pineapple. For those desiring natural exfoliants, scrubs containing oatmeal, powdered almond, and rice bran are used. Below are some examples of components of homemade manual scrubs used for exfoliation of the skin:
2. Jojoba beads, aspirin, and baking soda
3. Baking soda and water
4. Ground Steel oatmeal, yogurt (plain) and lemon juice
5. Milk, honey, ground almonds
6. Honey and sugar (brown or cane)
7. Coconut oil and sugar
8. Brown sugar, cocoa powder, and olive oil

You can look up many more, for example on the internet by googling "natural facial scrubs" or go to www.homemadeforelle.com.

Bleaching Creams

Women of color sometimes want lighter skin color or even tone, and so use skin lightening creams or bleaching creams. Skin lightening creams are safer and most health care providers will recommend bleaching creams only to treat small areas with sun spots or age spots. The commonest ingredient in these creams is HYDROQUINONE in high concentrations (up to 8%). Frequent use of these creams, coupled with sun exposure can lead to skin damage. They are often used alone or may be mixed with topical steroids and retinoids like Tretinoin. Initially, they cause skin lightening but may result later in darkening of the skin (exogenous ochronosis), or development of raised bumps or spots on the face. It is best to avoid bleaching creams since sometimes prescription strength hydroquinone may be sold as an over the counter bleaching cream and may result in lightening of skin but followed by darkening or hyperpigmented skin. Use of prescription strength should be under the care of a health professional who will monitor its effects.

Large Pores On Face
What are Pores?

Pores are the spaces around the hair follicles and help sweat, skin oils, and sebum (oily liquid secreted by the sebaceous gland) get up to the surface and keep the skin soft and protect it from drying up. However, they can be clogged by dead skin, sebum, and bacteria and in doing so cause the pores to enlarge; and so women with oily or combination skin tend to have larger pores.

Treatment

There is no treatment that will make large pores go away, but there are ways to make them appear smaller. These include:

1. Washing the face twice a day to empty pores of oil
2. Exfoliating with scrubs containing apricot, other coarse substances, or crystals will empty the pores (mechanical exfoliation) of oil, dead skin, and bacteria
3. Wash off make up at night so they do not clog the pores and enlarge them
4. Use sun screen to prevent sun damage and sagging skin
5. Eat healthy, plenty of fruits, and vegetables and avoid foods high in fat
6. Medications that act like exfoliating agents (chemical exfoliation) include Salicylic acid, Beta-hydroxy acid, Lactic acid, and Retinoid all help unclog pores
7. It is always good to start at medicines at low strengths and increase doses as needed. They may sometimes produce redness and irritation if they are too strong

Complementary Products Used for Large Facial Pores

Several have been suggested and these include:

1. Zinc and Magnesium present in skin products
2. Lemon and pineapple juices are rich in Vitamin C (antioxidant) and pineapple is rich in Bromelain which is an enzyme that can break down old skin giving a smoother skin
3. Use of a clay mask or blotting paper will act as a wick and remove excess oil

4. You can make your own mechanical/manual exfoliating scrub as outlined above
5. Use of a facial brush can also help remove dead cells etc

Dark Circles Around The Eyes

All women may have darker circles around the eyes which may be caused by fatigue, allergies, eczema, aging, hereditary, and exposure to sun which increases melanin production. It may also be due to the shadows cast by puffy eyelids or the loss of collagen and fat as one ages make the blood vessels under the skin stand out. Rest and sleep may clear the dark circles. Cold compress to area, cucumber slices, green tea bags, may be helpful. In those with dark complexion, It can be lightened with lightening creams containing hydroquinone, retinol, Vitamin C, and green tea.

Puffy Eyes (Bags Under The Eyes)

With age, lower eye lid areas get puffy as muscles become weak and skin loses its support, becoming saggy. Fat cells and fluid then accumulate leading to bags under the eyes.

Treatment

Reducing salt intake, getting enough rest/sleep, cool compresses, and use of cool cucumber slices may help. If severe, then chemical fillers and peels as well as laser surgery are used to improve them. Cosmetic eyelid surgery (blepharoplasty) can be done to redistribute the fat under the eyelids, tighten the skin, and strengthen muscles with elimination of the baggy look.

Complementary Treatment
Jade Rolling

This is an Ancient Chinese Medical treatment which uses the green Jade stone to roll over the face. It is believed to massage the facial skin to stimulate it, increase circulation, improve the lymphatic drainage to reduce puffy lower eyes and help decrease wrinkles.

Derma Roller

This is a roller with small needles attached and it is rolled over the face, in a process termed microneedling. It is believed that the small holes created in the skin stimulate the formation of collagen leading to increased tone and rejuvenation of skin by making it firmer. The holes allow penetration of anti-aging or anti-wrinkle serum or lotions into the skin. It may be used on other parts of the body as well.

There may be some bleeding especially if the needles are one millimeter or longer. It is used to treat wrinkles, acne scars, and stretchmarks.

Wrinkles

What are Wrinkles?

These are lines, creases and furrows which appear on the skin due to the normal aging process. Areas exposed to sun like face, arms, and neck are mostly affected. Other factors contributing to their formation include sun exposure and damage, genetics, and smoking. People who have dark pigmentation (increase melanin) like blacks tend to have less wrinkles and sun damage because melanin protects skin from ultraviolet rays. Like everything else, prevention is essential.

Prevention of Wrinkles

1. Stay out of the sun during the peak sunny times of 10 am to 2 pm
2. Use broad rim hats to protect face and neck
3. Wear sunglasses with Ultraviolet protection lenses
4. Reduce facial muscle contraction by less frowning and squinting. Forehead muscle contraction can lead to more wrinkles
5. Get an eye exam if you cannot see well and use reading glasses, if needed
6. Wear broad spectrum sun screen which protects against both UVA (main cause of wrinkles and sun damage) and UVB (causes sun burn) rays from the sun
7. Use moisturizers on face and exposed parts of your body
8. Wear clothing that covers the arms and legs when you will be in the sun for a long time
9. Breathable materials like linen and cotton minimize the sweating and heat
10. Stop smoking if you are a smoker. Most smokers produce wrinkles at an earlier age and they may appear after only ten years of smoking
11. Sleeping on your back prevents wrinkles because sleeping on your side can cause lines to form on the cheeks and chin,and sleeping face down can lead to wrinkles on your forehead

Treatment of Wrinkles

There are ways to make wrinkles less prominent but there is no absolute cure for wrinkles.

1. Exfoliates like alpha and beta hydroxy acids remove dead skin and surface cells
2. Retinoid creams – These are also antioxidants and destroy free radicals which damage skin cells. Retinol is the mild OTC form and if it does not work, then

one may need the FDA-approved prescription Topical Tretinoin or Retin A. It is present in most anti-aging creams

3. Vitamin C – Another antioxidant which increases collagen production and reduces fine lines and wrinkles. Choose a product in a pump or tube since those in easily exposed containers react with oxygen in the air and make them ineffective

4. Botox – Botulinum toxin is injected under the skin to relax facial muscles that cause wrinkles. It is often used with facial fillers. Injection has to be repeated since it lasts for about 4 months

5. Facial fillers – Different fillers are injected under the skin, for example, collagen and hyaluronic acid to cause fullness and make the wrinkles less prominent

6. Dermabrasion – A device with a rotating brush or burr is used to remove top layer of old skin, leading to growth of smoother new skin. It's used to treat crow's feet, wrinkles, fine lines, or acne scars on face and the neck, and it's usually done by trained Dermatologist or Doctor

7. Microdermabrasion – A micro version of dermabrasion done at spas, doctor's offices, etc. which uses a wand that sprays tiny crystals under pressure on the face or neck to remove top skin layer and suction it away, allowing growth of new skin. Some also have diamond tips that do the abrasion. It is used to treat large pores, superficial acne scars, age spots, and fine lines. There are home version devices costing $80-$300 and some people do it at home since it's cheaper

8. Chemical peels – Use salicylic acid or glycolic peels (Alpha Hydroxy Acid from sugar cane) to remove top layer of skin so that new layer grows which is firmer and smoother with less wrinkles. Dermatologists may use more potent peelers like Trichloroacetic acid which also work on middle layer of skin and not just the superficial layer

9. Laser and Light resurfacing – Energy from a light or laser source is used to disrupt the top layer of skin, so collagen etc. are stimulated to grow

Alternative Methods to Reduce Wrinkles

Several CAM (Complementary and Alternative Medicine) products either orally or in anti-wrinkle creams/gels have been touted to help with wrinkles due to their properties as anti-oxidants, anti-Inflammatories, or exfoliating agents. These include:

Vitamin C, black, Green or oolong tea extracts, Coenzyme Q10, Soybean, Omega 3 fatty acids, grape seed extracts, Cocoa, Salmon and Cold water Fish, and Idebenone (related to CoQ10).

Stretch Marks (Striae Distensae)
What are They?

These are parallel reddish streaks in rapidly growing areas and where skin is con-tinuously stretched. These include the belly, breasts, shoulders, buttocks, and upper thighs. A stretch mark results from damage to collagen and elastin in the dermis as the upper surface stretches. They are harmless and with time become light colored scars. They tend to occur:

1. When there is rapid weight gain as in pregnant or obese women
2. In both sexes during growth spurts or puberty
3. On shoulders of body builders
4. Those with diseases associated with overproduction of cortisone (Cushing's disease)
5. In individuals who are on chronic steroid therapy (both topical and oral)

Treatment

They may become less visible with time but may not disappear. Treatment has not been found to be successful and many creams and topical treatments have been suggested. These include:

1. Retinoids like tretinoin
2. Chemical peels
3. Laser light

These do not usually cause them to disappear, however, using them earlier rather than later may give better results

Cellulite (Orange Peel Skin)
What is it?

This is the dimple appearance of the skin (depression) which makes it look like an orange peel. It is found especially around the hips, buttocks, thighs, and legs of women. It is uncommon in men, but up to 80% of women may develop it. It is a result of fat pushing up against the skin and connective tissue pulling down from below. It is thought that thinning of the skin which occurs when collagen breaks down causes the fat cells to increase and connective tissue bands within the fat pull the skin down giving the dimple effect, while fat cells push out giving the bump like appearance.

Risk Factors for Developing Cellulite

These include:

1. Obesity although thin individuals can also develop it
2. Dehydration

3. Poor diet
4. Family history or genetics
5. Stress
6. Caucasian race (dark skin individuals do not have as much cellulite)
7. Increased fat under skin
8. Lack of exercise
9. Hormonal changes. It is believed the female hormone estrogen is involved in its formation

Treatment

It is not a disease, but a cosmetic problem and unfortunately there is no cure; however, most women do not like the appearance and so will like to get rid of it. Many treatments have been suggested but these have not been scientifically proven.

General practices or supplements which are used:

1. Drinking lots of water
2. Eating water rich vegetables like cucumber, eating tomatoes which contain LYCOPENE, and pineapple stem which contain BROMELAIN, or taking INDIAN GINSENG may also help
3. Exercise may help decrease the look, because it causes the muscles underneath to be tighter and create a smoother appearance of skin. Both aerobic and strength training are useful
4. Weight loss will help reduce cellulite
5. Quitting smoking helps keep the skin firm
6. Cellulite reducing creams: These may contain caffeine and aminophylline (used to treat asthma) and do not have lasting effects and could even be harmful
7. Retinol Creams: Some Dermatologists have suggested creams containing Retinol 4% to be used one to three times a day on affected areas
8. Mesotherapy: This involves injecting chemicals, Vitamins, enzymes under the skin to break down the fat under the skin. May help at times but carries with it some risks
9. Laser therapy: This is a new treatment being used. Liposuction may aggravate cellulite because it is ideally used to remove deep seated fat and not superficial fat under the skin
10. Spa and Massage therapy: Massage is believed to help cellulite by shifting mainly blood and lymph fluids around, stretch and relax the connective tissue to give a smoother surface to the skin. Massage types like Swedish, deep tissue, and lymphatic drainage are believed to work best. However, others think massage does not treat cellulite
11. Some spas may treat clients with special brushes that are supposed to open up the pores and cleanse the body of accumulated toxins in the skin. This is

followed by use of chemicals containing anti-cellulite creams, herbal preparations etc. which penetrate the skin

12. Cellfina treatment: This is an FDA approved procedure which is performed in a doctor's office. The procedure treats the connective tissue bands and releases them from pulling the skin down and so the dimpling effect is removed. It is expensive costing between $3000 and $6000 depending on number of areas treated. Studies show it's still effective a year after treatment

Hypo Or Depigmentation (White Or Lighter Skin Spots)
What is it?

Hypopigmentation is when there is loss or decreased pigmentation of the skin and occurs when melanin is decreased. This results in light, milky white, or creamy colored areas of the skin in various areas and of different shapes.

Conditions causing it include:

1. Ultraviolet light can result in damage to pigment producing cells
2. Medical conditions include Vitiligo, Eczema, Fungal infection, Lupus, Seborrheic Dermatitis, Chronic Lichen Sclerosus, and Pityriasis Alba
3. Post Inflammatory Hypopigmentation (occurs after inflammation of the skin)
4. Idiopathic Guttate Hypomelanosis (IGH – depigmentation associated with aging). We will discuss a few of them in details

Depigmentation Associated With Normal Aging (IGH)
What is it?

This is also known as Idiopathic Guttate Hypomelanosis (IGH). This is common in older fair skinned black women. Its exact cause is unknown but it is thought to be due to effect of the sun on the pigment producing cells causing loss of pigment in parts of the skin.

Signs and Symptoms

The condition produces several light colored or milky small round or oval spots of varying sizes flush to the skin surface of the legs, thighs, and arms. They do not itch, are not harmful, and is just cosmetic.

Treatment

Various treatments have been used with varying results and these include:

1. Freezing with liquid Nitrogen (Cryotherapy)
2. Topical steroids
3. Retinoids

4. Dermabrasion (removal of uppermost layer of skin by exfoliating with a device and crystals)
5. Minigrafting of the skin (placing normal skin from another area on it)

Dermatosis Papulosa Nigra (DPN)
What is it?

Dermatosis Papulosa Nigra (DPN) is a condition affecting mostly people with dark skin color, with about 40% of blacks or African Americans affected, and lower numbers in Hispanics and Asians. They present as multiple dark papules (raised bumps) or small mole-like bumps on the face, neck, and upper back. They may range in color from dark brown to black. The exact cause of DPN is not known although they tend to run in families and may start in adolescents but are more prominent after the age of 30 years.

Signs and Symptoms

They may be smooth, round, flat, and found mainly on the face, neck, upper back, and chest. They are not painful or itchy and look like warts but are not caused by viruses.

Treatment

It usually does not cause any symptoms but cosmetically may be unacceptable for some individuals. In that case, it is treated by excision of the lesions. Destruction can be by cutting off (excision), scooping out (curettage), burning by use of heat (electrocautery), laser, or freezing with liquid Nitrogen (cryotherapy). Occasionally, scarring could be a problem after removal especially if the process goes into deeper layers of skin.

Pityriasis Alba
What is it?

This is found mostly in young children and teenagers of black ancestry. It usually starts as small scaly red spots on the face or upper arms. This rash then progress into smooth light colored, whitish areas either oval or round in shape. People sometimes mistake them for fungal infections and treat them with antifungal medicines. The cause is unknown but they may be associated with a skin condition called Atopic Dermatitis or Eczema.

Treatment

They eventually go away and the skin color returns to normal. During the red scaly stage, redness and itching if present could be treated with a mild steroid cream like Hydrocortisone.

VITILIGO: (Vit-e-lie-go)
What is it?

This is a condition in which the cells which produce melanin or skin color are destroyed or stop working, and results in patchy loss of skin color with lighter skin color (hypo or depigmentation) interspersed with normal skin color. This can occur in all races but is more prominent in people of color or blacks. Exact cause is not known but it's believed that the body's immune system destroys the pigment making cells.

Treatment

There is no cure but there are treatments which may darken the depigmented area. These include:

1. Steroids which darken the area, but once it is discontinued the white area may return
2. UV Phototherapy is supposed to stimulate the growth of melanocytes
3. Skin grafting surgery is sometimes used to cover the depigmented area
4. Cosmetics to cover up the white areas of the skin is also used but has to be reapplied each day

Reminders on Your Radar

There are many diseases affecting the skin and presentation may differ depending on one's skin pigment color. In people of color inflammation presents as a dark or black color, while in caucasians inflammation appears as red or pink. Acne or pimples can affect adults, and the earlier it's treated the less likely scarring and pigmentation changes will develop.

Hair Structure

. . . .

Hair has already been described as a component of skin, (p. 84) and it can be divided into three, with the first two parts being under the skin and the outer part which projects out of the skin. It is made out mainly of Keratin, which is a tough protein present in hair, nails and skin. The structure is also known as "Hair Follicle" and it goes through a cycle of growth which is in three parts: Anagen, Catagen, and Telogen.

1. Anagen is when there is active growth, and this can last between three to six years
2. Catagen involves regression of the lower part of the follicle and cessation of hair growth and this lasts between two to three weeks
3. Telogen phase which is the rest phase, and lasts about three months. At any one time about 10% of the hair on one's head is in a resting phase. Most scalp hair are in Anagen phase at any particular time

Types of Hair According to Race

Hair can be classified into three types according to race, and these can each have subclassifications. These are African, Asian and Caucasian (European).

African type the follicles are elliptical or oval and growth is spiral, or thick curls. They have the lowest density but the spiral shape may give a denser look. This hair has the lowest growth rate as well as being more fragile.

Asian hair type has round follicles resulting in straight type hair and the density is higher than African type. The hair strands are thicker and the strongest due to thick cuticles (outer layer of hair), and give an appearance of fuller hair on the scalp.

Caucasian hair type is oval or round in shape and is very dense, it can be straight, wavy or curly. Hair color depends on melanin pigments produced in the follicle, and caucasian hair has more variety of colors than the other two.

Back to Natural African Hair

Many African American and blacks in Africa have over the past 20 years or so, opted to keep their hair natural or chemical free, which is a good idea because chemical relaxers have been found to be "hormone disrupting chemicals" which mimic female estrogens and contribute to the increased incidence of fibroids in females of African descent. The internet has many videos and blog sites where women give ideas of how to manage natural black hair. There are also specific shampoos, conditioners, styling products, and moisturizers which are more suited for hair in women of color. This is important given the fragility of African hair.

Hair Conditions And Diseases
Gray (Grey) Hair

Gray hair in older years is due to decreased melanin production by the melanin producing cells. The lack of melanin may appear as grey, silver or white and "graying" of hair is not reversible. Some women chose to maintain their grays while others will color their hair to conceal their grays Caucasians tend to gray earlier with Africans being the last in their 40s. What age one starts developing gray hairs is determined mostly by one's genes, and so we have our parents to blame!, however, certain medical conditions can cause early graying like Vitiligo, hormonal problems of the thyroid and Pituitary gland, Alopecia Areata and even Vitamin B12 deficiency. Some research say Chronic Stress may lead to premature graying while others debunk that, and are of the opinion that stress hormones may affect the activity of melanin cells, but not cause graying.

Alopecia (A-lo-pea-cia) Loss of Scalp Hair or Baldness

What is it?

Alopecia is the loss or hair from the scalp. It is also referred to as baldness. Normally, everyone sheds some hair on a regular basis, because hair goes through a cycle of growth and shedding. Each person may lose up to one hundred strands of hair on a daily basis, because hair in resting phase mentioned above fall out and new hair grow in its place. However, this normal cycle of growth and shedding can be disrupted by certain situations and this leads to alopecia or baldness.

It has many causes but the common ones are discussed below:

1. HORMONAL CHANGES

Hormones are chemicals produced in the body that control the function of a specific organ. Changes in estrogen and progesterone levels in females may cause alopecia. Examples are:

POST PARTUM: (After delivery) About 3 months after childbirth, the female hormones levels which were high suddenly decrease, and it affects hair causing large amounts to fall out

DISCONTINUATION OF BIRTH CONTROL PILL: When one stops taking birth control pills, the sudden drop in the female hormones may cause the hair to fall off diffusely from the scalp

MENOPAUSE (when women go through the change and stop having periods): The decreasing levels of female hormones lead to thinning of the hair mostly in the front but can affect the whole of the scalp

TREATMENT:

This depends on whether the hormonal change is temporary or permanent. If temporary as in discontinuation of oral contraceptives and post partum time, then hair will grow back. If permanent as in menopause, then use of hormone replacement therapy will help with that, however, one would not use hormone replacement therapy just for this purpose

2. **DISEASES**

Diseases include:

1. Low thyroid or overactive thyroid activity. The thyroid is a small gland at the front of your neck which produces an important hormone called thyroxine. If there is disease such that too much or too little thyroxine is being produced, hair loss can occur.
2. Infections of the scalp like fungal infection.
3. Skin problems like seborrheic dermatitis (serious dandruff).
4. Diabetes (sugar diabetes).
5. Kidney Failure.
6. Autoimmune conditions like Lupus and Psoriasis.
7. Iron deficiency anemia and Protein deficiency.
8. Eating disorders e.g. Anorexia Nervosa may result in hair loss.

TREATMENT:

This depends on the underlying disease. For most, once treated the hair loss will improve. All the above diseases and how they are treated are discussed in their respective chapters

3. **STRESS OF A MAJOR ILLNESS**

The stress of an illness or major surgery with sudden weight loss may result in hair loss at that moment or a few weeks later

TREATMENT:

This is temporary and the hair will grow back after recovery

Traction Alopecia
What is it?

This is hair loss caused by pulling the hair as a result of the type of treatment of the scalp and hair. Treatments like chemicals, hot combing, plaiting, corn rolling, use of rollers, and even perming can cause the roots of hair to be pulled out from the scalp. All of these tend to occur in black women.

Signs and Symptoms

A few bumps may be seen on the scalp and this can result in scarring of the hair root. The hot comb type may start at the center or middle of scalp and extends outwards. If it results in scarring of the scalp then the hair will not grow over that area of the scalp and there will be permanent loss of hair over that spot. Braiding or use of rollers may cause the hair loss from the front or temples of the scalp causing a receding hair line.

Treatment

Hair transplant treatment may help restore hair growth. If there is no scarring then discontinuing the various types of hair care mentioned above will restore the hair.

Medications Causing Hair Loss

Some medicines which can cause hair loss include:

1. Anti-hypertension (BP) e.g Metoprolol
2. Cholesterol medications e.g Gemfibrozil
3. Blood thinners e.g.Warfarin and Heparin
4. Birth control pills
5. Medicines for treating gout e.g. Allopurinol
6. Medicines for heart disease e.g. Metoprolol, Atenolol
7. Epilepsy (seizure or fits) medicines e.g. Valproic acid
8. HIV medicines
9. Antidepressants e.g. Amitriptyline, Paroxetine and Fluoxetine, Sertraline
10. Steroids e.g. Prednisone

Stopping the medicines will help restore the hair loss. In the case of birth control pills (BCP) using those with low androgen index (Progesterones with low androgen effects) may help, as excess androgens can affect the hair follicles and cause hair loss.

Androgenetic Alopecia (Female pattern baldness)
What is it?

This is genetically determined and is known as male pattern baldness in males (common baldness) and female pattern baldness in women.

This is the most common type of hair loss in women. It occurs earlier in males but can occur in women usually after the age of 40 years.

It may affect up to 40% of females at some time in their lives.

It is believed to have a genetic predisposition and usually females in a family may experience similar hair loss.

It is thought to be due to androgen (male) hormones. These male hormones are normally present in females but in lower amounts. It is believed that Dihydro-testosterone (DHT) which is usually produced from breakdown of testosterone, by an enzyme called 5 alpha reductase, has the capability to harm hair follicles causing them to shrink and die.

Signs and Symptoms

The hair follicle's hole shrinks producing thinner, shorter hair, and generalized thinning of hair especially in the crown or top of the head, leading to varying sizes of the follicles when observed under magnification by a health care provider. The hair then easily falls off

<h3 style="text-align:center">Treatment</h3>

To find out the cause of hair loss, a doctor will take a careful history and physical examination, followed by initial tests which will include blood work to check for thyroid disease, levels of male and female hormones, anemia, iron levels, and even check for syphilis and lupus (autoimmune disease) which can cause patchy hair loss. If needed, a scalp biopsy may be done to investigate further the cause of the hair loss.

The FDA of the USA, has approved one topical medicine for female androgenetic alopecia and that is MINOXIDIL 2% (the tablet form is used to treat blood pressure) which is applied to the scalp as a foam or lotion. It stimulates hair growth and slows down the hair loss.

In men the 5 alpha reductase inhibitor called FINASTERIDE (Propecia) is also used orally, but it is not approved for women.

Off Label Medicines Used to Treat Female Androgenetic Alopecia

Other medicines with anti-androgen effects used off label (not approved by FDA specifically to treat this condition) to treat female androgenetic hair loss include:

1. SPIRONOLACTONE (a diuretic which decreases testosterone – antiandrogen – and increases estrogen)
2. CIMETIDINE (an antacid which decreases DHT)
3. HORMONE REPLACEMENT THERAPY (estrogen and progestin) in post-menopausal women
4. BIRTH CONTROL PILLS (BCP) with low androgen activity. The different progestins in BCP each have a certain androgen activity. Those with least androgenic activity include Norgestimate, Norethindrone and Desogestrel, or Ethynodiol Diacetate. Examples are Desogen (desogestrel–ethinyl estradiol), Ortho-Cept, Emoquette, Apri (desogestrel and ethinyl estradiol), Ortho-Cyclen (ethinyl estradiol and norgestimate), Ortho Tri-Cyclen, Micronor (Norethindrone). The BCP Diane 35 and Diane 50 contain the progestin cyproterone which blocks the action of DHT and help with female pattern baldness
5. KETOCONAZOLE 2% shampoo used to treat fungal infections also has antiandrogen properties and can be used for hair loss. (American Hair Loss Association – Americanhairloss.org)
   OTHER TREATMENT OPTIONS
6. HAIR REPLACEMENT: With wigs, weaves and hair pieces, have helped several women avoid emotional distress due to hair loss

7. HAIR TRANSPLANT: Unlike most men who may qualify for surgical hair transplant, only 2 to 5 % of females with genetic hair loss may have successful hair transplant or grafting because female hair loss tends to be diffuse and not concentrated at one area

Supplements and Alternative Methods for Treating Hair Loss

It is thought that genetic hair loss may not be helped by supplements because of the hormonal basis for the hair loss. However, for the many other causes like dietary reasons, diseases, major illnesses etc. it is possible Vitamins and Mineral supplements may help. Good studies to prove they do help with hair loss are not available, but anectdotal reports have been made about their effectiveness.

Vitamins and Minerals

1. Biotin
2. B Vitamins: Niacin (Vitamin B3), Vitamin B12
3. Vitamin C
4. Zinc, Iron, CoQ10 and Lysine

Low Level Light Therapy (LLLT)

The laser comb and laser caps and helmets use cold laser red light to slow down hair loss by increasing blood flow to the scalp and improving the thickness and strength of follicles. These combs and devices are used in the home and are FDA approved to treat hair loss. They are sold online and in some dermatology clinics.

Cancer Treatment Alopecia (Chemotherapy induced Alopecia)
What is This?

This is hair loss associated with use of chemotherapy to treat cancer. In breast cancer treatment Taxanes (Docetaxel and Paclitaxel) and Anthracyclines (Doxorubicin and Epirubicin) are commonly used chemotherapy regimens which all cause hair loss.

'It may take from three to six months after therapy is completed or it may start growing back while you are still receiving chemotherapy. Be prepared for your "new" hair to possibly have a slightly different color, texture, or curl'

(Chemocare.com — Hair loss and Chemotherapy).

Signs and Symptoms

It can affect women physically, either by thinning of the hair or the hairs fall out in big clumps. Emotionally, it can cause a lot of mental distress for some women since a woman's hair is often thought of as her "beauty". However, although the saying goes, "beauty is more than skin deep", the emotional and cultural implications have to be considered by those who are not going through this distressful situation and empathy can go a long way to alleviate some of the distress.

Treatment of Hair Loss Associated With Breast Cancer Therapy

Hair loss from cancer chemotherapy treatment is temporary and usually grows back after treatment. Methods used include:

Do Nothing

Some women chose not to do anything about the hair loss and that is perfectly fine. They instead shave off their hair and wait to see it grow after they finish chemotherapy.

Treatment to Prevent Excessive Hair Loss

Some treatments to prevent excessive hair loss include:

Scalp Cooling

SCALP COLD CAP: These are used during infusion of the chemo drug to minimize hair loss. Cold caps and scalp cooling systems are tightly fitting, strap-on, helmet-type hats filled with a gel coolant that's chilled to between −15 to −40 degrees Fahrenheit, and worn 20–50 minutes before, during, and after the chemotherapy (Breastcancer.org). One such Cold Cap Therapy device was approved by the USA Food and Drug Administration for use (Zosia, Chustecka Medscape medical news, Dec. 8th, 2015)

How it works: Scalp cooling causes the blood vessels to constrict; resulting in decreased blood flow to the scalp and therefore hair is exposed to less chemotherapy and so less hair falls out. The cold temperature also causes the hair follicles to decrease multiplication

Other Ways to Cover Up the Alopecia

Wigs: These can be worn so that the hair loss is not seen by those outside the home

Caps and scarves: People may use these during the hair loss period. American Cancer Society, for example, sponsors a program called "Look Good, Feel Better" which has live or scheduled online workshops about skin care, makeup, or wigs and head coverings for cancer patients (https://lookgoodfeelbetter.org)

Alopecia Areata
What is This?

This is hair loss believed to be due to an autoimmune condition. Basically, this means your body is fighting against one of its own organs and in this case it is the hair follicles on the scalp and other parts of the body. It has also been found that some individuals with alopecia areata have a high incidence of other autoimmune diseases like Diabetes mellitus, Rheumatoid arthritis (a disabling form of arthritis or inflammation of joints), and Thyroid diseases. Many may have family members with autoimmune conditions as well.

Signs and Symptoms

The hair will fall out from any area of the body where hair grows; scalp, eye brows and lashes, pubic area, and axillae (arm pits). It may grow back and fall off again with repetition of the cycle.

Treatment of Alopecia Areata

See a doctor who will take a history and examine your scalp and skin. She may have to do tests like scalp biopsy etc. and blood work to come to the right diagnosis. There may be spontaneous improvements and then recurrences. Treatment is to stimulate hair growth and stop the immune attack. Several treatments have been used with varying success. Some may work for one person and not for others. The earlier the treatment, and the smaller the area involved, the better the results. These treatments include:

1. Steroids, topical, or intralesional (injected into lesion – this is used when area is small)
2. Minoxidil 5% topical cream
3. Topical anthralin
4. Topical immunotherapy (latter is a form of contact allergen which have been used for years but not cleared by FDA for use in alopecia)
5. Psoralen plus Ultraviolet A light (PUVA) topical and oral treatment. Psoralen is a light sensitive drug that makes the skin more sensitive to UV light and aids its absorption. Patients first have the Psoralen applied or taken orally and then one is exposed to the UVA light. PUVA is known as photo chemotherapy. This improves scalp blood circulation but like all other treatments there are risks involved
6. For those with extensive or complete scalp involvement (alopecia universalis or totalis) oral steroids or Immunomodulators are used. The Immunomodulators affect the immune systems and are being used in clinical trials. They are medicines used for treating some blood cancers and Rheumatoid Arthritis. They are not FDA approved for Alopecia areta
7. Some women just shave their hair and are comfortable with bald heads if they already have most of the hair off. There are support groups available on line

where patients discuss their condition, give emotional support, and offer advice on what works for them

---

Reminders on Your Radar

The commonest cause of female hair loss is female androgenetic alopecia or female pattern baldness which is related to the androgen hormone. It has a genetic predisposition and about 40% of women may be affected. Both prescription and OTC medicines have been used to treat it. Cancer therapy related alopecia is common during therapy but the hair grows back after cancer therapy ends. Wigs, caps, and scarves are available to wear during therapy if one wants to use them. Cooling the scalp before and during therapy may minimize the hair loss.

Hirsutism – Excessive Hair on Body
(Reference: Medscape.com)

. . . .

What Is This?

This is excessive unwanted hair in women in areas of the body where hair usually grow in men. The scientific name is HIRSUTISM (HER-SOO-T-SIM) and means excessive hair on the body. It is due to excessive male sex hormones collectively called ANDROGENS. Hirsutism is commonly found when there is:

1. Rapid weight gain
2. After cessation of oral contraceptive pill use
3. In women with polycystic ovarian syndrome (PCOS – see more on this in chapter on Diseases of Pelvic Organs)

Other causes of Hirsutism
Idiopathic Hirsutism

In certain cases, the cause of hirsutism is unknown and no reason is found. This is known as idiopathic hirsutism and it often starts around puberty and runs in families.

Ovarian and Adrenal Tumors

Rare causes are due to tumors (abnormal growth of cells) in the ovaries or adrenal glands. The adrenals are two glands situated on top of the kidneys and produce special chemicals called adrenal hormones which the body uses for various important functions.

Postmenopausal Hair Growth

In postmenopausal women (those who have gone through the change and have stopped menstruation) there are changes in levels of sex hormones mainly estrogen, progesterone, and testosterone, and the estradiol levels decrease significantly as production from ovaries decrease. This leads to the typical menopausal symptoms women at this age experience. The shift in the balance between androgen and estrogen levels can also lead to excessive hair growth (hirsutism) in areas of the body where hair follicles are especially sensitive to androgen, such as the chin, upper lip, and cheeks.

Medicines Which Cause Hirsutism

Sometimes some medications can also cause hirsutism, but the excess hairs caused by these medicines are thinner, finer, and lighter in color and occur all over the body. They do not depend on androgens or male hormones. Some of these medicines are Phenytoin (for Epilepsy), Diazoxide, Minoxidil (for Blood Pressure), Acetazolamide (for Glaucoma) Glucocorticoids (Steroids), and Cyclosporine (used after organ transplant surgery).

Signs and Symptoms

Excess hair occurs on the face, chin, upper lip, and chest. The symptoms associated with the underlying cause may also be present. For example, women with PCOS may be overweight or obese, may have irregular periods or no periods at all. If there is rapid weight gain or a medicine is causing this, these clues will be noted in the history.

Treatment

Your doctor after taking your medical history and examining you may do some blood work and treat you depending on the cause.

1. The treatment may include **oral medications** or **mechanical removal of hairs**. Some hair removal treatments need a trained person like an Esthetician or health professional to do them while others can be done at home using over the counter (OTC) products
2. Hirsutism caused by drugs will resolve when the offending drug is discontinued

3. For those who have hormonal imbalance like in polycystic ovarian syndrome, excess hair growth may be treated with hormone therapy, e.g. Birth Control Pills (oral contraceptives) or a drug called Spironolactone which has anti androgen effects

4. One cream that does a good job of minimizing the regrowth of removed hair and is by prescription is EFLORNITHINE HYDROCHLORIDE 13.9% (VANIQA) CREAM. After plucking, shaving, or laser treatment the cream is applied two times daily for a few weeks and the effect can last for about 4 weeks by preventing regrowth of hair. Note that it does not remove hair by itself

5. Mechanical removal of the hairs is known as mechanical depilation and examples of these include shaving, plucking (tweezing), and waxing. Depilatory creams or lotions bought over the counter act by dissolving protein in the hair. They do not work too well on the face. Shaving sometimes causes ingrown hairs in which the short curly hair reenters the skin leading to irritation, bumps on the skin, and inflammation. This result of shaving can be seen mostly in black men, but occurs in women as well

6. Electrolysis is the process by which an electric current is introduced to the root of the hair to destroy it

7. Laser or pulsed light which destroy the root of the hair produce more permanent or lasting results. These work well on coarse hair and facial hair, but do not work well on blond or grey hairs for which electrolysis may be a better choice

Each method has its advantages and possible side effects. Some are effective for only a few days e.g. shaving, while others may have lasting effects like laser therapy. See your doctor and discuss excessive hair growth if that affects you.

Hyperhidrosis (Excessive Sweating)

What is This?

Sweating is a natural process which occurs in our bodies for a number of reasons, including cooling our bodies, and regulate our body temperature. Excessive sweating occurs in some individuals and this is known as Hyperhidrosis which may be primary or secondary.

Primary Hyperhidrosis

This usually starts in childhood or adolescent years. It may be brought on by anxious situations or can just happen anytime. It may occur in families indicating that there may be a genetic disposition. There is no identifiable cause for it.

Secondary Hyperhidrosis

This is a result of other conditions like:

Diseases

1. Hyperthyroid, low blood sugar, Diabetes, Parkinson's disease, Stroke
2. Gustatory sweating (related to food)
3. Infection, fever, tuberculosis (TB)
4. Cancers like leukemia and lymphoma

Medications

1. These include psychiatric medicines called antipsychotics and antidepressants e.g. Haloperidol, Nortriptyline, Buspirone, Trazodone, Desipramine
2. Zinc supplements
3. Birth Control Pills may cause night sweats and day time sweats and may probably be due to the progestin component

Signs and Symptoms

The excessive sweating may involve the axillae (armpit), palms, and feet and in the inner thighs areas, all of which are areas with a lot of sweat glands. Individuals may be very self-conscious and may not want to be with others. Some individuals will wear dark or black clothes so the sweating is not obvious. Contact a doctor and be bold enough to bring up this issue if it bothers you and affects your socialization. Fear, anxiety, embarrassment, and isolation can all be avoided by being treated for this condition.

Treatment of Hyperhidrosis

The doctor should take a careful history and go over the medicines you are taking. Some blood work may need to be done to make sure it is not a result of a medical condition. For example, thyroid blood work, blood sugar level, and your white blood cells levels will be checked for any abnormality.

Primary

Many treatments have been used and may be topical or oral or a combination of both.

The most common is prescription strength topical antiperspirant containing Aluminum chloride called DRYSOL or HYPERCARE solution. This is applied to affected areas at night and washed off in the morning.

ANTICHOLINERGICS: These blunt sweating causing dryness of the skin. Common oral prescription medications include:

1. Propantheline Bromide, Glycopyrrolate (also comes topically), Oxybutynin, and Benztropine
2. The main problems which may arise with these medicines are some of their side effects which include dry mouth, urine retention, constipation, blurred vision, and even affect memory if taken over a long time (the anticholinergics). However, lower doses may not cause these problems. Alternating the oral ones with topical medicines may be more appropriate and have less side effects
3. Surgery and injections which are used for cases that are difficult to treat with the simpler methods

Secondary

Treatment or correction of underlying medical condition will get rid of the sweating. Let your doctor review your medicines if you think one of your medicines is causing the problem. If due to medications, lowering the dose, or discontinuation of the medicine may lead to resolution of the problem.

Moles (Nevi)
What are Moles?

Moles also known as Nevi are dark growths or raised bumps on the skin. They are areas of the skin where melanin producing cells accumulate and form a lump. Melanin is what produces the dark pigment seen in black and brown skin. A mole or nevus is produced by specialized cells called MELANOCYTES and can be produced in all types of skin color. Some moles are present at birth or develop during childhood or early adult years.

Signs and Symptoms

Most moles are dark in color and may be brown or black; they do not usually cause itching or pain. They may grow bigger with time and the benign or non-cancerous ones are usually less than 1cm in size, have smooth edges, and maintain the same shape. If they change, a few may change into skin cancer.

The ones that are suspicious are those:

1. Which change in shape and size
2. Surface becomes scaly and irregular
3. Itches
4. Become swollen, hard or lumpy

Diagnosis and Treatment

If you have a mole that has changed or any of the above occur, it is important to let a dermatologist (skin specialist) or any doctor have a look at it to determine if it looks benign or is of concern. If there is concern or it looks suspicious then a BIOPSY is done. This is when a small part or all of it is removed and sent for examination and identification at a lab.

Treatment

Most moles, if benign do not need any treatment, just watching them (periodic examination by a doctor) is all that is required, however; some people for cosmetic reasons would like them removed. They can be excised (cut off), frozen (cryotherapy), or removed with heat or laser.

Cancerous Moles

If they are cancerous, then they have to be completely excised together with some of the normal skin and tissue around them.

Fungal Infections of the Skin (Dermatophytosis or Tinea)
What are They?

Fungal skin infections are a group of different skin infections caused by organisms belonging to a broad group called FUNGUS. These are not bacterial or viral organisms. Groups within this included Tinea and Candida. They can cause infections on skin, hair, nails, and even on mucosa which are cells that line internal tissues like inside the mouth and the intestines.

Tinea

Tinea causes infections of dead keratin of skin, hair, body, and scalp, and they can thrive when immune state is decreased as with HIV infection, and diabetes mellitus; or if one is on chronic steroid medications. Some of them are discussed below.

Tinea Versicolor
What is it?

Tinea Versicolor is a type of fungal infection which causes hypopigmented lesions on the body. This forms oval or round light colored lesions especially on the face, upper shoulders, back, and chest. It is common especially in teenagers and it is usually associated with hot, humid conditions.

Signs and Symptoms

It presents as a pale skin color or light brown rash with itching especially after sweating and there maybe some white flakes of the skin involved.

Treatment

If there is any doubt, skin scraping can be taken and inspected under the microscope, but it tends to be easily recognized and diagnosed by health care providers. Antifungal treatment in oral, topical or spray forms are used depending on extent of rash and where it is present.

1. If on the scalp or skin, then the shampoo form may also be used together with oral medicines. The shampoo is used as soap and can be put on the skin for about 15 minutes before showering, and then rinsed off after lathering it all over the body. Shampoos include ketoconazole and selenium sulfide (common dandruff shampoo)
2. If just a small area is involved, then creams or gels of ketoconazole, and selenium sulfide can be used
3. If extensive oral treatment using Terbinafine, Fluconazole and Itraconazole can be used for one to two weeks

Candida Infection of the Vagina and Vulva (Yeast)
What is it?

This is fungal infection affecting the female external genital – the vulva and the vaginal lining. It is also known as "yeast" infection or "white" in some communities. It thrives in damp, warm, moist, and dark areas and other areas commonly affected are under the breast, groin area, and in the mouth. It is very common and can occur if there is elimination of normal bacteria present in that area as one will find after taking oral antibiotics like Amoxicillin. Other risk factors include decreased immunity as in chronic Steroid therapy, HIV infection, and when one uses soap, antiseptic wipes, bubble baths, and perfumed sprays etc. in the vulva area. Babies and those on chronic inhaled steroids can have the same infection in the mucosa or lining of their mouths. It may spread down into the Esophagus and Intestines in those with compromised immune systems.

Signs and Symptoms

If the vagina and vulva are involved there is usually a white discharge causing itching, redness, and weeping of those areas. The discharge may have a "cottage cheese" or white clumpy appearance. If the skin around the groin is infected, these areas may be itchy, red, scaly or dark colored, and weepy.

Treatment

Treatment is by vaginal creams, suppositories, or tablets inserted nightly for 3 to 7 days, e.g. Clotrimazole, Miconazole, and Terconazole. An oral medication called Fluconazole (Diflucan) is a single dose pill which can be used, and the single pill continues to work in the body for about ten days. In groin area, same creams may be used as well as oral medications.

Fungal Infection of the Scalp (Ringworm)
What is it?

This is usually caused by the "Tinea" species of fungus and tends to occur in children, resulting from direct contact with someone who has the condition.

Signs and Symptoms

It can cause a scaly whitish ring hence the name "ring worm" or just a patchy white area with some raised bumps around it and the hair on affected part is broken off. It may itch. In children, the area may develop what looks like little boils and cause the lymph nodes behind or in front of the ears or back of scalp to swell up and become painful.

Treatment

This is treated with oral antifungals like Griseofulvin, Itraconazole, Terbinafine, and Fluconazole. Topical agents alone are ineffective since deeper layers are involved.

Fungal Infection of the Nails

This is called Onychomycosis (Oni-co-my-coo-sis) or Tinea unguium and can affect the nails of the toes and hands. It can be caused by various fungal species or groups.

Signs and Symptoms

It causes the affected nails to be discolored, thickened, crumbling, and abnormal in shape, loosened from the nail bed, or may have a whitish powder coming from under the nail. It is usually not painful, but looks unsightly and may be an embarrassment especially for women. It may co-exist with another fungal infection of foot or hand called Tinea Pedis (see below).

Ways of Acquiring Nail Infection

1. It may be common in states of decreased immunity and so may be common in HIV patients and people with Diabetes

2. One of the most common cause is from pedicure and manicure done at nail salons and spas. Sometimes, fungal elements are trapped in the water jet outlets and one can acquire infection during the foot spa treatment

3. Instruments if not cleaned and sterilized properly or are reused can cause infections

4. The constant removal of the cuticle and exposure of the nail matrix where dividing cells are present cause fungal cells if present to be deposited there and grow out together with the nail

5. To prevent salon acquired infections, some people take their own nail care instruments to the nail salon

6. One has to look out for foot baths or nail instruments that are not well cleaned, and be observant at these nail salons

7. It is okay to demand that footbaths or spas etc. be washed again with disinfectant when one sees that instruments being used are not clean or the basin or foot bath has dirt rings on the sides

8. Progressive nail salons cover the foot bath with a disposable liner which is removed after each client and have a new set of instruments for each client

9. One can do one's own manicure or pedicure at home

10. Some high end pedicure places use individual disposable foot basins and not the water jet type of foot spa or bath

Treatment

If the nails of hands and feet are involved it takes a long time to eradicate the fungus and topical ointments/creams do not usually work fast enough due to lack of penetration and the tendency to be wiped off, however, those painted on like Ciclopirox which is a nail lacquer topical solution may do better. Oral treatment works better and they include tablets like Terbinafine (Lamisil) or Itraconazole (Sporanox). Other treatments include surgical removal of the nails followed by some oral or topical medications, depending on extent of infection and location, and use of laser therapy heat followed by topical. Studies have not shown much success with laser therapy.

Nail infections of the fingers usually will require at least 4 weeks of daily oral treatment or 4 months of what is called intermittent or pulse dosing treatment. With the latter, you may be treated 7 to 10 days of the month, with three weeks rest, and the cycle is repeated for 4 months.

For the toes, cycle is repeated for 6 months, and when this is used, then the health professional does not have to do blood work to make sure your liver has not been affected by the medication. However, if daily continuous treatment is used, blood tests have to be done periodically to check the liver during the course of the treatment.

Athlete's Foot or Interdigital Fungal Infection (Tinea Pedis)
What is it?

Individuals can have fungal infection in between the toes (interdigital) and this is called ATHLETE'S FOOT or TINEA PEDIS. Showering in public showers or at public swimming pools, without flip flops (plastic/rubber slippers) may lead to this, and so it is important to wear footwear for showering in public baths. Also, activities that cause feet to sweat a lot like jogging or boxing makes one prone to it.

Signs and Symptoms

The skin becomes moist, white and mushy with cracking of the skin in between the toes. It may be sore or itchy. It can also occur at the sides and bottom of the foot as a white or red scaling rash. It may be associated with fungus of the toe nails described above.

Treatment

For Tinea Pedis, infection, an antifungal cream, spray, or powder could be used for about 2 to 4 weeks to clear the infection.

Prevention

Carefully drying the feet after a shower or bath and applying talc powder or antifungal powder will help prevent it in the first place or a recurrence. Keeping the inside of shoes aired and dry may also help.

Fungal Infection of Other Parts of The Body
Signs and Symptoms

1. Groin: (Jock Itch): Redness, itching, burning, cracking, and scaling of the groin
2. The crack of the buttocks (butt cheek): Redness, cracking, and pain
3. Under the breasts (inframammary area): Moist, red, itchy, scaly, and painful skin
4. Skin folds of the lower part of the belly in obese individuals: Weepy, itchy, redness under folds
5. Neck and beard area of men: Itchy and dry skin, loss of hair, and scaly rash
6. Hands: called Tinea Manuum causes itchy dry red skin with bumps or patches

Treatment

Treatment of the above include oral antifungal medication or creams, sprays or powders for 2 weeks to 6 months depending on the part and extent involved.

Complementary Herbal Treatment

Tea tree oil has been used topically for nail and athlete's foot infections and found to be somewhat effective. However, some people have developed skin rash or irritation after use. One may first need to do a skin patch test to check reaction to tea tree. Consult your doctor, if you wish to use this.

Prevention

1. To prevent this, moist dark areas have to be wiped dry after taking a bath or a shower
2. Use of a powder with Menthol or corn starch after thorough drying helps absorb moisture from sweating or residual water left after a bath or shower
3. Airing those areas like removing socks and letting a fan blow air in those areas will prevent fungal infections
4. In cases of recurrent infections in moist areas, antifungal powder or spray like e.g. nystatin, naftifine, or terbinafine will help prevent re-infection

Dry Skin (Xerosis)

Excessive dry skin may be a result of:

Dehydration by not drinking enough fluids
Losing abnormal amounts of fluid from the body
Dry weather
Malnutrition
Aging
Side effects of some medicines
Medical conditions: chronic diseases like Eczema, Diabetes, and Kidney failure are associated with dry skin

Treatment

To avoid cracking of skin associated with infection, itching, and ulcers, the skin has to be well moisturized.

The following may help:

1. It is important that substances known as moisturizers and emollients be used frequently on the skin. Emollients are creams or lotions that soften and sooth the skin
2. To improve this condition affected individuals should take short baths or showers using lukewarm as opposed to hot water which quickly dries up the skin

3. Use mild cleansers like unscented mild soap or baby soap so the skin is not irritated. Immediately after a shower, dry your skin quickly, and while it is still damp, apply a moisturizer to lock in the moisture

4. Baby oils can be put in bath water to lock in the moisture on the skin or right after getting out of the shower

5. Moisturizers have to be used liberally and several times a day. These include petroleum jelly or Vaseline based moisturizers, Lubriderm, Eucerin, Cetaphil, Aquaphor, Lac Hydrin, and Aveeno products for dry skin or Shea butter. All help maintain the moisture of the skin

6. The best ones are ointments, oils followed by creams then lotions. Remember good old petroleum is a good and cheap moisturizer

Reminders on Your Radar

There are different types of fungal infections affecting the external genitals, skin, nails, and scalp. One may need an oral anti-fungal pill to take along with prescribed antibiotics for bacteria infections if one is prone to genital yeast infection. The common ones affecting the skin tend to occur in moist dark areas like under the breast, groin, and buttock cheeks. After treatment, these areas can be kept dry with corn starch or Menthol containing powder and the use of an antifungal powder may prevent recurrence.

11

Endocrine System (En-do-crin)

What are endocrine Diseases?

....

The endocrine system of the body is made up of a number of glands that produce several hormones to help the body function effectively. Hormones can be considered as chemical messengers produced in the body and transported through the blood to affect specific cells, so as to help regulate or control different functions of the organ. They help in the area of glucose control, sexual and reproductive functions, metabolism (e.g. chemical processes that convert food to energy) and other functions. The major glands producing hormones are the pituitary (a gland in the brain), pancreas, thyroid, ovaries, testes, pineal, and adrenal glands. We would discuss some of these.

Organs Producing Endocrine Hormones

....

These organs are located in different areas of the body and the common ones are:

The Thyroid: Located close to the "Adams apple" at the front of the neck

The Pancreas: In the abdomen (gut) close to the stomach

The Adrenal glands: There are two and they sit on top of the kidneys in the back of the abdomen

The Ovaries: There is a pair and they form part of a woman's reproductive system and are located on either side of the uterus, close to the opening of the fallopian tubes

The Testes: There is a pair and are part of a man's reproductive system, located in the scrotum

The Brain: has 3 areas involved in production of hormones

Hypothalamus: Tells the Pituitary gland when to produce or stop making hormones

Pituitary: This is the "Master Endocrine Gland" and it directs other endocrine glands when to produce hormones. It produces Follicle Stimulating hormone, Prolactin, Growth Hormone, Luteinizing hormone, and Thyroid Stimulating Hormone

We will examine some of the diseases that can affect some of these glands due to underproduction or overproduction of the hormones they produce.

Diabetes Mellitus: (DM)

What is it?

This is also known as sugar diabetes or diabetes. The main problem is elevated blood sugar and that is because the hormones required to bring this down to normal levels are not functioning well. The main hormones involved with this disease are INSULIN and GLUCAGON and the absence, deficiency, or ineffectiveness of insulin leads to diabetes mellitus. Glucagon on the other hand raises blood sugar levels in the blood. Someone who is living with DM is often referred to as a DIABETIC patient. There are many types of diabetes but the 3 most common ones are:

> "Life is not over because you have diabetes. Make the most of what you have, be grateful".
> — Dale Evans Oct. 31, 1912 - Feb. 7, 2001, American actress, singer

1. TYPE 1 DIABETES MELLITUS (TYPE 1 DM or T1DM)
2. TYPE 2 DIABETES MELLITUS (TYPE 2 DM or T2DM)
3. GESTATIONAL DIABETES (GDM)

Some terms and abbreviations pertaining to Diabetes Mellitus

DM	Diabetes Mellitus
BS	Blood Sugar – same as Blood Glucose
FBS	Fasting Blood Sugar – BS measured after an overnight fast
RBS	Random Blood Sugar – BS measured at any time
Hypoglycemia	Low blood sugar
Hyperglycemia	High blood sugar

Background

To understand diabetes, we have to understand how the body breaks down and processes food for energy and different functions of the body.

Food we normally eat is made up mainly of Carbohydrates, Fats, Proteins and Fiber. After eating a meal, it is broken down to smaller simple particles called

GLUCOSE (sugar), amino acids or fatty acids and these go from our intestines into the blood stream. The blood eventually takes all of these into cells which use them for energy required for all the body's activities. It is INSULIN which helps glucose move from the blood stream into the cells, where it is used for energy, stored in the liver or muscles as glycogen or if in excess amounts, it is converted to fat.

What Happens in Diabetes?

Both insulin and glucagon are hormones produced by the PANCREAS, an organ that also produces chemicals called Lipase and Amylase which aid in digestion of food in the intestines. In diabetes, the pancreas either:

1. Does not make any insulin or not enough insulin (TYPE 1 DM) or
2. Produces insulin, but the body's cells are not sensitive or responding to the insulin and so they are not able to use it properly (TYPE 2 DM)

TYPE 2 DM and Insulin Resistance

In Insulin Resistance, insulin is present, but not being used effectively by the cells and is significant to the development of TYPE 2 DM. Initially, in an attempt to reduce the BS levels, the body produces more insulin to overcome the cells resistance but with time however, the pancreas is not able to make enough insulin to maintain the BS at normal levels (it gets overwhelmed). Therefore, glucose or sugar accumulates in the blood while the body's cells are "starving" for glucose to use.

TYPE 2 DM and Age

Although, Type 2 DM is mostly seen in adults in the last 10 to 15 years, Type 2 DM has been diagnosed more and more in children who are obese or overweight. Obesity has been linked to Diabetes and so the rise in obese or overweight individuals has led to an increased incidence of the disease. Increased junk, sugary foods, and drinks which children now eat and drink, coupled with the lack of exercise or activity have led to increased obesity in children and hence, TYPE 2 diabetes in children as well.

TYPE 2 DM Prevalence Globally

TYPE 2 DM is a common disease all over the world, and is increasing in all countries, especially in low resource countries where people are getting obese and are exercising less. According to WHO statistics on TYPE 2 DM,

1. The number of people with diabetes has risen from 108 million in 1980 to 422 million in 2014
2. The global prevalence of diabetes among adults over 18 years of age has risen from 4.7% in 1980 to 8.5% in 2014

3. Diabetes prevalence has been rising more rapidly in middle and low-income countries
4. In 2016, diabetes was the direct cause of 1.6 million deaths and in 2012, high blood glucose was the cause of another 2.2 million deaths

(https://www.who.int/news-room/fact-sheets/detail/diabetes). WHO Media Centre. Diabetes Fact sheet Updated October 2018.

Diabetes Mellitus and How it Affects Other Diseases

Diabetes Mellitus is a serious condition and it can cause an increased incidence of the following diseases:

Heart disease and Heart attacks
Heart failure
Strokes/Mini Strokes (TIA)
Kidney disease and failure
Nerve damage causing numbness, tingling and pain of the extremities (neuropathy)
Nerve damage causing slowing down of movement of food in the stomach (gastroparesis)
Eye disease, vision loss and blindness (retinopathy)
Non-healing ulcers on the legs or feet
Poor blood circulation
Amputation of feet and legs as a result on non healing ulcers or poor blood circulation

Definition of Diabetes Mellitus

The American Diabetes Association, (ADA), European Association for Study of Diabetes (EASD), American Association of Clinical Endocrinologists (AACE) and the International Diabetes Federation (IDF) are organizations which educate and provide important information about DM to both lay people and health professionals as well as do clinical studies on DM. They have established fasting blood sugar levels which define whether a person is in:

Normal, Pre-Diabetic and Diabetic Blood Sugar Ranges.

Unfortunately, each of these DM organizations has different "normal" values for HgbA1C, and other blood sugar parameters which are used to monitor DM. We will use the normal values of the American Diabetes Association in our discussions here unless otherwise stated.

Measurement Units of Blood Sugar

There are usually two broad measurement units used in the world:

1. International system of units (SI) used by most countries in the world, and for blood sugar levels, the SI system uses millimole per liter (mmol/l)
2. SAE is used in the USA. The SAE includes, inches, feet, miles, pounds, gallons. In measuring blood sugar levels, the SAE uses milligram per hundred milliliter (mg/dl)
3. One can easily convert values from one system to the other by using the formula below:

Formula for calculation of mg/dl from mmol/l: **mg/dl = 18 × mmol/l** (multiply)
Formula for calculation of mmol/l from mg/dl: **mmol/l = mg/dl ÷ 18** (divide)

Fasting Blood Sugar or Glucose Levels

NORMAL	PRE DIABETES	DIABETES
70–100 mg/dl	100–125 mg/dl	greater or equal to 126 mg/dl
Less than 5.5 mmol/l	5.5–6.9 mmol/l	greater than 7.0 mmol/l (> 7.0)

Diagnosis of Diabetes Mellitus Based On Blood Sugar Levels

Several ways of diagnosing DM have been developed based on different types of blood sugar measurements. These include:

1. Fasting blood sugar (taken after at least 8 hours of fast without food or liquids – just water)
2. Random blood sugar (taken anytime of the day in the non-fasting state)
3. Hemoglobin A1C or A1C (A one C)

Usually 2 positive tests at 2 different times are needed to diagnose DM, however, if you have one positive test as well as symptoms of high blood sugar then the diagnosis can be made.

The values below are those of the American Diabetes Association (www.diabetes.org).

Fasting Blood Sugar

A person is defined as having Diabetes Mellitus when the fasting blood sugar measured on 2 (two) different occasions are greater than 126 milligrams per deciliter (mg/dl), or greater than 7.0 mmol/l. Normal fasting blood sugar is between 70–100 mg/dl (3.9–5.5 mmol/l) and Prediabetes is 100–125mg/dl (5.5–6.9 mmol/l).

Random Blood Sugar

This is when blood sugar is measured in the non-fasting state so it could be anytime of the day. It's also known as casual glucose test. Diabetes Mellitus is also defined as having a measured random blood sugar of greater than or equal to 200 mg/dl or 11.11 mmol/l associated with symptoms of high sugar like thirst, excessive urination, weight loss and excessive fluid intake.

Oral Glucose Tolerance Test (GTT)

This is when blood glucose is measured before and 2 hours after ingestion of 75-g glucose or sugar drink at a lab. It is similar to the test women take when they are being screened for diabetes during pregnancy. Diagnosis is made when the 2 hour glucose is greater or equal to 200.

Less than 140 mg/dl	normal
140–199	impaired glucose tolerance (Prediabetes)
Greater or equal to 200	Diabetes. It is confirmed by another repeated test

Hemoglobin A1C (A1C)

Hemoglobin A1C is a measurement which tells what one's average blood sugar has been over the last three to four months. It gives a better picture of blood sugar since the measurement does not describe a one-time (real time) blood sugar reading. There is no need to fast for the test. It is not a very accurate test in people who have sickle cell disease or other abnormalities of their red blood cells, because it gives a falsely decreased level. On the other hand those with high triglycerides and chronic kidney disease may get a falsely increased reading.

Diabetes Mellitus is diagnosed by a Hemoglobin A1C (HgbA1c) equal or greater than 6.5%.

HgbA1c	4.8–5.6%	Normal
HgbA1c	5.7–6.4%	Prediabetes
HgbA1c	>6.5%	Diabetes (Must be confirmed by a 2nd test)

Pre Diabetes (Impaired Fasting Glucose), Pre DM
What is it?

This is a state in which an individual's blood sugar is above normal reading but is not at the diabetes level yet. World wide more than 300 million may have prediabetes and about 30% of Americans have Pre DMs. It is also referred to as Impaired Glucose Tolerance (IGT) or Impaired Fasting Glucose (IFG). This is defined as a blood sugar level between 100 and 125 mg/dl or 5.5 to 6.9 mmol/l and HgbA1c between 5.7 and 6.4%. People with prediabetes can either revert back to normal, continue to stay at that level or go on to develop diabetes with time.

Treatment of Prediabetes

It is at this stage that risk factors for developing diabetes have to be vigorously controlled because over the next 3 to 5 years these changes may occur:

1. 25% of people with prediabetes will develop diabetes
2. Another 25% will revert to normal blood sugar levels
3. 50% will continue to be prediabetic

Treatment for Prediabetes include

Lifestyle changes with healthy diet, eating more vegetables and high fiber foods
Exercise most days of the week like walking, jogging, and gardening
Weight loss (target 7% of body weight)
Reduction of medications which may be causing the increased blood sugar
Counseling with respect to alcohol intake and smoking cessation
Use of medications

Medications like METFORMIN and ACARBOSE may be prescribed by a doctor to slow the progression to full-blown diabetes. They have both been found to lower cardiovascular risks.

Dietary Supplements (CAM Medicines) for Prediabetes

Dietary supplements like CHROMIUM PICOLINATE or CHROMIUM POLYNICO-TINATE and FENUGREEK have been used by some to improve blood sugar levels and make the body tissues more sensitive to insulin already present in the blood. However, these are not advocated by all health professionals, and according to the NCCIH National institute of health, there is no strong evidence that dietary supplements can prevent or treat Diabetes Mellitus. (Diabetes and Dietary Supplements – NCCIH nccih.nih.gov/sites/nccam.nih.gov/files/Diabetes. 11-08-2015).

VINEGAR: Research with vinegar taken before meals reduced blood sugar levels about 20 to 30%. It has been suggested that those who want to use this, limit it to 1–2 tablespoons of vinegar diluted with water to be taken twice a day.

Side effects of vinegar especially if consumed in large amounts include:
Low blood sugar if one is on other diabetes medicines, irritation of the stomach, nausea, erosion of dental enamel and even low potassium with long term use. (Andrea Scott. Vinegar and Diabetes: Dos and Don'ts-Medscape-May 12, 2016) Medscape Pharmacist
Consult with your doctor before starting any OTC medicines for prediabetes

Type 1 Diabetes Mellitus
What is it?

This usually occurs early in life and is usually diagnosed in children; however, the many variations of the condition have resulted in older folks being diagnosed in their 30s and 40s or even in elderly patients. In type I DM there is basically a destruction of the beta cells in the pancreas that produce insulin. It is believed to be a result of autoimmune destruction of the beta cells, resulting in the inability of the pancreas to make any insulin.

Signs and Symptoms

The main symptoms or presentation include frequent urination, thirst, weight loss, tiredness, weakness, and drinking a lot of water and fluids.

Treatment

Treatment is with insulin injections to replace what is not being produced by the body. Children are taught how to give themselves insulin shots or injections and how to check their blood sugar levels several times a day. Some use insulin pumps which give continuous insulin (basal dose) and boluses at meal times; instead of the intermittent shots, and also some use continuous glucose monitoring devices attached to their skin by small needles.

Type 2 Diabetes Mellitus (T2DM)
What is it?

This is mostly due to the inability of the body's cells to properly use the insulin it makes, but sometimes the situation is such that the body is also not making enough of its own insulin. Experts believe that by the time an individual is diagnosed with Type 2 diabetes, he or she has already lost over 50% of the function of the pancreatic cells called the "beta cells" which produce insulin. In fact most recent studies indicate that as much as 80% of the insulin producing capacity of the pancreas is lost over the previous 10 years, before the time of diagnosis of Type 2 diabetes. Unfortunately, this decline in pancreatic function continues relentlessly and the disease progresses until the pancreas may not produce much insulin at all. More and more obese or overweight individuals are developing diabetes and researchers have found an inter relationship between diabetes and obesity.

Signs and Symptoms

The symptoms present in Type 2 DM include:

1. Frequent urination, thirst, and drinking a lot of water and fluids

2. Blurred vision, and dry mouth
3. Unintentional weight loss, tiredness, weakness
4. Vaginal yeast infections in women, urinary tract or bladder infections
5. Numbness and tingling in the extremities

When you have several of these symptoms occurring together, it is important to consult a health professional, who will do blood and urine tests to make the diagnosis.

Treatment

Once a diagnosis of Type 2 DM is made, it is important to have it managed well. DM diagnosis is not a death sentence. Many people are living full, active and fulfilled lives with DM Type 2. The management of DM involves the patient and their health care provider. The patient has to take some charge to get it well controlled. Treatment is by diet, medications and non medication means to get the blood sugars in optimum range.

Healthy Eating

This will be discussed in details later on, but low carbohydrates, and moderation in both fatty meals and protein has been suggested.

Medications

TYPE 2 DM is treated with medications and these include:
1. Oral medications: several different classes of medicines, with newer ones being developed more recently
2. Insulin injections: several different types of insulin. Short acting, median and long acting types exist. They may be drawn from a vial or come in a convenient Pen form
3. Non insulin Injections: These are injections but are NOT insulin. Some of these are given daily or even once a week

CAM Medications for Treating DM

Complementary and alternative medications have been used to decrease blood sugar by people. However, just like in the case of Prediabetes, according to the NCCIH /National institute of health, there is no strong evidence that dietary supplements can prevent or treat DM. (Diabetes and Dietary Supplements – NCCIH nccih.nih.gov/sites/nccam.nih.gov/files/Diabetes.   11-08-2015).   Several small research studies have been done on Apple Cider Vinegar and the evidence suggests that about two tablespoons of it with water 2–3 x daily with meals may improve postprandial (2 hours or more after meals) and fasting glucose levels in people with diabetes mellitus. (www.medscape.com, Desiree Lie, Does a spoonful or 2 of Vinegar make the sugar go down?, Feb 16, 2012). However, there may be side effects of stomach irritation, and nausea, erosion of dental enamel. Vinegar containing 5–6% acetic acid is what should be used, as higher concentrations sometimes seen in Vinegar tablets can cause damage to the esophagus or even lower one's potassium level. Using balsamic vinegar or any other vinegar (wine, apple cider) with olive oil and spices as home made salad dressing will serve the same purpose, and make one avoid the high calorie commercial salad dressings.

Managing Type 2 Diabetes

The key to successful management of diabetes mellitus, and living a healthy full life in spite of the disease is rooted in the patient being actively involved in the management of her condition. Therefore the idea of self-management of one's condition is being advocated more and more by health care providers and this means the patient is actively involved in monitoring and knowing about their disease. No patient should be ignorant about their medical condition. An informed patient is usually a responsible one who is compliant with their medications, doctor's appointments and following the other principles listed below.

Principles of Self Management of Diabetes Mellitus

As a diabetic patient, one has to take control of their disease and co-manage their condition alongside their health care provider. One must be a team player who is actively involved in one's own care and not ignorant of what is going on. To do this:

1. One has to understand their disease. Read information about it and research it
2. Do self-monitoring of blood sugar with a glucometer
3. Know what one's Hemoglobin A1C (HgbA1c or A1C) is
4. Eat healthy
5. Be active and exercise regularly
6. Lose weight if one is overweight or obese
7. Take one's medicines as prescribed
8. Manage other conditions associated with diabetes well
9. Follow up regularly with one's health care provider
10. Have regular eye examinations
11. Take good care of one's feet to avoid injury or cuts
12. Reduce stress in one's life
13. Keep up to date with preventive screening tests to prevent other diseases

Some of the above measures will be discussed in more detail below.

Monitoring One's Blood Sugar (BS)

Self-monitoring of blood glucose by pricking one's finger is important to keep one within predetermined goals of blood sugar levels the patient and their health care provider have decided on. However, the importance of this routine tracking of BS has been shown not to be too significant for those who are not on insulin or a type of oral medications known as Sulfonylureas, because these two may cause low blood sugar and so closer monitoring is required. It's probably good to also check blood sugar when there has been recent changes in medicines or during an illness. One can check their blood sugar level at home using a glucometer, and if one is on a medicine like Metformin alone, one could routinely check it once a week. It is important to discuss what a glucometer is because it helps patients at home keep a watch on their blood sugar and be able to control their diabetes better.

Glucometer
What is it?

A glucometer kit is made up of:

1. A meter or small device (of which there are several types and sizes)
2. Test stripes: only to be used with a particular glucometer and so are not interchangeable
3. Lancets: sharp edge used to prick the skin and get a sample of blood from finger/arm
4. Control solution and alcohol pads for cleaning the skin
5. Instruction booklet, read this, since each meter works in a slightly different way
6. Booklet for recording your blood sugar
7. Lancing device may take 6 lancets and some have variable depth setting and so one can adjust how far it stabs your finger. Some use vacuum to draw blood and so give less discomfort

Using A Glucometer

Each one has its own instructions but generally, after washing and drying hands, the correct end of stripe is inserted into the test port of the device, The finger tip is cleaned with alcohol and the lancet is used to prick the finger (better to prick the side – less painful). The blood then goes on the edge of the stripe which is in the meter. Over the years, the newer glucometers are more advanced; some need smaller amounts of blood, others allow testing of other places apart from finger tips, and have other features which make the blood testing experience more comfortable. There are others that do continuous blood glucose monitoring (CGM) and about 345,000 Americans currently use those. They cause users to monitor glucose levels in real time and also readings over a period of time. One gets a better picture of BS trends with these, but they measure sugar in interstitial fluid which is the fluid between cells. A sensor has a tip inserted under the skin and its in contact with interstitial fluids, therefore it is able to send a message to a transmitter which transmits message to the meter, and they allow for less fingersticks. One has to prick the finger when sugar readings show too low or too high. The FDA, in 2017, approved the first of a CGM system which does not require backup finger pricking. A sensor is placed on the skin and it is changed every 10 days. One waves a reader device over it to see the current blood sugar levels and it can also tell what the trends have been over the past 8 hours.

Whatever way BS is measured, the recording of one's blood sugar at home will let one know how one's blood sugar control is doing in between one's clinic and doctor visits.

What are Optimal Blood Sugar Values?

The values below are what one should aim at, according to the American Diabetes Association. These are "plasma glucose values" which are obtained when blood is drawn by the lab and the cells are removed before the sugar content is measured. A glucometer measures whole blood values and these values are about 10% lower than plasma values. However, one's health care provider will let one know the values one should aim at. If one's readings are mostly above what has been agreed upon, then changes may be made to one's medication dosage, or another drug may have to be added so that one can get to the goal agreed upon.

Different diabetes organizations may have slightly different optimal numbers for the various parameters which are measured to monitor control of diabetes mellitus. For example, the American Association of Clinical Endocrinology recommendation has slightly different plasma values than the American Diabetes Association, and the latter's values are more generous while the Clinical endocrinology numbers aim for tighter control.

Blood Sugar Goals and Age

In general, the older one is (60 years and above), the more slack one is given (goal will be at higher number of the range) so one does not end up with hypoglycemia (low blood sugar below 70 mg/dl) and the problems associated with it.

Low Blood Sugar (Hypoglycemia)

The following can cause your blood sugar to go down when one:

1. Eats too little food or skips a meal
2. Takes too much Insulin or Sulfonylurea medicines without a meal

3. Lacks adequate carbohydrate intake
4. Exercises excessively without eating adequately
5. Drinks excess alcohol which can lower the liver's production of glucose

Signs and Symptoms Of Low Blood Sugar (Hypoglycemia)

1. It makes one feel shaky and sweaty, dizzy, nervous, and have palpitations
2. Nausea or vomiting, hunger, weakness and fatigue
3. One cannot think clearly, headache, sleepy, confusion, or seizures
4. Become comatose (unresponsive or passout)

It is a very scary or frightening situation and because of the symptoms most diabetics would prefer their blood sugars to run high in order to avoid an episode.

Prevention of Hypoglycemia

1. Wear a medical alert bracelet that says one is diabetic
2. Check one's blood sugar regularly, eat before exercising, and make sure diabetic medicines are not taken when meals are missed
3. Carry a sugar rich food or snack to use if needed. These include juice or regular soda (not diet), glucose tablets, and hard candies one can chew quickly . Wait 15 minutes and recheck one's sugar, if still low, repeat any of above foods again
4. If drinking alcohol, no more than 2 drinks/day for men and one drink for women. Drink alcohol only with food. Alcohol can inhibit the liver's function of constantly releasing glucose to keep blood sugar levels regulated and therefore that can lead to hypoglycemia

Glucose Normal Values for Diabetics

Glucose Plasma values: (American Diabetes Association).

Time	Value mmol/l	Value mg/dl
Before breakfast (fasting)	3.9–7.2 mmol/l	70–130 mg/dl
Peak Post prandial (about 60–120 minutes) after starting a meal	less than 10 mmol/l	Below 180 mg/dl

Glucose Plasma values: (Am. Assoc. of Clinical Endocrinology).

Time	Value mmol/l	Value mg/dl
Before breakfast (fasting)	Less than 6.1 mmol/l	Less than 110 mg/dl
Two hours after a meal	less than 7.8 mmol/l	Below 140 mg/dl

Know One's Hemoglobin A1C (HGBA1C)

HgbA1c is a more accurate reflection of blood sugar or glucose control since it gives one an idea of what one's average blood sugar has been over the last three or four months. So it is important to know what one's number is. Below is how it correlates with blood sugar or glucose values. It can be measured every three to six months (2 to 4 times a year).

Normal HgbA1c   A1C levels of 5.6% and lower are in the healthy range
Prediabetic range   A1C levels of between 5.7% and 6.4%
Diabetes range   A1C levels of 6.5% and higher

Optimal control in Diabetes: A1C levels of between 6.5% and 7% for most people with diabetes. (American Diabetes Association)

How HGBA1C Approximates to the Average Glucose Level

According to "UpToDate" which is an online medical journal (http://www.uptodate. com, Wolters Kluwer Health), the mean glucose level associated with various A1c values are:

A1C (%)	Mean Glucose (mg/dl)	Mean glucose (mmol/l)	*Approx
5	97	5.4	90
6	126	7	120
7	154	8.6	150
8	183	10.2	180
9	212	11.8	210
10	240	13.3	240
11	269	15	270
12	298	16.5	300
13	326	18.1	330

Note: * Approx values (last row) are much easier to remember because they are rounded up. Each A1c number is 30mg/dl more than the previous one. This is not in the "uptodate" article.

Lifestyle Changes That Help With Controlling Diabetes

Healthy eating, weight loss, and exercise are an integral part of diabetes care or treatment. Individuals may control their diabetes with these alone or in combination with medications.

Healthy Eating

Below are some suggestions about healthy eating:

1. Eat more vegetables, fish, whole grain bread (brown bread), less sugary drinks and less desserts high in sugar or fatty foods
2. Drinking sugary drinks is linked to development of type 2 diabetes according to research. One can have regular sugar but it's the amount that needs to be checked since like any other carbohydrate (carb) it can quickly raise blood sugar levels
3. Sugar is present in desserts and hidden in other foods, so it's best to avoid regular sugar or other sugars like honey, high fructose corn syrup, molasses, brown sugar, cane sugar etc. and use sugar substitutes especially the natural ones like Stevia, and Monk fruit
4. If one has to eat a dessert one can use it to replace another carb like bread in that meal
5. Try and trim fats from meats and poultry, and remove the skin from chicken before cooking it
6. An easy way to eat is to make sure one's plate is half filled with vegetables of any kind, a quarter with some type of protein and a quarter with carbohydrates (rice, pasta, sweet potato, potato, bread, corn, cassava, yam, yucca, etc.)
7. Cooking methods like baking, grilling, roasting, boiling, and steaming are preferred to frying. Excessive breading of chicken and meat should be avoided
8. Red meats should be eaten in moderation and fish should be eaten about two or more times a week if possible

Exercise and Keep Active

Try and do some exercise almost every day. This can be walking, gardening, dancing, running, jogging or working out at a gym (any muscle that you move is good EXCEPT one's jaw muscles for eating). Exercising and eating a healthy diet/meals will lead to weight loss and reduction in blood sugar. Other easy ways to get one's exercise done, is by doing simple things like using the stairs instead of the elevator or lift, parking one's car a little further from the entrance of where one is going and walking, going to the mall or park to walk around, and anything else that will keep one moving. Another way to motivate one to move is to use a step counter app on one's phone or a pedometer, FIT BIT, Apple watch, etc. to count the number of steps one walks daily. Aim at walking between 8000 and 10,000 steps a day which is approximately between four and five miles.

Lose Weight If You are Overweight Or Obese

Exercising and eating a healthy diet will lead to weight loss and reduction in blood sugar. Some individuals who lose weight end up getting off diabetes medicines after a while. Studies have also shown that weight loss in diabetes results in decreased rate of death, while weight gain results in increased incidence of coronary heart disease (disease of the blood vessels which supply the heart). There are approved weight loss medications one can go on in order to jumpstart one's weight loss, however, it is still important to eat healthy and exercise when on these. After weight loss it's important to continue exercising to maintain the weight lost.

Take Your Medications As Prescribed

When healthy eating, weight loss and exercise do not control one's blood sugar, one may be started on medications to help control one's blood sugar levels.

1. One may have several medicines to take and so make sure one is taking one's medicines as ordered. Medicines used to treat diabetes include oral medications, insulin and other non-insulin injectable medications

2. Compliance with medicines or taking one's medicines as prescribed is important to keep one healthy and prevent the complications associated with DM. Diet and exercise are important parts of treatment of diabetes. When one is not controlled with just diet and exercise, one may be started on a common medication called Metformin. This has been used for over 50 years and it is a safe medicine. Recent reports show it helps with decreasing cardiovascular risk as well as being safe for people with heart failure and even those with mild or moderate kidney failure

3. There are many other oral medications belonging to other classes which may be used along with Metformin. The other additions may depend on how one's blood sugar is doing. However, whether one is on oral medicines or injections, or both, they all play an important part in managing the disease, and preventing complications from excess blood sugar or hyperglycemia

4. Two of the new classes of drugs called SGLT2 inhibitors (oral) and GLP-1 RAs (injectables and oral) have been found to reduce risk of cardiovascular diseases like stroke, heart attacks, and cardiovascular death. These may therefore be used in patients with high risk of cardiovascular disease. The SGLT2i drugs may also lower kidney disease and risk of dying from kidney diseases. They work through the kidneys causing one to eliminate the sugar out in the urine

Manage Other Chronic Medical Conditions Well

Diabetes and any other medical conditions that one may have like hypertension (high blood pressure or BP), high cholesterol, and heart disease have to be well controlled. One should have regular follow ups with one's doctor or health care provider to assess how one is doing, to refill one's medicines, do blood work, and go over or review one's blood work results. Visits for DM are usually every 3 to 4 months, and more frequent if required. If new symptoms come up, like numbness and tingling in one's legs, yeast infections in women, vision problems, dizziness etc. one needs to let their health provider know. When all the other medical conditions are well controlled it helps decrease or delay the complications associated with diabetes.

Have Regular Eye Examinations

"I think that the greatest gift God ever gave man is not the gift of sight but the gift of vision. Sight is a function of the eyes, but vision is a function of the heart".

— Dr. Myles Munroe, Bahamian Pastor, evangelist, author, leadership consultant (20th April 1954—9th Nov. 2014).

Have one's eyes checked at least every year by an eye doctor to make sure the diabetes is not affecting one's eyes adversely. Diabetes is one of the common causes of blindness, and vision impairment, and the exam will enable any damage to the retina (light sensitive layer at the back of the eye) to be quickly identified and treated. Retinal damage (Diabetic Retinopathy) is the most common cause of eye problems resulting in blindness in diabetics.

Take Care of One's Feet and Inspect Them Daily

It is very important that a diabetic person takes very good care of their feet and skin in general. One of the unfortunate things that happen to some people with diabetes is they may develop cuts, sores or wounds on their feet or legs which do not heal, leading to amputation of a foot, toe or a leg. To avoid this do the following:

1. It is important to inspect one's feet every evening before getting into bed
2. A hand mirror is a good aid to use to inspect one's feet
3. If the skin on the legs is too dry, it leads to cracks in the skin of the feet or in between the toes and this can result in infection of the skin; which, if not treated aggressively can grow into a non-healing ulcer
4. Use of any moisturizer cream or lotion will prevent dry or cracked skin of legs and feet
5. Avoid tight or uncomfortable shoes to prevent injury to the feet
6. Any small sore, ulcer or scratch on the skin of the feet or legs should be brought to the attention of a health care professional as soon as possible

7. After a shower or bath, it is important to dry the area in between one's toes very well to minimize the development of fungal infection or athlete's foot

8. Some people who sweat a lot in between their toes find that use of menthol containing talc powder helps keep them dry

9. Walking bare foot is not a good idea, since one can step on a sharp object or glass and cut the foot leading to complications of non-healing ulcer

10. A diabetic should always wear shoes which are not tight and with good soles. There are special shoes for diabetics which tend to have wider fronts and are well padded with diabetic insoles. However, any pair of shoes that do not squeeze the toes should work well, and one can get the insoles at pharmacy shops or online

11. The fact that most diabetics may experience numbness with or without tingling (neuropathy) in the legs, feet and toes can result in the individual not feeling a cut in those areas, and so a small ulcer can develop and if not treated aggressively, can result in a big non healing ulcer, with subsequent amputation of part of lower leg

12. Some people who had started with a small insignificant cut on the foot have unfortunately had amputation of an entire leg due to non-healing of the wound which resulted, and underlying cause is from damaged nerves or decreased blood flow.

Try to Minimize Stress in One's Life

Stress in our lives leads to increased release of stress hormones and this can lead to increase in one's blood sugar levels. It is impossible to live without any stress at all; however, one can choose to minimize stress in one's life. Good choices may offend others but sometimes one just has to do that in order not to be overwhelmed. Sometimes we fail to delegate work or responsibilities to others and try to do everything by ourselves (micro manage). This can make us too busy and hassled, bringing unnecessary stress into one's life.

Some Tips on Minimizing Stress

Spend time relaxing by frequently doing things one enjoys.

Get some leisure time by oneself or with friends and family, in effect make sure one has a social life. Take vacations, and go on trips, sightseeing, get together with friends and also enjoy some "me" time.

Delegate some of the responsibilities to others; Trust others and stop micro-managing.

There will be more discussion about this in the second part of the book which discusses emotional and mental health.

Complications of Diabetes Mellitus

Complications due to Diabetes mellitus occur frequently when there is not tight control of blood sugar levels and neglect to treat other chronic diseases like hypertension and high cholesterol. Common complications affecting various organs in the body include:

EYE PROBLEMS: the blood vessels behind the eyes (retina) can be affected by diabetes leading to decreased vision or blindness. That is why regular eye exams and treatment of eye complications must be quickly attended to. The commonest eye problem is called Diabetic Retinopathy in which the retina, where an image registers during vision is damaged. Diabetes mellitus is the major cause of blindness in adults in the USA and around the world

KIDNEY PROBLEMS: The kidney is a very important organ as it filters blood and removes waste produced by cells in the body through the urine. Damaged kidneys may result in what is called chronic renal or kidney failure and patients may need to go on dialysis. This involves using an external filter to filter the blood, because the natural kidneys are not working well, and therefore there is accumulation of body waste products. One goes for dialysis two to three times a week, or do dialysis at home, or have a kidney transplant – receive a new donated kidney from someone. Diabetes mellitus is the leading cause of chronic kidney failure and need for dialysis when filtration by the natural kidneys are very low and there is dangerously high levels of body waste products

AMPUTATION OF LIMBS: Diabetes mellitus is the leading cause of amputation of legs, feet and toes due to nerve damage or circulation problems. Paying attention to proper care of the legs and skin, and good blood sugar control help prevent ulcers and subsequent amputations

HEART ATTACKS AND STROKES: More than 60% of people with Diabetes mellitus may die of either one of these two diseases. Women in particular have about 2–3x the risk of getting coronary heart disease compared to women without diabetes. Risk factors for these two conditions are discussed in the section on heart attacks and strokes. In recent studies, adding Acabose to Metformin has been found in the treatment of both Type 2 DM and Impaired Fasting BS to be associated with lower risks of major atherosclerotic events, ischemic stroke, and Hypoglycemia. (www.medpagetoday.com/reading-room/endocrine-society/diabetes)

CIRCULATION PROBLEMS: Decreased blood flow to the legs and to the neck vessels (Carotid arteries) results in Peripheral Vascular Disease or Peripheral Arterial Disease (PVD or PAD) which can result in pain in the lower legs especially with walking, and decreased blood flow to the brain resulting in mini strokes (TIAs) and strokes

NERVE CONDITIONS: The following are nerve complications of Diabetes

Peripheral Neuropathy
What is it?

Diabetic neuropathy is very common in both type I and type 2 DM. It affects up to 50% of patients with DM and results from either prolonged uncontrolled blood sugars or in those with long standing DM. The sugar affects nerves and damages them in the lower and upper limbs. Remember keeping blood sugars within target range helps prevent progression, and may decrease severity of the symptoms. One must talk to their doctor if one suffers from neuropathy.

Signs and Symptoms

These include burning, pain, numbness and tingling of arms, hands, legs and feet. This can be very debilitating and can lead to amputations of limbs if they are involved, as discussed above.

Treatment

1. There are medications that can help treat or reduce the symptoms of nerve damage. These include oral medications, creams and ointments
2. Examples are certain oral antidepressants like Amitriptyline, and Duloxetine, and other types like Pregabalin and Gabapentin
3. Pain relieving creams like Capsaicin cream and other creams that are compounded by pharmacists. These compounded creams may contain combination of some of the following: Gabapentin, Lidocaine, Ketamine, Amitriptyline, and Clonidine
4. Two Medical foods PoDiaPn (folate salt, ALA, Vitamin B12 and Pyridoxine) and Metanx (contains folate, Vit. B9, Vit. B12 and Vit. B6) have been approved by FDA for treating Diabetic Neuropathy

Complementary and Alternative Medicines for Neuropathy

Apart from prescription medications, there are some Complementary and Alternative therapies that may help. Not all research on these are conclusive but some patients have said they help. These include Vitamin B complex, Alpha lipoic acid (ALA), Biotin, Biofeedback, Acupuncture, and electric nerve stimulation.

Autonomic Neuropathy
What is it?

Apart from nerves supplying the extremities, uncontrolled or long standing DM can affect other nerves which supply organs that perform automatic functions of the body. This condition is known as autonomic neuropathy and affects nerves supplying the gut, reproductive system, and blood vessels. The functions they perform include: beating of the heart, maintaining blood pressure, process of digestion by the intestines, temperature control by sweat glands and sexual functions.

Signs and Symptoms

Some of the abnormalities in these affected functions and signs present as the following:

1. Lowered Blood Pressure: This may drop especially with standing up, and the lowered blood pressure may cause dizziness and faintness
2. Digestion: This is slowed and food does not move quickly through the stomach, which may feel full quickly, gassy or have bloated sensation, upper abdominal pain, nausea, vomiting, (this is called Gastroparesis) and Diarrhea or Constipation may occur frequently
3. Gustatory Sweating: Excessive sweating of face, scalp, chest and neck a few minutes after food ingestion due to stimulation of salivary glands (gustatory sweating). Foods commonly triggering this are chocolate and cheese
4. Sweat Glands: Temperature control is affected, with either excessive or decreased sweating
5. Sexual organs: The decreased nerve functions contribute to this, and may manifest as loss of libido and vaginal dryness in women, and erectile dysfunction in men. About a third of women with diabetes have sexual issues. Vaginal dryness can be treated with vaginal lubricant gels or creams, estrogen creams especially in postmenopausal women and Ospemifene a non-Estrogen pill which makes the vaginal walls thicker and helps with painful sex (Dyspareunia). Further treatment is discussed in the chapter on treating postmenopausal vaginal dryness. Discuss sexual concerns with one's doctor

Treatment

GASTROPARESIS (Decreased movement of food in the bowels)

There are medicines available to help keep food moving down the gut faster, e.g. Metoclopramide, Erythromycin (can develop resistant bacteria from prolonged use), and for nausea and vomiting one can take anti nausea medicines like Promethazine or Ondansetron.

Gustatory Sweating

This is rare, but if it is a bother, avoid those foods. There are oral and topical medicines that can be used to decrease sweating; and include topical creams containing Glycopyrrolate, oral Oxybutynin, Clonidine, or Scopolamine. These may have side effects of dry mouth and constipation.

Hypotension (Low blood Pressure)

One has to change body positions slowly, don't stand up too fast, and keep well hydrated.

Sweating Problems

Keep cool by having water with ice, and dressing in layers which can be removed if heat is a problem. If feeling too cold then dress in warm clothes.

Use of Insulin in the Adult With Type 2 Diabetes Mellitus

Most individuals who have Type 2 Diabetes will eventually go on insulin injections if they live long enough with the disease. Use of insulin or other injectables is not a sign of failure on one's part. This is because after a number of years, the body is unable to produce enough insulin to take care of the glucose the body produces from food one eats. Taking insulin shots or injections before meals and at bedtime may be what is needed in this case to keep the blood sugar in an acceptable range. It may seem to be a daunting task, but these days the needles used for giving injections are tiny and hardly hurt.

> "Use of insulin or other injectables is not a sign of failure on your part. This is because with time, the body is unable to produce enough insulin to regulate blood sugar."
>
> —Dr. Barbara Entsuah.

Insulin Pens and Pumps

Now, apart from insulin that is drawn from a vial or bottle with a syringe and needle, there are Insulin Pens that can be loaded with a cartridge filled with insulin, and dialed or twisted to give the precise amount of insulin required at a time. The needles attached to the end of the pens are very tiny and therefore the shots are not painful at all. For others, the insulin is delivered into the body through an INSULIN PUMP which delivers the insulin through a small needle inserted under the skin. Sometimes people with Diabetes Type 2 may start insulin earlier on in the course of their illness because they are not well controlled by oral medications or pills. One's doctor will talk about what medicines are needed to give one good control of one's diabetes. Remember that good control leads to fewer complications associated with the disease.

Non Insulin Injectables Used to Treat Diabetes

The array of medications used to treat Diabetes mellitus are changing very rapidly, and new medications are being developed to help give better control of the disease. New medications which are non-insulin injections have also been introduced, and these are sometimes given as once a day or once a week injections that can be used with oral medications to treat the disease. Some are even combined with insulin. Make sure one asks their doctor about what other options are available. These act in totally different ways from insulin.

1. Some called GLP-1 Agonists act by stimulating insulin production, decrease appetite, and cause less glucose production by the liver. They are either daily or weekly. Examples of these injectables are Liraglutide (Victoza), Exenatide (Byrudeon), Dulaglutide (Trilucity), and Exenatide (Byetta)
2. There is another injectable called Pramlintide (Symlin), which is from a different group called Amylin Analogue and is used with insulin at mealtimes. It slows down food movement, decreases glucose production by the liver, and suppresses one's appetite and weight. (American Diabetes Association www.diabetes.org)

Reminders on Your Radar

Diabetes management involves the patient and the team of medical staff to maintain good control of blood sugar, since there are many complications. It may affect many organs like the heart, eyes, kidneys, nerves, circulation, feet, and sexual organs. Optimal blood sugar control will prevent many of these complications, and this can be achieved by taking medications as prescribed, eating a healthy diet, exercise and weight loss if obese. Regular eye and feet examinations are important. Most people with diabetes if they live long enough may eventually end up on insulin to control blood sugar. Being on insulin is not a sign of failure, and insulin does not cause death in people with diabetes. It is either excess or lack of insulin which may cause coma and death and so the right amount is needed to bring sugar levels down to optimal levels. Proper use of insulin rather prolongs life in most patients. Many oral and injectable medicines have been shown to decrease not only blood sugar but blood pressure weight and prevent death from cardiovascular disease.

Thyroid Diseases
(Reference: medscape.com)

....

The Thyroid Gland

There is a small gland or structure in front of the neck just below the "Adam's Apple" area called the THYROID GLAND. The thyroid is part of the endocrine system and it has two lobes with a bridge between them called the Isthmus, giving it a butterfly or bowtie shape. The thyroid gland plays a very important role in metabolism and functions of the body. Metabolism is the chemical processes which occur in the body's cells in order to maintain the different activities which keep you alive, e.g. like beating of one's heart, breathing, and brain functions.

> **The thyroid gland is the organ that secretes hormones that control the body's metabolism, and it is often referred to as the "conductor of the opera" or the engine controlling a car.**
> —Barbara Entsuah

Thyroid Hormones

The gland produces thyroid hormones called T4 (Thyroxine) & T3 (Triiodothyronine) after receiving instructions from the brain. Iodine is an important component of these hormones. The thyroid gland has sometimes been referred to as the "conductor of the opera" because the hormones it produces affect so many organs like,

1. Heart
2. Gut or intestines
3. Kidneys
4. Skin
5. Female reproductive systems (affects fertility, menses, and puberty)
6. Brain maturation and function including mood and memory
7. Affects cholesterol, and other body fats
8. Glucose production and break down by insulin in the body

There are two broad diseases associated with the thyroid gland that can affect both women and men and these are HYPOTHYROIDISM and HYPERTHYROIDISM. There are also many types of these two conditions but the general effects of the conditions will be discussed.

The Thyroid Gland

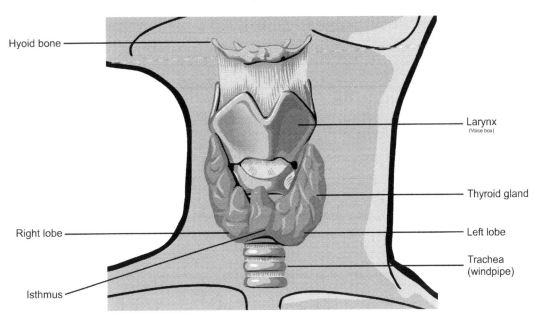

Hyoid bone

Larynx
(Voice box)

Thyroid gland

Right lobe

Left lobe

Trachea
(windpipe)

Isthmus

Hypothyroidism
What is it?

This is when the gland is underactive or sluggish and is not producing enough of the hormones to be used by the cells. It affects mostly women or those in their middle age, however Hypothyroid can affect all ages and sexes and there is even a congenital form in which newborns or infants are affected. In developed countries, newborns are routinely tested for Congenital Hypothyroid. Why the gland is sluggish and not producing thyroid hormones is due to many factors.

Causes of Hypothyroidism

1. In countries like the US, Hypothyroid is mostly due to an autoimmune condition called Hashimoto's disease, when the body produces antibodies to fight the thyroid gland because the body perceives the thyroid gland as foreign, and so wants to get rid of it. Hashimoto's disease will be discussed in detail below

2. In other parts of the world, it is mostly due to deficiency of Iodine, which is used to produce T4 and T3, resulting in a Goiter and Hypothyroid

3. After surgery to remove all or part of the thyroid gland

4. Following treatment of someone who previously had Hyperthyroid and had gland removed by surgery or destroyed by radioactive iodine

5. Certain medicines (e.g. Lithium and Amiodarone)

6. Radiation treatment to the neck and chest area for cancer treatment

7. Congenital (one is born with the disease at birth)

8. Viral infections may also affect the gland leading to destruction of cells and resultant hypothyroid

Hashimoto's Disease (Autoimmune thyroiditis, Chronic lymphocyte thyroiditis)
What is it?

This is also called Hashimoto's thyroiditis, and it is an autoimmune disease affecting the thyroid gland. There is production of antibodies or immune cells against the thyroid cells by the body, resulting in inflammation of the thyroid gland, and its gradual destruction. It's the most common thyroid disorder in America and about 14 million people are affected, with women being affected seven times more than men. The thyroid may become enlarged (Goiter) and inflamed and early on in the disease the enlarged gland produces more thyroid hormones and may initially present with symptoms of HYPERTHYROIDISM described below. However, as more cells are destroyed, the blood tests will give a picture of HYPOTHYROIDISM which is what most patients end up with or present with.

Signs and Symptoms of Hypothyroidism

Hypothyroid may present with one or several of these symptoms and if one feels a number of these for a while, without any improvement, it may be a good idea to ask one's health care provider to do blood work to check one's thyroid hormones. Some of the symptoms hypothyroid may present with include:

1. Feeling cold when everyone is fine or even warm
2. Slow heart rate
3. Weight gain
4. Hair falling out, dry hair, and skin
5. Feeling fatigue, sluggish, slow, or forgetful
6. Feeling depressed
7. Irregular heavy periods or no periods
8. Deep voice
9. Swelling of the thyroid gland (Goiter)
10. Pain where the gland is located
11. Lethargy

Tests and Examination

Important information one's doctor should know include one's past medical history (e.g. radiation to one's neck and chest), medications one takes or has taken, and even one's family history because thyroid problems can run in families. All these help her know what tests to order after one's physical examination.

Tests to check one's thyroid hormone and other chemicals to see if one suffers from this condition will be ordered. The main blood work done are called TSH and Free T4, but others may also be done. If needed, one may also be ordered to have a thyroid gland ultrasound to look at the gland. If found to have abnormal test results, which confirm a diagnosis of Hypothyroid, one will be treated. Non treatment of hypothyroid can cause complications as noted below:

Treatment

One will be given a form of the thyroid hormone THYROXINE to replace what one's gland is not producing. The regular thyroid hormone replacement is Levothyroxine, but there are brand and generic forms as mentioned below. It is important to take the same generic form or brand name that has been prescribed. Using different generics may affect the levels in the blood and may cause the medicine not to be very effective.

Examples of replacement medicines are:

Levothyroxine: Brand names are: Synthroid, Levoxyl, Levoxine, Levothroid, Tirosint, and Unithroid

Desiccated (dried) natural thyroid hormone: from pork called ARMOUR THYROID or Nature-Thyroid, which contains both T4 and T3. Some endocrinologists do not recommend Armour thyroid because it may effect bone health and may cause irregular heartbeat; besides the ratio between the two (T4 and T3) may vary from batch to batch during production

Pure T3 Liothyronine: Examples are Cytomel, or Triostat may be combined with T4 to treat hypothyroidism when patients complain they are not feeling better on just T4. Now T3 is the more active form of thyroid hormone and is what affects metabolism. In the cells of the body, T4 is converted to T3

After treatment of Hypothyroid with thyroid replacement medicines, it is very remarkable to see the change in patients once the thyroid hormone is replaced. Some say they feel like a new person and describe increased energy, clearer thinking, a sense of well-being, and even weight loss. Abnormal periods or irregular menses may normalize and hair will grow normally.

Medications That Interfere With Thyroid Medicine

Some medications taken at the same time as Levothyroxine may impair its absorption from the stomach causing lower levels in the blood. These medications include:

Calcium and Iron supplements
Medicines used for acid reflux like Omeprazole, Pantoprazole, and Esomeprazole

Cholesterol medicines known as statins—Simvastatin and Atorvastatin, Female hormone called Estrogen

When to Take One's Thyroid Medicine

Thyroid replacement medication must be taken first thing in the morning on an empty stomach. One has to wait at least 30 minutes before eating or taking any other medications. This is very important in order to get the maximum benefit from the medicine. They can also be taken at other times as long as one has not eaten for at least 3–4 hours. To avoid missing doses, one must make it a habit to take the medicine at the same time each day or set a reminder on one's phone.

Complications of Hypothyroidism

If untreated or undertreated, hypothyroid may lead to complications of weight gain, heart disease, joint pains, enlarged thyroid gland, depression, high Lipids and in very severe cases coma or loss of consciousness.

Hyperthyroidism
What is it?

This is when there is overproduction of the thyroid hormone by the gland. Very rarely, the excess thyroid hormone may be produced from a tumor that contains thyroid tissue in the ovaries. In hyperthyroidism, the gland becomes hyperactive and there is excess amount of thyroxine circulating in the blood stream. Several causes are known, however it is mainly a result of an autoimmune condition of the body producing antibodies that stimulate the thyroid gland to grow and produce more thyroid hormone. This antibody is called "Thyroid Stimulating Immunoglobulin" and the condition is called Grave's Disease. The thyroid hormones circulate in the blood producing the symptoms mentioned below.

Signs and Symptoms

Some of them will include:

1. Feeling hot when everyone is fine or cold
2. Rapid heart rate, palpitations, or irregular heart beats
3. Weight loss, fatigue
4. Inability to sleep (insomnia)
5. Bulging of the eyes
6. Increased sweating/perspiration
7. Irregular or lighter menses

8. Anxiety
9. Trembling or shaking of hands

Treatment of Hyperthyroidism

Once the appropriate tests are done and the diagnosis is confirmed, it can be treated by:

Medicines
Surgery
Radiation to the gland using a nuclear containing oral iodine pill.

After some forms of treatment like the nuclear therapy, a patient may end up becoming HYPOTHYROID (low thyroid state) because most of the hormone producing cells have been destroyed, and so may need to be on thyroid replacement medication (Levothyroxine).

Goiter

What is it?

This is the swelling of the thyroid gland at the front of the neck. Sometimes, the enlarged gland may be smooth and is known as a Diffuse Goiter, while at other times, it may consist of multiple lumps and nodules and is then known as a Multinodular Goiter.

It can be a result of:

Deficiency of iodine
Hypothyroidism (underactive or sluggish)
Hyperthyroidism (hyperactive or overactive)
Cancer of the thyroid gland
Eating large amount of foods that block the absorption of iodine like Pearl Millet

Signs and Symptoms

It can present as a swelling, which may or may not be painful
It may compress structures behind it, causing difficulty in swallowing
Hoarseness due to the vocal cords being compressed
If large enough, it can be obvious at the front of the neck making it unsightly
Depending on whether the goiter is associated with hypothyroidism or hyperthyroidism, the other symptoms associated with them and described previously (see above) may occur

Treatment

An ultrasound of the thyroid is needed to make the diagnosis and also show if there are any discrete lumps or masses called nodules within the swollen gland. One may need to have a biopsy of the thyroid gland as well as blood work, and then the doctor will decide what the best course of action to take. This may be medical or surgical depending on the cause.

1. If it is a result of hypo or hyperthyroidism, the size of the goiter will decrease with treatment
2. The size of goiters which have normal thyroid blood work may be reduced by giving Levothyroxine
3. Due to the unattractive cosmetic effects of a large swelling, surgery is often performed to remove it, especially if it is compressing structures in the neck and affecting swallowing. After surgery, as a result of the removal of the gland, one may have to go on thyroid hormone replacement medicine to supplement lower amounts that the body is producing
4. In cases were only part of the thyroid gland is removed, some patients may not need thyroid hormone replacement, if the remaining thyroid gland is able to produce sufficient amounts of hormones to meet the body's needs
5. Cancer of thyroid with a goiter is treated with surgery and radioactive iodine which destroys the gland. Replacement with thyroid hormone is needed after that

Reminders on Your Radar

The thyroid gland produces two important hormones needed for various metabolic and growth processes by the body. Two main thyroid conditions are HYPO-thyroid and HYPERthyroid; low and high levels of thyroid hormones respectively. In hypothyroidism one has to replace the hormone(s) through medications that have to be taken daily, and it may have to be taken for life. Hyperthyroidism treatment may involve medications, nuclear iodine treatment or surgery, after which one may have to be on thyroid replacement medicine(s). Iodine is very important in thyroid hormone production and table salt is usually iodized to give people a ready source. If one prefers other sources of salt, make sure they contain enough iodine. Worldwide many individuals suffer from iodine deficiency which results in a goiter or swelling of thyroid gland in front of the neck.

Obesity (Adipose Based Chronic Disease)
What is It?

This is a condition caused by excessive amount of body fat and its storage; leading to increase in weight. Traditionally, it has been defined as weight of at least 20% above one's ideal body weight for height, age and sex/gender. It is also defined as a Body Mass Index (BMI) of 30 and above. It has a negative effect on the individual's health, and may result in physical, emotional, psychological and social difficulties for the person.

"Obesity is a worldwide problem, and in the US more than 30% of the adult population is obese (72 million); and worldwide it's estimated that 1.5 billion adults are overweight, and 500 million are obese"

(WHO estimates 2008).

Body Mass Index

To determine obesity, a scale or measurement called BODY MASS INDEX (BMI) is used. This is calculated from the ratio between weight and height (body mass divided by the square of the height). Mass/ht^2 kg/m^2 or; if in pounds: lbs/in^2 x 703. BMI is more accurate than weight alone, however, it has the disadvantage of not taking body fat percentage into account and so some people do not think it's a good measure of obesity. Depending on BMI, weight is classified as:

Underweight
Normal
Overweight
Obese
Morbid obese (extremely obese)

Prevalence of Obesity

Obesity or excess body weight is a worldwide disease and since it's a chronic disease, it has recently been given a new name: **Adipose Based Chronic Disease (ABCD).** Individuals from both resource rich and resource poor countries have problems with obesity. In the US more than 39.8% of the adult population is obese (93.3 million) (CDC health statistics 2015–2016) and worldwide it's estimated that 1.5 billion adults are overweight, and 500 million are obese (WHO estimates 2008-WHO obesity and overweight: Fact sheet 311 Updated march 2011). The definition of who is overweight or obese is by use of BMI which is explained below.

CAUSES:
The etiology or causes of obesity are multifactorial. Weight is determined by:
Genetics (genes one inherits from one's parents which control body weight)

Environment (one's surroundings like access to food/drinks, parks, open spaces)
Habits and attitudes regarding food
Sedentary lifestyle

One cannot change the genes one inherits, however everyone can influence their environment, behavior and habits.

How Energy Translates to Weight

Normally, one uses part of the energy which is released from the breakdown of fats, protein and carbohydrates to fuel the various processes that take place in their bodies (metabolism); for example the work of breathing, digestion, and functioning of other systems. Whatever energy is left over is stored as fat, unless it is used for other activities like exercise. On the other hand, if one's energy use is increased by extra activities like exercise, running, walking, aerobics etc. then stored energy in the form of fat is broken down and this leads to weight loss.

How Socialization Affects Food Intake

We live in societies where socialization is done around food, and unlike our forefathers, food is not only eaten to give energy and for survival, but it is used for many other reasons. One sometimes eats when one is bored, happy, sad, depressed and the list goes on. Sometimes it is hard to say "No" to food, and so one may increase intake of food, not because one is hungry but maybe because it is present and others are eating it. This leads to increased energy intake and the excess amount is stored as fat.

Obesity and Associated Diseases and Conditions

It is important to try and achieve a healthy weight, and then maintain it because being overweight or obese is associated with many diseases. These include:

Type 2 Diabetes mellitus, Impaired blood sugar, prediabetes
Heart disease, hypertension (high blood pressure), heart failure, hyperlipidemia
Gallstones and fatty liver
Breathing problems including asthma and obstructive sleep apnea
Swelling of the feet, joint pains or arthritis
Depression, low self esteem, social isolation

Relationship Between Obesity and Cancer

Through large clinical studies, there is evidence that higher body fat is associated with at least nine types of cancers. These include:

Female organs: Uterus, breast, endometrium
Digestive organs: Stomach, liver, pancreas, colon and rectum
Kidney
Blood cells: Multiple myeloma
Brain cancer: meningioma

Weight Classification Based on Body Mass Index

BMI	WEIGHT CLASSIFICATION
<18.5	Underweight
18.5–24.9	Normal weight
25–29.9	Overweight
30–39.9	Obese
>40	Morbid Obesity

It has been studied and documented that weight loss from exercise and healthy eating, use of pharmacological drugs and Bariatric (stomach reduction) surgery can lead to reversal or improvement of medical conditions like:

Hypertension, Diabetes mellitus, high cholesterol, Metabolic syndrome and minimize pain in joints from arthritis and low back pain. Others include sexual problems, Obstructive sleep apnea, and even irregular heart beat known as Atrial Fibrillation (Afib). The effects on heart structure leads to Afib.

Central Obesity
What is it?

This represents visceral fat, or fat in the internal organs instead of just under the skin or in the subcutaneous layer. It is a measure of one's cardiovascular disease (CVD) risk, and the larger the central obesity the higher the risk of CVD.

It is measured by:

1. Waist circumference: For men greater than 102cm (40") and for women greater than 88cm (35") puts one at increased risk
2. Waist/hip ratio: Ratio of the circumference of the waist to that of the hips (W/H); Men – greater than 0.95; and Women – greater than 0.8 means increased risk
3. The shape of the body or area where the fat is deposited – People with pear shape bodies, where the fat is more in the hip area below the waist line have less risk of heart disease, diabetes, and metabolic syndrome compared to those who are apple

shaped – where the fat is located in the abdominal or central section of the body above the waist line

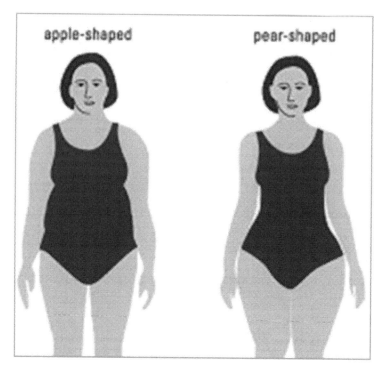

https://www.womenshealth.gov/healthy-weight/weight-and-obesity

Sugary Drinks and Obesity
How bad are they?

According to the American Heart Association, sugary drinks and beverages are linked to:

1. Obesity, diabetes, high triglycerides, heart disease and hypertension
2. They have a lot of "empty calories" meaning they contain hardly any vitamins, minerals and proteins
3. For example, one 12 ounces (12 oz.) can of most beverages/sodas e.g. Coca Cola or Pepsi contains about 10 teaspoons of sugar, and one teaspoon is equivalent to about 4 grams of sugar. If converted to energy one gram of sugar is equivalent to about 4 Calories (Cals). So it contains a total of 160 Cals from sugar
4. The 20 oz. size has about 65 gm of sugar or 260 calories. If one considers that if one drinks one can of soda a day that means an additional 140 calories every day. In a year, that will be 365 days multiplied by 140 equals 51,100 calories each year. Since there's 3500 calories per pound, that one soda per day adds 14.6 pounds per year

5. Not all drinks with "juice" written on the bottle are pure juices. One has to look out for drinks that say "fruit drink". These have added sugar mostly in the form of high fructose corn syrup in them

6. Even pure juices like orange or apple juice have to be in moderation since 8 oz. of orange juice contains about 24gm of sugar and 96 calories

7. Unfortunately, drinking these sugary drinks become a habit and stopping them becomes more difficult with time. One has to adopt drinking water with ice, and some lemon or with a little bit of juice mixed with it, or a "drink enhancer" drops to give it flavor

8. When one eats out, to cut down on further caloric intake, order water with ice and lemon instead of a soda/pop or soft drink which could add about 160 calories a glass to one's total intake

9. Drinking soda once in a while should be the norm rather than drinking it daily or regularly. Maybe once a week or so

Challenges to Maintaining a Healthy Weight

To combat overweight, or obesity and its complications, one has to have a renewal of mind with regards to food and this is called BEHAVIORAL CHANGE. How one regards food and what one uses it for have been embedded in their minds or psyche and may not be conducive to maintaining a healthy lifestyle. Examples include eating when bored or stressed, eating to socialize, eating while watching sports on TV and many others that one does even unconsciously.

Behavioral Changes Needed to Maintain a Healthy Weight

Some problems which may lead to unhealthy eating and some helpful solutions will be discussed.

1. PROBLEM: DEALING WITH STRESS IN ONE'S LIFE
   Chronic stress leads to chronic elevation of stress hormones, mainly Cortisol, in one's body. This, over a long time, can contribute to chronic diseases like obesity, diabetes, hypertension, stroke and even heart attacks. Cortisol leads to deposition of fat especially in the abdominal area. Along with stress, one then goes on and eats high caloric foods like sugary foods or junk food to "de stress" or reduce one's stress level
   SOLUTION: HEALTHIER COPING SKILLS
   To reverse this, one has to learn to deal with stress by using other healthier coping skills. These may include calling a friend on the phone to talk to, going for a walk, doing some gardening, doing deep breathing exercises, watching a funny movie on a DVD, having sex, and doing meditation and prayer. These are a few ways to deal with stress instead of eating and gaining weight.

Therapy with a psychologist may be helpful, to help one use better coping skills to manage problems

2. PROBLEM: LACK OF SLEEP

    Sleeping fewer number of hours (quantity) and poorly e.g. restless, frequent waking up (quality) have both been attributed to weight gain in studies that have been done. This is due to alternated energy balance and increase in some hormones that regulate weight according to studies done in Holland by Dr. Femke Rutters and associates (Oct. 2015)

    SOLUTION: IMPROVE SLEEP

    One can try the suggestions under the topic "Insomnia" in the chapter "Brain Problems". One may need a sleep study to find out if Obstructive sleep apnea of leg movement are the problem

3. PROBLEM: FREQUENT CONSUMPTION OF JUNK AND FAST FOODS

    It is a challenge for many individuals to eat healthy due to the increased advertising of junk or fast foods, and cheap and readily available foods or sweetened drinks and beverages. These foods often contain what is termed "empty calories". This is a term used to describe food and drinks containing a lot of added sugar and solid fats which contribute high calories but not much of other nutrients or vitamins. They make one gain excess weight especially if exercise is not part of one's regular lifestyle. All around the world, in both prosperous and resource poor nations, the rate of obesity and chronic diseases related to obesity have been steadily rising over the last 20 to 30 years in both children and adults. For example, a country like India was formerly known for its slim or healthy weight individuals; however, with the arrival of fast foods and western style foods like hamburgers, French fries, and fried chicken, obesity has increased and even kids are getting gastric bypass surgery.

    SOLUTION: LIFESTYLE CHANGES

    These are deliberate and permanent or ongoing changes one makes in order to stay healthy. They include healthy eating and exercising regularly. Lifestyle changes help us maintain a good weight or even lose weight, and should always accompany any weight loss method, be it special diet, medication or surgery. These changes are not easy because the "bad" habits have been going on for years, but determination and taking things one day at a time helps. Dietary counseling from a dietitian/nutritionist may be helpful.

Tips On Healthy Eating and Drinking

There are some simple ways in which we can increase our consumption of healthy foods and drinks, and decrease amounts of the not too healthy drinks and foods. These include:

1. Drink more water – it fills one up and lets one feel less hungry
2. Drink flavored water instead of sweetened beverages. Add fruit juice
3. Limit sweetened beverages – these make up a lot of empty calories
4. Limit pure juices to no more than 4oz a day. These including pure or unsweetened apple or orange juice which can add on calories if drunk in large amounts
5. Eating the whole fruit is even better since it would give one both the juice and the fiber it contains. The presence of fiber slows down the rapid absorption of sugar from the fruit
6. Use a tall thin glass instead of short wide one. It will make you drink less
7. Limit white carbohydrates. These include white rice, white flour, white sugar, white bread and pasta. These have been refined, and complex carbohydrates or fibers have been removed. Use their non refined equivalent
8. Limit other simple carbohydrates like table sugar, high fructose corn syrup, candy, cakes, soda/pop and some packaged cereals which are sweetened
9. Bread is enjoyed by most people and eating whole wheat bread slows the rise in glucose due to the higher fiber content. One should eat it toward the end of the meal and then the blood sugar spike is lower, making one feel fuller for a longer time. One still needs to limit amount of bread

Eating and Cooking Tips

1. Chew food slowly so it takes a long time to finish eating
2. Use a smaller plate or bowl so the total amount of food is reduced
3. Add vegetables to one's meals, filling most of the plate with vegetables
4. Limit frying, instead try baking, sauteing, grilling, stir frying, broiling or boiling
5. Eat more home cooked meals. There is a lot of hidden fat and carbohydrates in restaurant meals and one also saves money by cooking and eating at home
6. If one eats out, and the food portions are large, do a take away box to eat later at home
7. If portion sizes are large at a restaurant then one can share a serving with a spouse or companion
8. Eat proteins and vegetables first, or the bread can be eaten with the vegetables if possible
9. Eat more fish and chicken and limit the amount of red meat (beef, pork, lamb, goat or mutton)
10. Remove skin and fatty portions off meat and chicken before cooking. Skin tends to have fat stored under it
11. Increase fiber in one's diet. (See detailed discussion of fiber below)

4. PROBLEM: BEHAVIOR AND ATTITUDE TOWARD FOOD

One's behavior and how one regards the role of food determines their intake of food. Certain practices which one grows up with or have been accepted as the norm in societies across the world determine some of their attitudes toward food. These include:

1. "Cleaning up one's plate" and not leaving any food on it or it will be "wasted". So even when an individual is full up, one will try and finish the food on one's plate
2. One uses food as a reward for children and adults alike
3. When one is stressed, one may eat more sugary and fatty foods like desserts, chocolates as a means of "de-stressing". These are known as comfort foods, and studies have confirmed one tends to eat these when stressed
4. One will go straight to the fridge and look for something to eat when one is bored

SOLUTION: CHANGE OF BEHAVIOR TOWARD FOOD

These attitudes and behavior toward food would need to change and one consciously has to make an effort not to let food rule one's lives. One should not always use food as reward, and should try to have less "comfort" foods around the house. If full, the rest of the meal can be put away for a later date and there is no need to force kids to finish their food if they are full. Smaller portion sizes should be served.

5. PROBLEM: LACK OF EXERCISE

Exercise plays an important role in maintaining a healthy weight or losing weight. Excessive amounts of food intake which is not balanced with excessive output or energy spent through exercise will lead to excess stores of energy as fat. Healthy eating coupled with exercise as a lifestyle will help avert this.

SOLUTION: GET INVOLVED IN SOME TYPE OF EXERCISE

All exercises can help with weight loss if done adequately enough. Simple Exercises and activities which will make one lose calories and lose 10 pounds in a year without dieting by burning an extra 100 calories every day include the following activities:

Walk 1 mile for about 20 minutes
Pull weeds or plant flowers in the garden for 20 minutes
Mow the lawn with a push mower for 20 minutes
Clean house for 30 minutes

Jog for 10 minutes

Use stairs instead of the elevator/lift

Park one's car a little further from one's destination and walk

Walk to pick up something in the room instead of asking one's kids to bring it to them

Walking about 10,000 steps a day is equivalent to a distance of about 4 to 5 miles

Put on some music and dance to it at home

To MAINTAIN weight, one has to do about 30 minutes of moderate level exercise daily. This is important for those who have lost weight through medicines, surgery etc. If one does not exercise weight lost can be regained because with loss of muscle one's basic metabolic rate goes down and one does not burn as much energy; and energy not used is stored.

Foods or Other Substances Which Are Important in Obesity

....

The Importance of Fiber

What is it?

Fiber is a carbohydrate found in plants mainly fruits, vegetables and whole grains and is also known as roughage or bulk. Part of it is not absorbed by the body during digestion and so produces bulk and helps stool move through the intestines to be eliminated.

The other advantages of fiber are:

1. Plays a role in weight loss because it helps one feel full, sending messages from the stomach to brain to make one stop eating, and so less calories are consumed

2. Affects sugar levels in the body by slowing the rapid absorption of glucose from the intestines into the blood due to its role of thickening food. This causes less insulin to be released to push glucose into cells, and so less fat and less weight gain

3. Fiber, especially soluble type lowers cholesterol levels by reducing amount of bile acids (made from cholesterol) reabsorbed from the intestine. It reduces the LDL (lousy/bad cholesterol)

4. It causes one to have regular bowel movements as it helps stool move through the intestines

5. It helps prevent conditions and diseases like constipation, diverticulitis (inflammation and infection of pockets in the large bowel wall), hemorrhoids and colon cancer

Types of Fiber

There are 2 types of fiber, insoluble and soluble fiber and both play an important role in our digestive system and other ways mentioned above.

Insoluble Fiber

What is it?

Found in leafy vegetables, skins of fruits and vegetables, bran of corn and wheat, beans and roots or tubers like yams, cassava or yucca.

How it Works

It is not absorbed but passes through the intestine, drawing water into the bowels and thus helps stool move through the gut swiftly, promoting regularity and preventing constipation and other conditions mentioned above. It also helps the bowel maintain certain acidity (pH) such that some types of bacteria or organisms will not flourish and encourage production of particular cells which may become cancer cells later on.

Soluble Fiber

What is it?

This is found in oats, peas, beans, berries, seeds, mangos, apples, sweet potatoes, pears, plums, flax seeds, dried beans, brown rice, barley, and lentils.

How it Works

Unlike insoluble fiber which cannot be digested, soluble fiber absorbs water and mixes with food, forming a gel which is then digested slowly, prolonging the digestive process and causing a sense of fullness in the stomach and so one does not get hungry quickly. It also causes slower absorption of carbohydrates and glucose into the body and so rise in blood sugar occurs slowly.

Bottom Line

Eat more plant foods which are high in fiber and they will fill one up quickly. Apart from fiber, these foods are rich in vitamins and minerals and these are important for one's body's energy production.

Rice

Rice is a popular staple grain eaten by more than 50% of the world population, so we will discuss it in a bit more detail.

1. Eat whole grain or "brown" rice instead of regular polished white rice. It is healthier than white rice as it has bran which is full of fiber, minerals vitamins and antioxidants
2. Brown rice requires more cooking time and more water, and it needs to be "doctored" with a little coconut or olive oil, seasoning like seasoned salt, garlic, onion etc. to make it more palatable
3. Different types of polished rice have different starch content. Long grain rice has a lower starch content and when any type of oil is added to rice during cooking, the oil converts the starch present into a resistant starch which is absorbed slowly
4. Adding other ingredients to rice like beans, lentils, quinoa, spinach, sesame seeds etc. slow absorption of the starches and lowers rice's Glycemic Index
5. Chilling rice after cooking with oil helps with conversion to resistant starches
6. Wild rice is not actually rice but is made up of grain from grasses which resemble rice. It is higher in fiber and protein and so it is more nutritious
7. Black rice has higher amounts of nutrients, proteins, antioxidants and fiber than brown or white rice. It is supposed to lower bad cholesterol and help prevent heart disease per researchers. It is eaten mostly in Asia and is also known as "Forbidden rice" or purple rice and turns a deep purple when cooked because it contains anthocyanins which are same phytochemicals found in blueberries

Vegetables (Veggies)

Vegetables are good for providing needed vitamins, nutrients and fiber as well as "filling up the stomach" and helping one feel full and so would not continue eating. It is good to add vegetables to every meal if possible, especially to lunch and dinner. Some of them are low in calories and carbohydrates while others are higher.

LOW CALORIE VEGGIES: Generally green leafy veggies like spinach, collard green, kale, broccoli, watercress, red veggies like raw tomatoes, red onion, red cabbage, and white vegetables like garlic, turnips, mushrooms, onions, scallions are low in calories. Others low in calories include celery, avocado, asparagus, okra, cucumbers, green or wax beans, peppers, bamboo shoots, zucchini, Brussels sprouts, herbs, snow peas, snap peas, eggplant, tomatillos, pumpkins, and spaghetti squash

HIGH CALORIE VEGGIES: These are usually starchy and high in carbohydrates and include: beets, peas, butternut squash, parsnips, potatoes, sweet potatoes, corn, plantains and carrots. Remember it is the amount per serving that counts, so portion size is important

Grains and Seeds

There are "new" grains that are being used more by health conscious individuals instead of white rice and some of these are also quite high in protein and fiber. Some are actually seeds and have been used in other countries for generations. Examples are:

Bulgur: It's made from wheat kernels, dried and cracked. It's low in calories and high in fiber

Quinoa: This is actually a seed and its gluten free. It is high in fiber and protein

Farro: This is an ancient grain which is a type of wheat

Couscous: Mediterranean grain which is low in fiber but has moderate amounts of protein

Freekeh: Is also called Farik and is made from green durum wheat which is roasted

Buckwheat: Is a seed and not wheat grain. It is gluten free. It is used to make flour and noodles

Millet: It is a grass seed with many varieties, high in minerals and vitamins and originally from Africa. However, some species e.g. Pearl millet blocks the absorption of iodine and high consumption may lead to goiter in those who consume low levels of iodine in their diet

Fatty Acids

One may have heard a lot about Fatty Acids – some being good and others bad. Fats are needed by our bodies for many functions which will be discussed under the individual types.

There are 3 important ones one should know about and these are

1. Saturated fatty acids
2. Unsaturated (monounsaturated and polyunsaturated) fatty acids
3. Trans fatty acids (Trans fat or trans-unsaturated fatty acids)

Almost all natural sources of fat are a mixture of saturated, unsaturated (mono and polyunsaturated) fats, but the ratios differ. For example fat in chicken has a higher ratio of unsaturated fats compared to beef which has about 50%. All vegetable oils contain a combination of saturated, monounsaturated and polyunsaturated fatty acids. In order to preserve and prolong the shelf life of these oils in foods, they have been partially hydrogenated by the food industry making them semi solid at room temperature. For example, hydrogenated soybean oil is used to produce margarine and shortening for baking and frying.

Saturated Fatty Acids

Saturated Fatty Acids are fat molecules without any double bonds between the carbon atoms and are unable to accommodate any more hydrogen atoms. They are usually solid at room temperature. Most saturated fats and are found in products like dairy products (whole milk, cream cheese, cheese, butter) and animal products – meats (pork, lamb, beef chicken with skin); but they are also high in some plants like coconut oil, palm oil and palm kernel oils. Fats of most other plants and fish are high in unsaturated fats. Although saturated fats increase LDL, it has been shown in studies that they increase the particle size of LDL, and the larger sized LDL particles do not increase risk for heart disease. It has also been found that "not all saturated fats are created equal" For example:

  Coconut oil contains lauric acid which raises LDL cholesterol as well as HDL, and raises LDL more than, palm oil does.

  Meats contain Palmitic acid and butter Myristic acid and both raise LDL substantially

  Chocolate contains stearic acid which does not raise LDL

  Saturated fats had been thought to be worse than Trans fatty acids in the past; however, recent studies show they are better than Trans fats which were used to replace them in foods in the past

Unsaturated Fatty Acids (monounsaturated-MUFA and polyunsaturated – PUFA)

Polyunsaturated Fatty Acids

The major classes of PUFA are Omega 3 and Omega 6 found in both plants and animals. They are called "essential fatty acids because they cannot be produced by the body and have to be taken in the diet or as supplements.
  There are 3 main types of Omega 3 and these are:

1. Alpha linolenic acid (ALA): Found in nuts, seeds, and plants oils for example, chia, flaxseed, walnuts, rapeseed, soybean, canola oil, sunflower, and flaxseed oil. It is an essential Fatty acid (means cannot be produced by the body)

and is obtained in the diet. A small amount of ALA can be converted to EPA and DHA in the body

2. Eicosapentaenoic acid (EPA) and (Docosahexaenoic acid (DHA): These are animal Omega 3s and are found mainly in fish like salmon, sardine, tuna, trout, mackerel, sardines and herring, krill oil, foods fortified with omega 3 like eggs, juices, milk, infant formulas and Omega 3 dietary supplements. Farm raised fish have higher levels of mercury or PCBs and other toxins, and some fish like king mackerel, tuna and shark tend to have higher levels because they are bigger, live longer and are up on the food chain. All this is due to polluted water. Pregnant and nursing mothers should avoid these

3. Omega 3 dietary supplements include fish oil, krill oil, algal oil and cod liver oil, however the latter contains Vitamin A, of which excessive amounts can lead to toxicity

Benefits of Omega 3

Omega 3 fatty acids especially DHA are found in high amounts in cells of the brain, retina (eye) and sperms. They, like other fatty acids, provide energy for the body. Some studies show that Omega 3 mostly from food sources do the following:

Lower triglycerides
Help protect the heart from cardiovascular diseases
Lower risk of breast and colon cancer
Help with a baby's brain and vision development
Lower risk of developing macular degeneration
Lower risk of Alzheimer's disease
Some people think it may help with ADHD symptoms, but more studies are needed
Help with joint stiffness and pain
Lower risk of depression and boost the effects of antidepressants
Lowers inflammation in asthma

Studies on Effect of Omega 3 on Patients at Risk for CV Events

A recent multinational four years study showed that giving high doses of Omega 3 EPA (4grams) to patients who were at high risk of a cardiovascular (CV) event, or high risk diabetics with raised triglyceride levels had risk reduction of a CV event (e.g. stroke, heart attack, angina) compared to patients on a placebo (sugar pill). Everyone was already taking statins like Atorvastatin (REDUCE-IT: 25% Reduction in MACE with high dose EPA-Medscape-Sept. 25, 2018).

MACE – Major adverse cardiovascular event

Omega 6

The 2 main types of omega 6 are Linoleic acid and Arachidonic acid. Linoleic acid is an essential fatty acid and so has to be derived from the diet. The oils, nuts and seeds with high omega 6 are Safflower, Grape Seed Oil, Sunflower Oil, Corn Oil, Cottonseed, Wheat Germ Oil, Soybean Oil and their seeds. If eaten in moderation and used to replace saturated fats (which we get mostly from animal fats), they can help one's heart. It is believed that getting more Omega 3 compared to Omega 6 is better since Omega 6 may result in inflammation if levels are too high.

MONOUNSATURATED FATS – MUFA (e.g. oleic acid)

These are found mostly in plant oils like olive oil, hazel nut, macadamia nuts, almonds, canola oil, sesame oil, peanut oil, avocado, nuts and seeds. They help lower bad cholesterol, and reduce risk of heart attacks and strokes. Olive oil is an important part of the Mediterranean diet and is high in monounsaturated fats.

Trans Fatty Acids (Trans Fat)

What are These?

These are mainly produced by adding hydrogen to polysaturated fatty acids and are made from vegetable oils, but some are found naturally in dairy products, beef and pork fat. They were thought to be better than saturated fats because they were from vegetable oils, but lately have been found to be worse than saturated fats for cardiovascular health.

They are in solid forms at room temperature, and do not become rancid so give foods a longer shelf life. They however increase total cholesterol and LDL, but also lower HDL (good cholesterol) and interfere with how the body uses Omega 3.

Industry produced Trans fat products include stick margarine and shortening like Crisco. One tablespoon of stick margarine may contain 2.1gm of trans fat and same amount of butter will have 0.5gm. Trans fatty acids are often present in baked goods like doughnuts, cakes, cookies, chips and crackers. The margarine stick which is solid has more Trans fat than the semi-solid soft ones. Hydrogenated oils which are solid at room temperature may contain about 15–25% of Trans fatty acids. Any food with "partial hydrogenated vegetable oil" on the label has Trans fat.

Margarines that are made with olive oil are soft and have no Trans fats. Other tub margarines have little or no trans fat. Interestingly, animals like sheep and cattle have stomachs which naturally produce Trans fats and so their body fat may contain up to 11% of Trans fats.

However, hydrogenated vegetable oils are the major source of Trans fats and that is why there is the push to eliminate them in foods, with United States FDA mandating that foods be labeled with the content of Trans fats. Most foods currently have "no trans fats" written on the label, showing that industry is listening to public opinion and keeping levels below 0.5gms per serving. They have replaced them with oils that have high monounsaturated fatty acids like corn, sunflower, and soybean.

Reminders on Your Radar

Saturated fats raise LDL cholesterol the most (but can raise HDL), Trans fats raise them moderately (but lower HDL) and Unsaturated fats do not raise LDL. To lower cholesterol, Trans fats are to be avoided or reduced in intake, and some saturated fats may be bad, others neutral and some beneficial. The MUFA and PUFA (omega fatty acids) are beneficial for lowering bad cholesterol and they protect against heart disease. Choose to eat all types of fats in moderation, however avoid foods which are high in saturated fats and trans fats and do less frying. Do remember most foods contain a combination of different fats but the ratio of good to bad "fats" is what is important.

Fad Diets

. . . .

There are several diets that have been toted for weight loss. They include:

Atkins: Low carbohydrates (Carb) diet

Ornish: Low fat diet

South Beach: Modified low carbohydrate diet, lower in carbs and higher in protein/good fats

Gluten Free: Replacement of gluten by eliminating wheat, barley and Rye from the diet

Ketogenic (Keto) Diet: High fat, adequate protein and low carb diet

Commercial weight loss programs: Jenny craig, Weight Watchers, Nutrisystem

We will examine the science behind some of these

Gluten Free Diet
Gluten Free Diet (GFD) and Weight Loss

Many people think a gluten-free diet leads to weight loss, but that may not be the case. GFDs tend to be high in fat, calories and sugar and low in fiber, minerals, and vitamins. Any weight loss is due to decreased caloric intake and not the gluten-free foods. For example a slice of regular whole wheat bread which contains gluten contains about 69 calories, 2 grams of fiber and less than 1 gram of fat. A slice of gluten free bread may have 20 to 30 more calories, double the fat and half the fiber. For some dieters, their gluten-free efforts makes them eat more lean protein, fruits and vegetables and so this kind of diet can produce some initial weight loss.

The gluten-free diet leads to decreased white flour, sugar, junk food and so less calories resulting in weight loss.

Gluten free does not mean fat free or calorie free, and some people indulge in a lot of gluten-free snacks and fried foods. Therefore, a gluten-free diet may not be healthier than regular diet or result in weight loss. Many gluten-free foods may contain just as many or more grams of carbohydrates, sugars and fats as foods containing gluten. A similar situation is sometimes encountered in people on a vegetarian diet who are obese because they consume a lot of calories which do not come from animal products but from carbohydrates.

Atkins Diet

This was introduced by Dr. Robert Atkins. This is an example of a low carbohydrate diet, with a high protein and or high fat diet. A typical American diet consists of 50% of calories from carbohydrate, 35% from fat and 15% from protein. The Atkin's diet has been modified over the years and the standard one now is Atkins 20, based on eating 20 grams of carbs as high-fiber vegetables daily, high protein and fat in the form of lean proteins, healthy fats. Proteins include meat, chicken, salmon, sardines, trout, dairy, like full fat cheese, butter, yogurt and cream. Also, nuts and seeds and healthy fats like olive oil, coconut, avocado oil, those with omega 3 Fatty acids, MUFA and PUFA, as well as eggs. The 20 Atkins is divided into four phases and foods differ depending on the phase. A newer version Atkins 40 starts with 40 grams of carbs and is less restrictive compared to 20 version.

The low carbs (lower than 50 g) forces the body to burn fat as fuel. The liver changes fat to fatty acids and produces ketone bodies (KB) which are used for energy and this causes sodium and water to be excreted causing weight loss. Ketosis also suppresses hunger. People on this diet can get recipes on the Atkins website and books are available to guide one.

Ketogenic (KETO) Diet

This is also a low carb diet, with high fat and adequate amounts of protein. It has been around since the 1920s, and has been used in many clinical situations including resistant epilepsy, obesity, diabetes, metabolic syndrome, traumatic brain injury, Non alcoholic fatty liver to name a few. The fat content is about 65 to 80% of daily calories while protein makes up 15 to 25% and carbs 5 to 15%, which is about 30g carbs. Just like the Atkins diet, the Keto diet leads to ketosis or production of KB. It is difficult to adhere to this diet for a long time, however a recent study of a ketogenic diet in obese patients for 24 weeks concluded that there were benefits from long term ketogenic diet without significant side effects. The benefits include: weight loss and decrease in total cholesterol, with increase HDL and lower levels of LDL, TG and blood glucose. (Hussein M.D, et al. Exp. Clinical Cardiol. 2004, 9(3) 200–205). A few people, however, do see increase of LDL-C of about

10% as a result of the high fat content. Increase in uric acid also occurs. Due to the limitation of foods like milk, whole grains, potatoes, beans, there are deficiencies of nutrients like calcium, Vitamin D, magnesium, zinc, phosphorus and selenium, fiber and potassium. Hydration is important on this diet, and it is advised to drink half one's body weight in ounces, e.g. if one weighs 150 Lbs one will need to drink 75 oz of fluids/day.

Adverse Effects: These may be short or long term

Short term: constipation, dehydration, loss of appetite, nausea and vomiting. "Keto flu" – this is feelings of headache, fatigue as a result of fluid loss through the kidneys

Long term: mineral deficiencies, fatty liver, kidney stones, increased levels of LDL and TG

It is important that those who embark on this diet, choose healthy fats like PUFA and MUFA found in nuts, almonds, sesame oil, seeds, olive oil, and avocados.

Commercial Weight Loss Plans

These are mostly balanced reduced portion size and low calorie diets and seem to be effective for short term weight loss and not necessarily sustained long term weight loss. Examples include Weight Watchers, Jenny Craig, and Nutrisystem. The meals may be based on regular everyday foods for portion control as in some of the above or purchasing of their own prepacked meals sent to them. Meal replacement shakes, frozen entrees, are also available for purchase in grocery or supermarkets and examples are Slim Fast, Lean Cuisine, Healthy Choice etc.

Low Carbohydrate (Carb) Foods and Snacks

The following can be substitutes for high carb foods or snacks

High to Mod. Carbs	Low Carbohydrates	High to Mod. Carbs	Low Carbs
Reg. Milk	Almond or coconut milk	Cane or brown sugar	Monk fruit, Stevia
Ice cream	Halo top ice cream	Bread	Lettuce wrap
Rice	Cauliflower/broccoli rice	Reg. Yogurt	Plain Greek Yogurt
Pancake	Almond flour pancake	Pizza crust	Coconut flour crust
Reg. flour	Coconut or Almond flour	Potato chips	Parsnip chips
Mashed potato	Mashed cauliflower	Potato chips	Turnip chips
French fries	Zucchini fries	French Fries	Cauliflower crisp

Examples of low carb snacks are below. Note they may be high in 'good fat'. They include:

Nuts like almonds, cashew walnuts, pecans, hazelnuts, macadamia
Fruits like: blackberries, raspberries
Vegetables: spinach, broccoli, asparagus, kale, Guacamole, tomatoes, lettuce, cucumber
Protein and high fat foods: bacon, boiled eggs, sardines, salmon and tuna fish

For more information on weight loss see: https://medlineplus.gov/diets.html; health.clevelandclinic.org/weight loss; familydoctor.org/prevention-and-wellness/food-and-nutrition/weight-loss.

Remember, that whatever one choses to use, it's important to exercise at least 150 minutes a week, and this should be both aerobic/cardio and strength training. This is because with weight loss, there is also loss of lean body mass and muscle mass loss.

In Conclusion

....

We often want a quick fix or a quick way to lose weight and so may go on fad or popular diets which promise rapid weight loss; however, most people gain the weight back because either the diet is so extreme or not practical, or they do not incorporate healthy eating and regular exercises into their daily life after initial weight loss. Without behavior changes (TLC – of exercise, healthy eating, portion control etc.), it is quicker to go back into one's former unhealthy eating and lifestyle (e.g. sitting in front of the TV for many hours, snacking on junk, empty calorie foods or unhealthy foods) and gain all the weight which was rapidly lost on some fad diet.

Environmental Factors Contributing to Obesity

....

Apart from factors which have to do with the individual's own behavior, attitudes and eating habits, there are general environmental factors contributing to a community's increased obesity rate. These include the following:

Sedentary lifestyle with restriction to the indoors – not much movement such as walking, jogging, or physical activity
Sitting down at work without moving around much

Criminal activity in some areas keeping people sedentary behind closed doors

Reduction in structured physical activity like organized sports

Increased television viewing

Computer use for games and social media

Cell phones and other devices which are often used when sedentary

Communities with no close by grocery shops, but neighborhood stores selling cheap sugar-sweetened drinks and high caloric-dense fast foods

Reduction in number of parks, and open green spaces where physical activities can take place

No affordable gyms or exercise facilities that people can go and use

No farmers markets selling fresh vegetables and fruits

Use of Medications and Surgery to Treat Obesity

....

Introduction

When conscious lifestyle changes and weight loss attempts mentioned above do not lead to significant weight loss and an individual also has other medical conditions, then weight loss medications and weight loss surgery may have to be incorporated in the obesity treatment. When medications or surgery are used to treat obesity, the use of lifestyle changes has to continue otherwise an individual can gain back most of the lost weight. I have seen individuals who have had weight loss surgery and

> I do not believe that using medicines to assist in maintaining a healthy weight is a sign of failure, especially if the individual is trying hard at lifestyle changes. There is no "magic diet pill", they just help one jumpstart or continue with weight loss based on healthy eating and regular exercise.
>
> —Dr. Barbara Entsuah. MD.

gained back an enormous amount of weight because they did not take care to continue with behavior changes (TLC). This leads to frustration, depression, resignation or "giving up" and so it is important to continue with lifestyle changes when other treatment methods are used.

Medications for Weight Loss

Several weight loss medications used in the past, had led to serious side effects including heart problems and had to be withdrawn from the market (Dexfenfluramine and Sibutramine). However, better and safer medicines are now available and approved by the FDA (Food and Drug Administration of the USA) for treatment of obesity.

When are Medicines Appropriate

They can be used if an individual has a BMI of greater or equal to 30 with no other medical issues, or even with a lower BMI of 27 with medical problems like diabetes, hypertension or impaired fasting blood sugar. The use of a dietitian or nutritionist is a valuable tool and I encourage that resource to help anyone whose treatment has gone beyond lifestyle changes. I cannot overemphasize that lifestyle changes of healthy eating, and exercise should be continued, otherwise the weight is gained back, resulting in frustrations. I have seen patients who had gastric bypass but have gained back most of the weight they lost. There is no quick fix to maintaining a healthy weight.

Oral Medications

There are four oral medications as of 2017 approved by the FDA and include

Orlistat (Xenical, Alli)
Lorcaserin (Belviq)
Phentermine/topiramate (Qsymia)
Bupropion/naltrexone (Contrave)

Injectable Medications

Liraglutide injection (Saxenda), for obese patients with weight-related problems is injected once daily and has been approved by USA and other countries for weight loss.

Complementary and Alternative Medications for Weight Loss

There is a long list of supplements that have been toted for weight loss. Unfortunately, most have not withstood the rigors of scientific studies and their claimed successes have been based on anecdotal reports from individuals. It has also been shown that some supplements are adulterated with stimulants and sold as weight loss medicines. Some stimulants may affect the heart and cause problems. These include: DMBA, Ephedra, BMPEA, DMAA (1, 3-dimethylamylamine), AMP (2-amino-4-methylpentane) which have been banned by the FDA and have been found in weight loss supplements. Some supplements are adulterated with added medicines like thyroid hormone, laxatives, diuretics, or drugs to mask the effects of stimulants (e.g. Propranolol), but these are not listed as components. It is important to check with one's doctor before starting any weight loss supplement. Just because it be advertised as "natural" does not mean they are safe.

Cam Weight Loss Supplements

NAME	POSSIBLE SIDE EFFECTS/NOTES
Apple cider vinegar	lowered blood sugar and potassium levels
Garcinia cambogia	stomach upset, nausea, and headache
CLA (Conjugated linoleic acids)	constipation or diarrhea
African mango	headache, dry mouth, sleep problems and stomach aches
Bitter orange	rapid heart rate. It's similar to ephedrine
White kidney bean (Phazyme 2)	heartburn, excessive gas, and diarrhea.
Green Tea	insomnia, palpitations from caffeine
Green coffee bean	insomnia, headache, palpitations from the caffeine
Cissus quadrangularis	no significant side effects
Chitin/chitosan and glucomannan	diarrhea, constipation, bloating
*HCG	ovarian stimulation, multiple pregnancies, blood clots
Acai berry	appears to be relatively safe
Raspberry ketone	increased heart rate and increased blood pressure
Hoodia Gordonii (P57)	thirst suppression, (lots of fake pills available)
Fenugreek	Allergic reactions, gas, bloating and diarrhea
Hydroxycitric Acid (HCA)	dizziness, dry mouth, liver problems Found in Garcinia
Litramine	(Fat burner from cactus) may cause newborn defects.

*HCG stands for Human Chorionic Gonadotropin

Surgery for Weight Loss (Bariatric Surgery)

This is also an option for weight loss. There are many benefits associated with weight loss following gastric surgery. These include reduction in incidence of:

Medical conditions: Hypertension, diabetes, joint pain from arthritis especially in the knees, sleep apnea and high cholesterol levels

Mental health: Psychologically, some individuals feel good about themselves and have a more positive outlook of life after losing a lot of weight from the surgery. There is also more social interaction with others

Types of Bariatric Surgery

The three common surgeries are

Gastric bypass, Gastric Sleeve and adjustable Gastric Banding.

Requirements

1. Individuals have to meet certain requirements before having bariatric surgery
2. These include BMI of 40 or more, or BMI of 35 with medical conditions like Diabetes mellitus, Hypertension, or Sleep Apnea
3. Documented failure to achieve weight loss goal with diet and exercise
4. Appointments with a psychologist, dietitian, family medicine or internist physicians for evaluation of the individual's physical, mental and motivation prior to the surgery

Weight loss surgery is just a tool to help with weight loss, and it is important the person has the desire to continue to achieve and maintain weight loss goals. Exercise, and healthy eating are essential, otherwise most weight will be gained back after the surgery.

A brief description of the different types will be given here, however more information can be acquired at internet sites like WebMD, Familydoctor.org, emedicine-health.com etc.

Gastric Bypass

Roux-en-Y procedure creates a small pouch in the stomach which is connected directly to the second part of the small intestine, with the stomach separated into two, and so food bypasses most of the stomach. It limits the amount of food one can eat at a time and also the area of stomach that food can be absorbed from. Food has to be chewed very well before swallowing.

Complications

Too much food: results in stomach problems like, nausea, vomiting and abdominal pain

Physical problems: Abdominal pain, hypoglycemia (low blood sugar), bloating, anemia, kidney stones, and gall stones

Dumping syndrome: Food moves quickly from stomach to the small intestines without being digested well and high amounts of glucose quickly enter the small intestines and the blood. High levels of insulin is released resulting in rapid drop of blood sugar (hypoglycemia) leading to symptoms like dizziness, palpitations, sweating, nausea and vomiting and even fainting right after a meal

Prolonged Recovery Time: The surgery is more difficult with longer recovery time compared to other procedures. Many foods which are fibrous like meat, breads, pasta, rice, raw vegetables have to be avoided

Gastric Sleeve

It is believed to be effective as the Roux-en-Y with regards to the amount of weight that can be lost. A part of the stomach – about 80% is removed, leaving a sleeve which looks like a banana, and this causes only small amounts of food to be eaten at a time. It is not as complex as the gastric bypass, and recovery time is shorter. The gastric sleeve is connected to the upper small intestine (duodenum) as is normally, and so there is no dumping. Digestion occurs naturally and hunger is decreased as area of stomach where the hunger hormone Ghrelin is produced is removed.

In both cases eating small meals, chewing properly, avoidance of high carbohydrate and fatty meals, and drinking fluid between meals may be helpful. Both procedures require nutritional supplements and these include multivitamin, calcium, and Vitamin B12. After Bypass one also requires Iron supplement.

Adjusting Gastric Banding

This is not as popular as the other two due to many side effects caused by the band, post surgically. By laparoscopic means a band with an inflatable balloon is placed around the upper part of the stomach creating a small pouch. The size of band can be changed or adjusted creating a small upper stomach pouch, limiting the amount of food that can be eaten or what the stomach can hold. Saline is used to inflate the band to tighten it and food moves slowly through the stomach. The saline is introduced through a port which is stitched beneath the skin. It is the simplest of all 3 procedures but has several troubling side effects.

Complications

These include erosion of the band, infection of the port, malfunction of the tube and port used to adjust the balloon or obstruction of the mouth of the pouch.

Intragastric Balloons

Intragastric balloons are newer non-surgical weight loss devices called ORBERA and ReShape Integrated Dual Balloon System which are balloons that are inserted into the stomach during short outpatient endoscopy procedures. The ReShape has two balloons while Orbera has one inserted balloon. The balloon's volume is meant to decrease amount of food one eats and assist in portion control. Both stay in the stomach for 6 months and are deflated and removed after that time, and so they are both temporary measures. There have been a few deaths after these procedures according to the United States FDA and so they are monitoring them closely.

Importance of Exercise to Maintain New Lower Weight

This is important because with weight loss, there is loss of lean body mass, and with this comes decreased basic metabolic rate. Exercise increases metabolic rate, so one needs to exercise regularly, to increase metabolic rate and total energy expenditure. Aging is associated with slower basic metabolic rate and that is why many people gain weight as they get older.

Reminders on Your Radar

Obesity is a major problem in both resource rich and poor countries. It is a multifactorial problem and can be tackled from many angles both individually and nationally. Lifestyle changes like healthy eating, exercise and weight loss measures like medicines and surgery may all be used to combat it. It takes years to become obese and so losing weight takes a long time to achieve desired weight, and so gradual loss of about 1 to 2 pounds a week or reduction of calories by 500 to 1000 calories per day is prudent. Behavior changes include – not using food to de-stress; and treatment of depression have to be addressed. Fad diets do not provide long term weight loss and maintenance of the lost weight, so it is best to avoid them.

12

Respiratory Diseases and Conditions

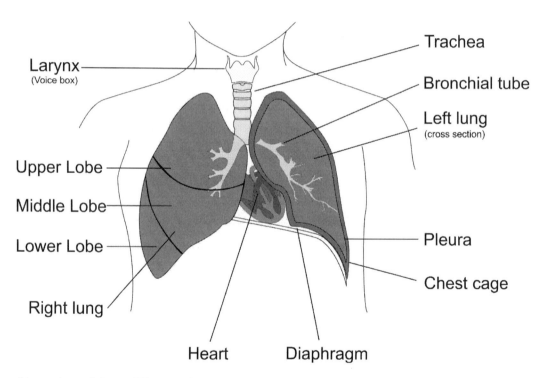

Larynx
(Voice box)

Trachea

Bronchial tube

Left lung
(cross section)

Upper Lobe

Middle Lobe

Lower Lobe

Pleura

Chest cage

Right lung

Heart

Diaphragm

Above is a picture of the respiratory system and the various parts involved in breathing

Respiratory System (Breathing system)

. . . .

Introduction

This is made up of organs or structures that assist with one's body's breathing system and exchange of gases. The respiratory system starts from the nostrils and ends in the lungs which are in one's chest cavity and surrounded by

"As long as you're breathing, it's never too late to do some good".

—Maya Angelou
American Poet, writer (April 4, 1928 – May 28, 2014).

one's ribs. The system allows air to move from nostrils or mouth into the lungs and out again. Air is very important because it is made up of many gases including the most important type called oxygen.

The Process of Breathing: (Getting oxygen in and removing carbon dioxide)

When we breathe in air and it gets into our lungs, it eventually travels to the tiny or terminal airways which end as round air sacs called alveoli. These sacs are like tiny balloons or grapes filled with air. These are surrounded by tiny blood vessels some of which carry carbon dioxide which is a by-product from cells. At this level, there is exchange of oxygen from the air we breathe in, with the carbon dioxide which is present in the tiny vessels or capillaries. The carbon dioxide is released into the air sacs and eventually breathed out (expiration) with the expired air. The oxygen rich air on the other hand gets into the blood and it is called oxygenated blood at this point because it has a high concentration of oxygen. This is then taken away by another set of vessels to supply the rest of our body's cells with oxygenated blood. All cells need oxygen to function normally, and without oxygen, cells will die and organs will not be able to perform their normal functions. Inhaled air contains about 20% oxygen and exhaled air contains about 14 to 16% oxygen. The normal level for blood oxygen is 95 to 100%. When one visits a clinic as part of the process to obtain one's vital signs, one may have a little device placed on one's finger called a Pulse Oximeter and this records the oxygen saturation in one's blood. Lower levels may mean that one does not have enough oxygen in one's blood or cells.

Diseases and Conditions of the Respiratory System

We will talk about a few diseases that can affect this complex system which is vital to our very existence. Not all conditions or diseases are covered here, and one can read about others not mentioned here. The respiratory system can be divided into two: Upper and Lower respiratory systems.

Upper respiratory: Include the nose, nasal passages, sinuses, pharynx, and the portion of the larynx (voice box) above the vocal cords. Common infections include: Common cold, catarrh (runny nose and mucus associated with inflamed airway), sore throat, ear infection (otitis media), tonsillitis, sinusitis and laryngitis (inflamed or infected voice box)

Lower respiratory: Include the trachea, bronchi, bronchioles, and the alveoli, which make up the lungs tiny airways. Common conditions include: Asthma, flu, pneumonia, acute and chronic bronchitis (COPD)

Noninfectious causes include allergic rhinitis (allergies, hay fever), asthma, and COPD

The ones caused by infections are mostly by microorganisms or germs. Germs are tiny living organisms which may be mainly BACTERIA OR VIRUSES. Fungal elements (fungus) may also cause these infections. When one gets an infection, it attacks a particular part of one's body and is manifested by certain symptoms. The 2020 corona virus infection COVID19 was a very contagious one causing a worldwide pandemic.

Upper Respiratory Infection or Common Cold
What is it?

Colds are caused by VIRUSES, and there are over two hundred viruses that can attack one's upper respiratory system resulting in inflammation of the upper respiratory system. A cold may present as nasal congestion, cough, sore throat and sometimes fullness and redness in the ears.

Signs and Symptoms

These include: cough, rarely mild fever, runny nose, sneezing, sore throat, headache, nasal discharge which may start off as clear but maybe yellow or green, some muscle ache, and watery eyes. It usually starts gradually and may last 3 to 14 days.

Treatment of the Common Cold

There are no specific medications to treat the common cold; however one can treat the symptoms using OTC (over the counter) medications while one's body's own immune system fights the germs and gets one better. Antibiotics do not help with viral illnesses, unless one develops a secondary bacteria infection.

FLUIDS: One has to drink plenty of fluids including water, tea, tea with lemon and honey, hot chocolate, soups etc. Fluids liquify the discharge so one can cough, blow, or spit it in a tissue

REST: To allow one's own body's defense or immune system to get rid of the infection

TOBACCO: Stop smoking if one is a smoker, and avoid contact with second hand smoke

PAIN RELIEF: For headache, achiness and sore throat one can use pain medications like Acetaminophen (brand name examples include Tylenol, Panadol, Paracetamol), Ibuprofen (brand names include Motrin, Advil, Bruffin), Naproxen (e.g. Aleve) or Diclofenac. The last 3 belong to a group of medications called NSAIDS (Non-steroidal anti-inflammatory drugs). They treat pain, fever and inflammation. Aspirin is also an NSAID, but most times, it is used for other conditions rather than pain. The non coated type may irritate the stomach if taken in large doses

SORE THROAT: Apart from taking pain medication, gargling with warm salt water, and sucking throat lozenges (cough drops) may relieve some of the pain. Spraying throat with chloraseptic spray or other similar throat sprays that numb the throat may also help. Sucking frozen lollipops, or treats may make sore throat feel better

NASAL CONGESTION (stuffy nose): One can use decongestants like Pseudo-ephedrine or Phenylephrine tablets or menthol nasal inhalants, which shrink the swollen tissues of the nasal cavity and also prevent excessive nasal discharge, making breathing through the nose relatively easier. Some come as nasal sprays (e.g. oxymetazoline, Afrin) but it is not advised to use these for more than 3 days, because they can cause what is called a "rebound effect" if used for a long period of time. This means they will shrink the swollen blood vessels but soon cause the swelling to come back

SIDE EFFECTS: Decongestants may increase blood pressure and are not usually advised in people with hypertension or heart disease unless cleared by one's physician

Salt water or saline nasal spray (e.g. Ocean spray) can be used in the nostrils as many times as needed to loosen the mucus, remove crusts, decrease postnasal drip, and decrease swelling inside the nostrils. One can make one's own and use a medicine dropper to instill into one's nostrils.

How to Make Saline Solution (salt water nasal rinse)

Take 1 teaspoon of salt (can add 1/2 teaspoon of baking soda – optional) and add it to 500–750 ml of boiled cooled water or bottled sterile water. Put a small amount in a disposable cup and instill it in one's nostrils using a medicine dropper.

Antihistamines: For runny nose and sneezing during a cold, an antihistamine can be used to help dry up the nostrils, make one breathe better, and help with itching. There are drowsy and non drowsy ones. Examples of drowsy ones are Diphenhydramine (Benadryl) or Chlorpheniramine and Brompheniramine, and non drowsy ones are Loratidine and Cetirizine. The non drowsy antihistamines do not work as well for colds

COUGH: This is mostly caused by drainage pouring down from the back of one's nostrils and down the back of one's throat and upper airways. The cough mechanism helps bring up the mucus/phlegm so that one can spit it into tissue paper or handkerchief. Remember not to cough into your hands as this can spread to others

Treatment: One can use a cough suppressant (diminishes or blocks the cough reflex) when the cough is dry, and examples of cough suppressants are Dextromethorphan (DM), Benzonatate, Diphenhydramine, and narcotics like Codeine (latter is a prescription medicine). A common cough expectorant is guaifenesin which is found in many cough syrups. It will cause thinning of the phlegm which can be coughed up. Sucking lozenges containing honey, lemon, vitamin C, or menthol may also help diminish the cough. Cough medicines are generally not recommended for kids

Combination Cold Medicines

Some cough and cold medicines come as a combination of all the above (multi-symptom cold medicine) and that can be used to treat all the symptoms, like congestion, pain and cough. It is important to read the label on any medicine container so one knows what it contains, and what it is intended to treat. Remember to always take medicines as directed. If a medicine package says to take up to three times a day, then so far as one has the symptoms, take it as directed because its duration of action is taken into account and it may be effective for only four to six hours at a time. One may not feel better quickly, if one doesn't follow the instructions.

Complementary and Alternative Medicines for Treating Colds

These include

Zinc tablets, mega doses of Vitamin C, Airborne, and Echinacea. Normal doses of Vitamin C is up to 2,000 mg daily. Mega doses may cause nausea, diarrhea, heart burn. Several studies have shown that megadoses of Vitamin C do not prevent the common cold in ordinary folks

A natural cough suppressant is honey and making tea with lemon and honey has been found to soothe the throat and calm the cough, and one gets vitamin C from the lemon

Natural substances like menthol in ointment form can be rubbed on the chest and throat to ease coughing and ease stuffy noses. Care has to be taken not to apply these close to the eyes or on broken skin

Some Vapor Rubs contain camphor and this can be toxic if sufficient amounts get into the circulation

There are also inhalation forms containing eucalyptus oil, menthol, camphor etc. which are mixed with steam to soothe stuffy nostrils and chest congestion

Some people recommend essential oils like lemon, eucalyptus, tea tree or Rosemary as a blend or alone in a bath or as a steam inhalation to help with congestion or cold symptoms. Check with one's health care provider if it is okay for one to use

Again, these may relieve some of one's symptoms as one's own body (one's immune system) clears out the infection

Flu (Influenza)
What is it?

Infection of the respiratory system with effects on the whole body, caused by specific viruses, but they are not as many as those which cause the common cold. In recent years, there have been epidemics of different types of flu viruses in various parts of the world. Each year different strains may affect different areas of the world. According to the CDC, about 80,000 Americans died of the flu and its complications during the 2017/18 flu season.

Symptoms and Signs

Most of flu illnesses will have symptoms which develop suddenly and include fever (greater than 102° F or 38.8° C), chills and shakes, fatigue, bodily aches, occasionally some runny nose, cough, mild sore throat, headaches, nausea or diarrhea.

Treatment

There are some flu-specific medicines but they help diminish symptoms and recovery by 1–2 days only, and are effective if started within 48 hours of symptoms onset. The dangerous flu types like H1N1 which cause epidemics are usually treated in the hospital but they are not what cause the seasonal flu. Most can be treated symptomatically as outlined under treatment of cold. The flu specific medicines are also used to prevent flu if one is exposed to it within 7 to 10 days.

When to See A Doctor

One may need to see a doctor if:

Symptoms like fever greater than 41° C (105.8° F) does not go down but continues for more than 3 days

Worsening of symptoms in spite of using OTC medications

Symptoms lasting more than 10 days

Increasing cough, chills and shakes

Earache or discharge

Severe pain in one's face

Swollen glands in one's neck or under the chin (inflamed lymph nodes or glands)

Shortness of breath, difficulty in breathing, or wheezing (whistling sounds in chest with breathing)

If one has several chronic medical conditions and are elderly

Complications

Complications may include ear infection, acute bronchitis, acute sinusitis or pneumonia depending on the symptoms. One will need a doctor to examine and give them appropriate medicines.

Prevention of Flu and Other Respiratory Illnesses

Respiratory illnesses are spread when droplets containing the viruses or bacteria (germs) are sneezed or coughed out by an infected person directly into another person's face, or when hands containing the germs contaminate other hands, door knobs or other surfaces, and used to touch the eyes, mouth and nose.

Washing hands frequently will stop the spread of the germs.

When one coughs, it is important to cough into a tissue to "COVER ONE'S COUGH" and then wash one's hands with soap and water.

Coughing into the bent elbow or sleeve instead of into the hands will also prevent the spread of germs.

When soap and water are not immediately available, use of hand sanitizers can help. It is a good idea to carry a small bottle of hand sanitizer in one's bag or purse at all times.

Social gatherings are places where people shake hands a lot and so it is important to use hand sanitizers discretely or wash one's hands when one has shaken hands with several individuals.

It is also a good habit to go straight to the bathroom to wash one's hands after coming home from church, work etc.

Cleaning one's own kitchen counter tops and bathroom surfaces with soap and water or some form of disinfectant will minimize the spread of viruses. However soap and water are very adequate for reducing the amount of germs one comes into contact with.

Avoiding close contact with someone who has a respiratory infection will prevent one from getting the infection. Advise them not to shake hands, cough into one's face and not to kiss or hug any one.

If one has a respiratory infection, don't shake hands and instead give an elbow bump, do a bow, wave or fist bump to avoid the spread of the germs.

Flu Immunization or Vaccination

1. Each year in developed countries a flu vaccine is produced based on types of flu strains authorities think will be out based on many factors they look at
2. It is recommended **for all individuals,** 6 months and older; but especially the elderly, children, and pregnant women and those with chronic medical conditions like diabetes, heart disease, and respiratory illnesses like asthma or chronic bronchitis (COPD)
3. It minimizes the risk of getting the flu and even if one gets the flu after being immunized, the disease is usually a milder form
4. Everyone should get vaccinated each year

COVID-19 Respiratory Illness

In December 2019, a new Coronavirus emerged from Wuhan in China called SARS-CoV-2 and caused a disease called COVID-19. Coronaviruses have been known for a long time with some causing infections in mammals and birds. In humans they cause mild infections like the common cold, but a more serious one in 2003 led to infections in Asia called Severe Acute Respiratory Syndrome associated with coronavirus (SARS-CoV). From Asia it had spread to Europe, South America and North America. In 2012, there was a similar Coronavirus called Middle East Respiratory Syndrome-related coronavirus (MERS-CoV) which started in the Middle East and spread to other countries like the USA and others in Europe. MERS CoV has infected more than 2,200 people and killed nearly 40% of those infected. Both of these were fairly contained, and vaccines for both are being developed as of 2019. The emergence of the novel coronavirus starting in Wuhan China has spread rapidly, and as of April 2020, there is a worldwide Pandemic of the disease COVID-19 caused by this new virus. All countries whether resource rich or resource poor are grappling with containing and treating the disease. This Novel Coronavirus has infected over 2 million people in over 180 countries and territories, as of mid-April over 137,000 people had died. Thousands are being infected and dying daily in the worse hit countries like USA, Italy, UK, Spain and France. Others are India, Brazil, Russia, and Germany. China used extreme methods to contain it, which many other countries are not doing, or cannot do.

Symptoms and Signs

May range from Asymptomatic: no symptoms, patient is perfectly fine but is infected

Mild illness: like an upper respiratory infection or common cold symptoms like runny nose, cough, sore throat, low grade fever, diarrhea, loss of smell or taste

Severe illness: all the above plus severe cough, fever, Shortness of breath, Pneumonia, difficulty in breathing, chest pain and headache. These can become worse and may lead to respiratory failure. In this situation, the individual cannot breathe well on their own and some need oxygen, and different breathing machines, with the most serious patients going on a ventilator to do the breathing for them.

Prevention

To mitigate the spread, the following have been recommended:
- Social Distancing by staying a minimum of six feet away from other people
- Stay home and isolate oneself if one has symptoms, and restrict contact with others
- Use of a face mask by infected individuals and those in close contact with them
- Frequent hand washing with soap and water for at least 20 seconds
- Use of a hand sanitizer that contains at least 60% alcohol if water and soap are not available.
- Cover your cough or sneeze with a tissue, then throw the tissue in the trash.
- Avoid touching your eyes, nose, and mouth with unwashed hands.
- Avoid close contact with people who are sick.
- Clean and disinfect frequently touched objects and surfaces.
- Use a face mask when going outside to crowded places even if you don't have symptoms
- Increased testing of individuals without symptoms to identify and isolate those who are infected
- Quarantining of those who have had close contact with sick individuals
- Increased testing to identify asymptomatic carriers so they can be isolated
- Vaccines to protect people from the infection are being developed but may not be ready until at least 12 to 18 months' time.
- The mantra of some world top clinicians has been TESTING, TRACING and TREATMENT

Treatment

There are no specific medicines for treating the infection as of now, however some have been used to treat the symptoms and a few of them have some antiviral activities. The medicines currently being used are:

Acetaminophen for pain and fever
Steroid at times if body's immune response is overwhelming the body
Remdesivir (a new antiviral medication being tried on compassionate grounds)
Oxygen, and breathing support with machines including ventilators
Hydroxychloroquine (Currently not recommended due to side effects)
Azithromycin or other antibiotics

However, the latter two can cause irregular heart beat on their own and may not be suitable for people with heart conditions. There are ongoing trials of use of Hydroxychloroquine and the new antiviral Remdesivir. The trials for use of Hydroxychloroquine and Remdesivir have approved the latter, but not Hydroxychloroquine.

The disease is a very new one so what specifically helps treat the infection has not been identified and so there is currently ongoing research on what drugs are best for the disease, and also its rapidly changing symptoms.

Sinus Infections (Acute Sinusitis)
What are the Sinuses?

There are four paired sinus cavities within the facial bones and those near the nose are called paranasal sinuses. They are located on the forehead, close to the nostrils and below the eye balls. They are filled with air and lined with a mucous membrane which produces secretions, and also have little hairs on the membrane. Together they trap bacteria and other foreign particles and move them out into the throat and nostrils through small openings. They also help reduce the weight of the head, humidify the air we breathe and help with vocalization.

What is A Sinus Infection?

Sometimes after a cold, catarrh or flu infection, the infection spreads and may settle in the sinuses resulting in inflammation, fluid and pus build up in the sinus cavities. Infection may be caused by bacteria, viruses and fungi. The infection is known as ACUTE SINUSITIS

Signs and Symptoms

These include:

Nasal congestion or drainage which is thick yellow, green or brown mucus
Smelly discharge coming from nostrils
Pain in the teeth and gums
Pain or pressure in the face
Swelling of the face and cheeks
Frontal headache
Pain under the eyes
Fever
Fatigue
Loss of smell or taste

Treatment

Immediately after acute sinusitis starts, the following measures started by one self, may help.

1. Use a decongestant like Phenylephrine, or Pseudoephedrine tablets
2. Use of saline nasal rinse (described above) to copiously irrigate the nasal passages several times a day. This helps unplug the openings into the sinuses so they can drain the accumulated fluid or mucus present. Use of steroid nasal spray after sinus rinse
3. Treat pain and inflammation with Ibuprofen or other NSAIDs. Use Acetaminophen if one cannot take NSAIDs
4. One will need to see a doctor if there is no improvement in 48 to 72 hours and one is taking them around the clock as the instructions indicate
5. The doctor will decide whether one needs antibiotics and may also give one a steroid nasal spray like Fluticasone (Flonase) or Triamcinolone (Nasacort) to use

To Use Or Not to Use Antibiotics In Sinus Infections?

Not all sinus infections require antibiotics, since most of them are caused by viruses, and antibiotics do not cure viral infections. There is a move to try and discourage doctors or health providers from immediately giving antibiotics, since using antibiotics when they are not needed causes antibiotic resistance to develop. This means certain bacteria become resistant to the antibiotics and they grow stronger and so cannot be easily killed by usual antibiotics. Antibiotics are not the cure for all infections. I often have to spend a whole lot of time explaining to people they do not need antibiotics for the common cold or the first few days of sinus congestion. Most doctors would use antibiotics after 7 to 10 days of symptoms with no improvement with the measures described above. Once symptoms start getting better one is on their way to recovery and should continue taking the medicines.

Chronic Sinusitis

Some individuals have chronic sinusitis and they keep having recurrent infections as well as persistent inflammation. An Ear, Nose and Throat (ENT) or otolaryngologist specialist may require a CT scan of the sinuses and may do a nasal endoscopy. Sometimes sinus surgery may be needed or long courses of antibiotics and oral steroids are given to bring it under control. They may need two to three times a week nasal irrigation with a steroid irrigation fluid prepared by using some saline and a vial of a steroid called Budesonide which is normally used in a nebulizer machine by asthma sufferers.

Asthma

What is it?

Asthma is a chronic disease affecting the airways of the lungs, causing them to be narrow, and swollen, preventing air from moving freely in or out. The narrowing is reversible and in between attacks the airways work well. In asthma, the airways are sensitive to certain things which cause them to become inflamed, resulting in swelling of the lining of the airways, increased production of mucus

Asthma kills more adults than children every year, because children tend to be well controlled and they attend routine office visits, urgent care and emergency room visits with their parents/guardians more readily than adults.

and tightening of the muscles around the airway tubes (constriction). Asthma causes are unknown but may have both environmental or genetic causes, and may run in families. Many may have asthma as kids but may grow out of it as they get older, however, some may have persistent asthma as adults and if not well controlled can lead to death. For example according to the CDC, in the United States, 185 children and 3,262 adults died from asthma in 2007 (www.cdc.gov/vitalsigns/asthma). These are preventable if one knows how to manage one's asthma and regularly visits their doctor.

Triggers of Asthma Attacks

There are many things in the environment that can trigger an asthma attack or flare up.

Allergies like dust, pollen, smoke, cigarette smoke
Animal dander and pet hairs
Cockroach saliva and feces
Cold air, changes in temperature, like very cold or very hot
Perfume fragrance, and hairspray
Plants and trees, flowers
Infections of respiratory systems like colds and flu and sinus infections
Medicines like Aspirin, beta blockers and Ibuprofen
Physical activity and exercise
Acid reflux may also cause an attack
Emotional upset e.g. strong emotions like anxiety, anger etc
Foods: these include eggs, peanuts, wheat, soy, tree nuts, food preservatives, fish, sea foods like shrimp and shellfish

Identifying Triggers

Each individual has to know what triggers or irritants make their asthma worse and then try and avoid them. However, triggers can be identified by testing for environmental allergens and doing allergy food tests. Those that are positive are then avoided by the person.

Occupational Asthma
What is it?

Occupational asthma is asthma related to the work place, and symptoms tend to appear when at work and they improve on days when one is away from work environment. Some sufferers may develop asthma later on in life as adults, having been previously fine in their younger days.

Common triggers of occupational or work related asthma include:

Smoke, mold, dust, chlorine, drugs, animals, plants, sea foods, dyes, wood dust, and certain metals

Signs and Symptoms

Symptoms include coughing, wheezing (which is like a whistling sound in the chest), shortness of breath, difficulty in breathing, fast breathing, tightness in the chest, and difficulty talking. In very severe dangerous attacks, lips may turn blue (lack of oxygen) and individual will pass out. Some may present with just coughing which is triggered by various allergens and just goes on and on. Treatment is discussed below.

Diagnosis of Asthma

After taking a medical and family history, a physical exam is performed by a health care provider who will determine the severity of asthma with airway tests like spirometry, pulmonary function tests and peak flow tests. A chest x-ray may be ordered and allergy skin tests and food allergy tests are done to determine the triggers of one's asthma attacks.

Treatment of Acute Asthma Attack

An acute attack may be triggered by a cold infection, allergic rhinitis or any of the triggers mentioned above. The symptoms mentioned above will be present. The medicines used are called fast acting or rescue medications. One can use inhalers, tablets and liquid forms which open up the airways and lungs to quickly provide relief if an acute attack is occurring. The inhalers known as rescue or fast acting inhalers are better than tablets because they go straight to the lungs and therefore bring quick relief. It is important to carry one's rescue inhaler with one at all times, since one does not know when breathing difficulties will occur.

Examples of these Inhaled fast acting, rescue medicines are:

1. Albuterol – Brand names are ProAir, Ventolin, Xopenex, and Salbutamol
2. Ipratropium – Brand name is Atrovent

These are also available as liquids to be used as aerosols (vaporized) in a nebulizer machine which propels the nebulized medications straight into the lungs as it is inhaled through a mask or mouth piece. Individuals with moderate or severe asthma may have their own nebulizer at home. In some countries one can buy it with a prescription from a pharmacy or medical store.

What next if no improvement?

If there is no improvement or symptoms get worse after using them for a few hours, one has to go and see a doctor or go to the Emergency Department (ED). However, if in the beginning breathing is difficult, and talking in sentences is hard, then one has to go straight to see a health care provider or go to the ED. One has to be put on oral or inhaled steroid medicines to help with the inflammation producing the symptoms, and antibiotics may also be needed if bacteria is thought to be the cause. One will also receive several rounds of nebulized albuterol until symptoms get better. In severe cases that end up in the emergency room, oxygen, Intravenous medications like steroids and nebulizer treatments are also needed.

Prevention of Acute Asthma Attack

Prevention of asthma attacks is vital in order for one to live and enjoy every day activities. Some of the ways to prevent attacks include:
1. Avoid triggers that bring on an attack. If exposure to allergy triggers are decreased, then asthma symptoms are reduced. For example, if smoke makes one's airways sensitive then avoid places where people are smoking or smoking grills and open air flames
2. Allergy triggers should be well controlled either with allergy medications or Immunotherapy. The latter comes as allergy shots (injections) or allergy liquid drops placed under the tongue (sublingual Immunotherapy)
3. Before Immunotherapy is started allergy skin testing or allergy blood work have to be done, to identify which allergens one is allergic to. Small amounts of these specific allergens are then purified and put in liquid drops form or as injections given under the skin every one to two weeks, and then at longer intervals. Over time, one reacts less to the allergens and so symptoms decrease. People may take allergy shots for up to 5 years and then have to stop them

4. Minimize stress in one's life as that can bring on acute attacks

Prevention Or Controller Medications

If one gets frequent acute attacks, then one is usually put on a prevention or long term controller medication. These have to be taken daily to prevent attacks, and they are used whether one has symptoms or not.

1. There are two main types of asthma controller medications: **Inhaled steroids** – for example, Fluticasone propionate (Flovent), Fluticasone furoate (Arnuity Ellipta) and inhalers called long acting **Beta 2 agonists** (non steroids) e.g. Salmeterol and Formoterol
2. However, the long-acting beta 2 agonists have been banned from being used as a single medicine by the FDA due to concerns about increased risk of asthma symptoms. They are however safe when combined with steroids
3. Combined inhalers include Fluticasone/Salmeterol (Advair), (Budesonide/Formoterol), (Symbicort), and Fluticasone/Vilanterol (Breo)
4. There are some oral medicines like Montelukast (Singular) or Zafirlukast which are also used as controller medications, either alone or with the above medications. Other medications like Theophylline and Cromolyn may also be added on for better control, but they are not first choices for preventing or controlling asthma. If you have depression on Montelukast talk to your doctor
5. In severe asthma, or in countries where inhalers are expensive or not available, one may be put on low dose oral steroids for control
6. New medicines called monoclonal antibodies e.g. Omalizumab (Xolaire), Mepolizumab and Resulizumab may be used instead of steroids for controlling severe asthma
7. If one has allergic rhinitis (hay fever) that has to be well controlled with oral medications e.g. Loratidine (Claritin), Fexofenadine (Allegra), Montelukast or Cetirizine (Zyrtec); or nasal sprays like Fluticasone (Flonase), Azelastine (Astelin), and Ipratropium (Atrovent)
8. Other diseases like acid reflux, sinus infections, and sleep apnea need to be treated if present, in order to keep asthma under good control

Every patient with asthma, has to know how to treat acute attacks when they start. Recording the number of attacks per month may help one's health care provider decide whether one needs to be a controller or prevention medicine.

Treatment of Occupational Asthma

Once occupational asthma is suspected, it can be confirmed with the usual tests done for ordinary asthma and there needs to be avoidance of the trigger, by changing the workplace or removing the trigger. Despite this, some individuals may still have symptoms even if away from the trigger, because their airways have become very sensitive to the trigger. Treatment is with the same medications used for ordinary asthma as described above.

Exercise Induced Asthma
What is it?

Exercise induced asthma is asthma symptoms which come on after physical exertion, playing sports or exercising. It is also known as exercise induced bronchospasm.

Signs and Symptoms

Patients will complain about chest pain, chest tightness, wheezing, shortness of breath, poor performance in their sport, and a long time to recover after running or being active. Symptoms may be brought on by cold weather, high pollen counts, poor air quality, aerobic exercises, especially high impact ones.

Treatment

Diagnosis is made by history and physical examination and no tests are needed when it is clearly related to only physical activities as described above. Treatment is to prevent onset of symptoms by giving treatment with a Beta 2 agonist like Albuterol inhaler prior to exercising. If this does not prevent the symptoms from occurring, then medicines from another class which acts on chemicals causing inflammation like Montelukast or Zafirlukast can be used. Others like Cromolyn and Nedocromil which prevent histamine and other chemicals which cause bronchi to contract when released can be added.

Acute Bronchitis
What is it?

Acute bronchitis is inflammation of the bronchial tubes of the lungs and it is usually caused by a virus or bacteria, lung irritants like tobacco, smoke, and dust, and even acid reflux from the stomach and esophagus into the breathing tubes. It is mostly caused by a viral infection and may start after a cold, flu or sinus infection which does not go away but moves from the head area into the respiratory tubes. The infection causes inflammation, swelling of the tubes and production of mucus.

Signs and Symptoms

Presents with cough, and chest tightness, excessive phlegm, difficulty in breathing, wheezing or whistling sounds in the chest. There may be fever, chills, and shortness of breath.

Treatment

One has to see a health care provider for diagnosis and treatment. It may resolve as one's immune system fights it and it may last up to 10 days. Symptoms will be treated depending on what is present. Albuterol inhaler, cough expectorant, pain or anti-inflammation medicines like Ibuprofen or even some steroids may be used. Drinking lots of fluid, tea with honey and bed rest all help in recovery. Antibiotics may also be used if it is believed bacteria are involved. The cough associated may take a few weeks to resolve. It may lead to pneumonia and serious lung problems in those who have weaker immune system and so follow one's health provider's advice.

Pneumonia
What is it?

Pneumonia (ne-mo-nia) is an infection of the tissues of the lungs mainly within the tiny air sacs at the distal end of the lungs. It is mostly caused by viruses or bacteria, but fungi and environmental substances can also cause pneumonia. There are different types of pneumonia but the commonest type is called community acquired pneumonia (CAP). This is acquired from someone in the community who is infected and is carrying the virus or bacteria. The infected person then transmits it through coughing and expelling the respiratory particles containing the germ, which are then inhaled by another person. It may also develop from a cold, bronchitis or flu, especially if one has a decreased immune system, chronic conditions like Diabetes or if one is elderly.

Other Types of Pneumonia

Apart from CAP, there are other types of pneumonia like aspiration pneumonia, hospital acquired pneumonia (HAP) and opportunistic pneumonia. Aspiration pneumonia occurs when there is swallowing difficulties and some fluid or food particles end up in the lungs and cause inflammation and pneumonia. A person with stroke whose ability to swallow is affected, or one who is very sick and bedbound, can develop this type of pneumonia. Opportunistic pneumonia occurs when one's immune system is down or decreased as in HIV/AIDS or other conditions which cause one's germ-fighting mechanism to be defective. These germs will not normally cause an infection in someone whose immune system is intact. HAP occurs during a hospital stay.

Signs and Symptoms of Pneumonia

Symptoms of pneumonia may start with cold-like symptoms with runny nose and cough and then extend to include, a productive cough (cough with phlegm or mucus), fever, chills, tiredness, shortness of breath, difficulty breathing and pain in the chest or rib areas. If a cold or flu does not get better, but gets worse with time, then one has to see a health care provider because it could turn into pneumonia.

Treatment

After taking a history and examination, one's doctor may order a chest x-ray and or blood work, and then treatment will depend on type of pneumonia. If it is a bacterial form, one will need to take antibiotics, pain medicines, and even an inhaler like Albuterol (Ventolin, ProAir etc.) to help open one's airways and make one breathe better. When CAP pneumonia is mild, it is referred to as walking pneumonia and may not require hospitalization. Severe cases with fever, difficulty in breathing, low oxygenation, and chest pain, need to be admitted to the hospital where intravenous antibiotics, oxygen and breathing treatments with medicines like Albuterol may be required. Aspiration pneumonia and opportunistic pneumonias tend to be serious and are treated in a similar manner in the hospital.

Chronic Obstructive Pulmonary Disease (COPD)
What is it?

COPD is a chronic lung disease which results in difficulty in breathing due to inflammation of the bronchial airways. It is made up of two main diseases: chronic bronchitis and emphysema. It is usually a result of prolonged exposure to cigarette smoking through personal smoking or second hand exposure, as well as smoke from wood burning in some countries. Some individuals have a genetic defect causing them to develop the disease.

Chronic bronchitis: There is inflammation, (swelling and redness) of the bronchial tubes with excess mucus formation and chronic cough

Emphysema: The air sacs at the end of the lung tubes called alveoli are enlarged and their walls are destroyed and so oxygen and carbon dioxide exchange is affected. Not only is there difficulty getting enough oxygen into the blood when one inhales, but there is also difficulty breathing out (exhaling)

Signs and Symptoms

Chronic cough, which produces mucus

Shortness of breath, difficulty in breathing and breathlessness

Excessive production of mucus

The airways become sensitive and try to close resulting in wheezing and harsh breathing

Swelling of the feet and blue coloration of the lips due to lack of oxygen

Heart failure from dysfunction in the right side of the heart

The last two symptoms are common in emphysema

Treatment

Most important thing is to STOP smoking or stay away from smoke

Use of inhalers or oral medications which open up the airways making breathing easier

Steroid inhalers are also used by patients in addition to the ones like Albuterol or Ipratropium

Severe cases may require continuous oxygen use and patients may be seen around carrying portable oxygen canisters with attached tubes in their nostrils

A patient may occasionally have an exacerbation of their symptoms if they have an infection, or are exposed to irritants. They would then need more intensive treatment, and if worse may need hospitalization, steroids, nebulizer treatments, antibiotics, and oxygen

It is important to get yearly flu shots to prevent the flu, and also periodically receive the pneumonia vaccine to prevent pneumonia

Regular visits to a doctor or health provider is important to prevent exacerbations

Nicotine and its Effects

Tobacco and its effects cause more deaths each year than from the combined deaths from HIV, illegal drug use, Motor Vehicle Accidents and firearm related deaths (www.cdc.gov/tobacco/data).

The leading cause of smoking related death is lung cancer and according to the CDC, cigarette smoking is the number one risk factor for lung cancer, being linked to about 80 to 90% of lung cancers. Tobacco contains a number of cancer causing chemicals (carcinogens) which change the cells in the lungs, and its been reported tobacco smoke has over 7,000 toxic chemicals. Smoking also causes other cancers like esophagus, larynx (voice box), throat, kidney, bladder, stomach, cervix, colon, mouth and a type of leukemia. Other effects are development of COPD and coronary heart disease, increased wrinkling and lines of the skin, and birth of small babies if mothers smoke during pregnancy (low birth weight).

Electronic Cigarettes (E-CIGARETTES)

The use of E-CIGARETTES or Electronic Cigarettes by some individuals who want to quit smoking is fine if they quit both cigarettes and the E cigarettes eventually, but some continue to smoke the e cigarettes thinking it's a good alternative. The e-cigarette is a vaporizer which vaporizes liquid-containing substances like nicotine, glycerin and different flavors into a smoke. It is not altogether harmless and may prevent people from completely quitting tobacco use. People may also use more nicotine when they smoke these and may also continue to smoke regular cigarettes.

Smokeless Nicotine

Smokeless nicotine can also cause cancer and is also a source of irregular heart rhythm. Cancers caused by smokeless nicotine e.g. chewing tobacco include those of the lip, throat, mouth, esophagus, stomach, pancreas, larynx (voice box), kidneys, bladder, liver, colon, rectum, cervix in women and acute myeloid leukemia (blood cancer).

Reminders on Your Radar

Diseases affecting the respiratory system range from those which affect the upper respiratory system and those that affect the lower respiratory system. Infections include viral and bacterial infections of upper and lower respiratory like the common cold and pneumonia respectively. Other diseases include inflammation and constriction of the lower respiratory systems like asthma and bronchitis. Uncontrolled asthma kills more adults than children, and if it is not controlled one has to be on a daily controller or prevention medicine. There are ways one can prevent respiratory infections and inflammation by not smoking, controlling one's environment by avoiding allergens, and smoke from second hand smoking. Avoid spread of viruses and bacterial by covering your cough and by handwashing or using hand sanitizer. Smoking cigarettes is the cause of several cancers of the mouth, throat and lungs and we should all encourage smokers to stop.

13

Diseases Affecting the Heart and Blood Vessels

Introduction

....

The heart and the blood vessels can be considered as a pump with pipes; with the heart pumping blood through blood vessels (the pipes) to supply important nutrients and oxygen to the body's cells and organs. Diseases can affect both the vessels and the heart. We will discuss a few of these. These will include:

The best and most beautiful things in the world cannot be seen or even touched – they must be felt with the heart.

— Helen Keller, American author, political activist, and lecturer (Jun 27, 1880–Jun 01, 1968).

1. Hypertension
2. High cholesterol or Hyperlipidemia (increased cholesterol and other lipids)
3. Coronary Artery Disease (CAD) – Blockage of the blood vessels that supply the heart
4. Heart attack – Myocardial Infarction (MI) – Sudden blockage of vessels around the heart
5. Peripheral vascular disease (PVD) – Blocked arteries in the neck, arms, or in the legs
6. Congestive heart failure (CHF) – Heart Failure – Heart not beating hard enough
7. Irregular heart beat
8. Varicose veins
9. Lymphatic system

How the Heart Pumps

The blood circulating in the body (4.5–5.5 liters in adult) does so at a certain force or pressure. Blood pressure (BP) is measured by 2 numbers; systolic (sis-to-lick) (SBP) (upper number) and diastolic (Di-a-sto-lic) (DBP) (lower number) pressure – SBP/ DBP. BP can be explained by a pump and pipes illustration. The systolic pressure is the pressure that is measured or generated when the heart (pump) squeezes or pushes blood through the blood vessels (pipes) to the various organs of the body. The squeezing action is also called contraction. Diastolic pressure is the pressure measured during the time that the heart relaxes and fills with blood. One's Blood Pressure is recorded as these 2 numbers: For example: 120/60 (SBP/DBP).

Classification of Blood Pressure

There are normal values or ranges depending on age. When one's pressure is chronically above the normal for age then one has Hypertension Disease. The definitions for normal or abnormal BP have been tightened since 2017 when the American College of Cardiology and the American Heart Association produced new Hypertension guidelines (www.acc.org). They lowered the blood pressure (BP) cutoff for hypertension diagnosis from 140/90 mm Hg to 130/80 mm Hg.

Below are the values:

Ages 18 Years and Older (> Means greater than; and < means less than)
NORMAL: (SBP/DBP) Less than 120/80 mmHg
ELEVATED: 120–129 / 80 and less (<80)
HYPERTENSION: High blood pressure – divided into 2 stages depending on
   the numbers

Stages of Hypertension

Stage 1 Hypertension (SBP/DBP) 130–139/80–89
Stage 2 Hypertension greater than or equal to 140 (SBP) or greater than or
   equal to 90 (DBP)
Hypertensive crisis: (SBP/DBP) >180/>120
Prior to 2019, 140/90 was stage 1, but now its Stage 2 with the new classification

Measuring Blood Pressure

Machine cuff size is important and select the right size cuff based on one's arm circumference measured at middle of arm around the biceps with a tape measure

Arm Circumference. (cm/ins)	Usual Cuff Size
22–26 cm 8.7–10.2 ins	Small adult
27–34 cm 10.6–13.4 ins	Adult
35–44 cm 13.8–17.3 ins	Large adult
45–52 cm 17.7–20.5 ins	Adult thigh

Generally, there is also a small difference in BP in the left and right arms, however; if the difference is more than 10 mm Hg then it means there may be vascular or blood vessel blockage in the arm with the higher reading; or even a condition like diabetes is present, and one's doctor should investigate it further.

Measurement of Blood Pressure

Unfortunately, BP is measured inaccurately even in a doctor's office most of the time. The errors include the following:

Legs crossed
Arm not at heart level
Feet not flat on the ground
Individual talking
Back unsupported
Wrong BP cuff size
Patient on the mobile phone
White coat hypertension – presence of medical personnel makes some people
    get elevated BP

High office readings for the first time, should be confirmed at home or outside office readings taken on different occasions. It is a good thing to invest in a BP Monitor/ Cuff so that one can take their BP measurements at home. Upper arm cuff should be used for readings, and wrist cuffs only if arm size is too large to fit a cuff or for medical reasons like lymphedema of the arm(s) due to mastectomy for breast cancer.

Tips on Getting Accurate Readings with an Arm Cuff

Patient should be relaxed, still and sitting down in a quiet place if at all possible
Cuff should not be over clothing, arm should be bare
Sit on a chair with back supported and feet on the floor or foot stool
Arm should be at heart level and supported on a table
Legs should not be cross at the knee or ankle
No talking on the phone or be distracted

(targetbp.org. TARGET BP American Heart Association and AMA)

Wrist BP Measurements

Wrist measurements tend to be inaccurate in older adults because the artery in the wrist is not well compressed to take the reading. However, if that is the only cuff available the proper way to measure is:

1. Apply the wrist device
2. Keep elbow on table or desk with forearm bent

3. Place the wrist at heart level on your chest
4. Keep arm relaxed and hand resting against one's body
5. Measure wrist blood pressure without moving arm from seated position
6. The forearm should not be above the heart, below the heart or level on the table

(2018 American Medical Association. 18-212522:4/18)

Hypertension

....

What is it?

Hypertension is the "silent killer". Most times it does not reveal it's presence until complications set in. Every adult from the age of 20 years needs their Blood Pressure checked one to two times a year, and more often if they have hypertension.

Hypertension also known as High Blood Pressure (HBP) is the condition of chronic elevated blood pressure and occurs when either one or both of the two numbers are constantly higher than normal. When the pressure has been too high for a long period of time, it can result in serious complications. It is the leading risk factor for death and disability worldwide. Hypertension can be present without the individual showing any symptoms like dizziness, headache or chest pain. In fact one may not feel anything in spite of high blood pressure, meanwhile it is causing damage to one's organs. When high blood pressure is treated and well controlled, the complications discussed below are unlikely to take place.

What Causes Hypertension

Hypertension may be classified as Primary and Secondary.

Primary Hypertension (Essential Hypertension)

Most people with high blood pressure have primary or essential hypertension. This type has no identifiable reason for the elevated BP and it may be due to environmental or genetic factors, and it is found in about 90% or more of people who have hypertension. About 10% of people with hypertension have Secondary Hypertension and for these, there is a cause or reason for the high blood pressure.

Secondary Hypertension

Most secondary hypertension are a result of abnormalities in endocrine, vascular (blood vessels) and renal (kidney) systems. Some of the reasons for Secondary Hypertension are:

Blockage of the arteries of the kidney (renal artery stenosis)
Thyroid conditions (overactive or hyperthyroidism)

Obstructive Sleep apnea (airway gets blocked and one stops breathing during sleep)

Medications: When taken on a regular or chronic basis, drugs like steroids (Prednisone), non-steroidal drugs like Ibuprofen, Naproxen, Birth control pills, some chemotherapy medications, decongestants, Fluoxetine, and tricyclic antidepressants can all cause elevation of BP

Chronic intake of alcohol and tobacco

Categories of Hypertension

New guidelines on stages of Hypertension and when to treat depending on age were released in 2017 by the American College of Cardiology. Other organizations have other guidelines and they do not all agree with the same categories of BP in adults. The categories are based on an average of 2 or more readings obtained on 2 or more occasions.

BP Category	SBP		DBP
NORMAL (mmHg)	<120	and	<80
ELEVATED	120–129	and	<80
HYPERTENSION			
Stage 1	130–139	or	80–89
Stage 2	>140	or	>90

(2017 ACC-AHA guidelines for prevention, detection, evaluation and management of high BP In adults. Hypertension (JACC Nov 2017)

This categorization causes more people to be diagnosed with hypertension because previous guidelines defined hypertension as greater or equal to 140/90.

Complications of High Blood Pressure (Hypertension)

High blood Pressure or hypertension, if untreated can lead to:

Heart attack (blockage of vessels)
Stroke (Brain Attack)
Congestive heart failure (defect in pumping ability of the heart)
Enlarged heart or disease of the heart muscle (cardiomyopathy)
Hypertensive heart disease
Conduction problems within the heart like irregular heartbeats
Kidney disease and chronic kidney failure
Blindness

*Hypertensive heart diseases include conditions that affect the heart and are attributable to the high BP. These include:

1. Ischemic heart disease: (decreased blood flow to heart and increased oxygen demand by heart muscles)
2. Coronary artery disease (blockage of arteries supplying the heart muscle)
3. Heart failure (heart not pumping blood to organs well – Pump failure)
4. Left ventricular hypertrophy (thickened left heart muscle)

More than 50% of heart failure is attributable to hypertension, and this is very common in African Americans, who may have genetic predisposition. People with chronically elevated blood pressure have been found to have double the risk of developing coronary artery disease. So treatment of Hypertension is very Important.

Treatment of Hypertension
Introduction

It has been suggested that medications for Stage 1 should only be prescribed if the individual has also had a major adverse cardiovascular event like a heart attack or stroke; or has a history of Diabetes Mellitus, Chronic Kidney Disease, or high risk for a major cardiovascular event. Medication should be started in all who have chronic kidney disease or diabetes no matter the age for stage 1 hypertension (130–139/80–89) with targets below 130/80.

Treatment of Hypertension

If one has hypertension one needs to see a health care provider or doctor to have a complete history and physical exam done. She/he may order some tests including blood work, chest x-ray and EKG, (ECG, electrocardiogram). For those with stage 1 hypertension, some doctors will use ASCVD risk assessment mentioned previously to decide if they need just non pharmacological treatment or addition of medications.

Taking Charge of One's Blood Pressure
Non Pharmacological Treatment

These include lifestyle changes each of which reduces SBP by 4 to 8 mm Hg. Everyone with high blood pressure should use lifestyle changes to help bring down their BP. Follow a healthy lifestyle which is a low salt diet like the DASH diet, diet rich in fruits and vegetables, and physical exercise whether they are on medication or not.

LIFESTYLE CHANGES: Referred to as Therapeutic Lifestyle Changes (TLC)

The following are things one can do to take charge of one's blood pressure and get it under control. Remember one does not want to get the complications listed above. Doing these things listed below may help one avoid them.

1. Exercise regularly
   This will lower one's blood pressure. Choose an exercise that one will enjoy doing, for example it could be walking, dancing, aerobics, biking, swimming, Zumba, salsa or join a gym. Exercise about 30 minutes for 4–5 days a week. One can divide the 30 minutes into 3 ten minute sessions per day. Exercise with a friend or relative if possible to make it more interesting if one finds it boring

2. DASH DIET (Dietary Approaches to Stop Hypertension)
   This has been recommended by the US National Heart, Lung, and Blood Institute for people to prevent and control high BP. It also reduces the risk of many diseases like cancers, stroke, heart disease, heart failure, Diabetes and kidney stones. It is a diet rich in fruits and vegetables, nuts, with low-fat and non-fat dairy, lean meats, fish, and poultry, and whole grains. It limits sweetened beverages, and foods that are high in saturated fats (www.nhlbi.nih.gov/health-topics/dash-eating-plan)

3. Decrease salt intake in one's diet
   Table salt is made up of Sodium and Chloride. It is needed by the body for different processes, and to do this, the body just needs about ¼ of a teaspoon of salt each day (500 mg of sodium). Too much of it causes high blood pressure because it holds excess fluid in the body, thereby increasing the blood pressure and causing the "pump" (heart) to overwork. The American dietary guidelines and American Heart Association both recommend that salt be limited to less than 2300mg a day, which is about one teaspoon. People who are very sensitive to salt include the elderly, those with kidney disease and those who are black or African American. For those mentioned above, daily salt intake should be about 1500 mg of sodium which is about 5/8 of a teaspoon – just a little over half.

Salt Content of Foods

Most of the salt we eat may come from canned or processed foods, or added salt during cooking or at the table. Most foods, even fruits and vegetables, naturally contain sodium; however that does not constitute the bulk of the sodium we eat. The foods which may have high salt content and need to be limited include canned foods which have salt added to preserve them, pickled fish or pickles, soy sauce, Worcestershire sauce, noodles, canned soups, processed cheese, potato chips, plantain chips, salted nuts, pretzels, and salted popcorn. To make food palatable, salt substitutes can be used instead of regular salt (some of the sodium is replaced by potassium), or other combination of spices and seasonings can be used. Salting food without tasting is a habit some people have acquired and this should be avoided. One should taste the food first.

Increased Intake of Dietary Potassium

Diets rich in potassium may lower BP by 4–5 mmHg in individuals with hypertension. Fruits and vegetables like green leafy vegetables, banana, avocado, kiwi, potatoes, beans, lentils, and meats like beef, pork, and fish are rich in potassium. Some people replace part of regular salt sodium with potassium.

Weight Loss

One should make attempts to lose weight if overweight or obese. Healthy eating, exercise, weight loss medications and surgery are some of the measures. Every 2 Lbs reduction may cause a 1mm Hg drop in BP.

Reduce Alcohol Consumption

Alcohol intake should be reduced to no more than 2 drinks daily if men and women, no more than 1 drink a day. Such measures can reduce BP by up to 4 mm Hg in those with hypertension.

Medications

There are many different classes of medicines used to treat high blood pressure if one's doctor decides by one's risk calculations that one should be on medications in ADDITION to TLC. One's health care provider will choose the medication they think is best for one, taking into consideration other diseases that one may have. Under the topic of "Medications", the various types of medicines that are used to treat hypertension were discussed. Examples of medications they may start with are:

> Diuretics: (called water pills – because they may initially cause one to urinate a lot) – Hydrochlorthiazide, Chlorthalidone, Bendroflumethiazide or Indapamide
> Calcium channel blockers: Amlodipine or Nifedipine, Diltiazem, Verapamil
> ACE Inhibitors: Lisinopril, Benazepril, Ramipril
> ARBs: Losartan, Valsartan, Irbesartan
> Beta blockers: Metoprolol, Atenolol, Carvedilol

When pressures are high, combinations of these may be used. If BP is not controlled on these first line medicines or there are other medical conditions present, then other classes may be added.

1. Take medicines as prescribed
    When one requires medicine to lower one's blood pressure, do not resist getting on blood pressure medications, because it's better to have a controlled BP than have the complications that can result from chronic elevated BP
2. Know the names of one's medicines and keep a list of them on oneself. Sometimes one may need 2 or 3 different blood pressure medications to get one's blood pressure under control. The aim is to get it down to goal so one does not develop complications. Set an alarm on one's phone to remind one to take them

Side Effects of Medicines

1. Discuss any side effects from one's medicines with one's health care provider, and remember to take one's medicine as prescribed
2. Blood pressure medicines may have side effects in some individuals and so make sure one reports and discuss any new symptoms one may feel after starting a new medication with one's health care provider

Not everyone may experience a side effect from a particular medicine. All medications, including common "over the counter" ones we take for simple illnesses have side effects but they do not affect everyone in the same way.

Schedule Regular Follow up Visits with One's Health Provider

It is important that one sees one's doctor or health provider regularly to have one's blood pressure checked, do regular blood work to check one's kidney function, blood sugar and cholesterol and one's medicines refilled. Since it is a chronic disease, medication is usually taken for life unless some circumstances cause the blood pressure to come down, for example weight loss, or if it is due to a secondary reason and that has been treated.

Therapeutic Lifestyle Changes

As discussed above, these lifestyle changes should also be practiced by anyone on medications for Hypertension. Briefly these include:

1. Maintain a healthy weight
2. Healthy eating
3. Limit alcohol intake
4. Avoid use of tobacco
5. Exercise regularly

Hyperlipidemia (Increased Cholesterol and Fats in the Blood)
What is it?

Cholesterol in the blood is a result of what you produce in the liver and intestines, which makes up about 85% of your total daily needs. This amount produced depends on your genes, and the other 15% comes from what you eat.

This is increase in cholesterol and other fatty substances in the blood which are known collectively as LIPIDS. The most important lipid is Cholesterol, and some of its characteristics are noted below.

We need to remember some abbreviations mentioned below:

HDL: Cholesterol: High density lipoprotein cholesterol (Healthy Cholesterol)

LDL: Cholesterol: Low density lipoprotein cholesterol (Lousy or bad Cholesterol)

ASCVD: Atherosclerotic Cardiovascular Disease

TIA: Transient Ischemic Attack (Mini stroke)

PVD: Peripheral Vascular Disease (blockage of vessels in the legs and carotids in the neck)

Remember ASCVD include Heart attack, CAD, Angina, Stroke, TIA (mini stroke) and PVD

Characteristics of Cholesterol

1. Cholesterol is a yellow waxy fat found in all cells, but mostly in liver, and it is needed to produce other chemical substances like male and female sex hormones (testosterone, progesterone and estrogen), bile acids, Vitamin D, cortisol and steroids. It is also an important part of the cell membrane or cell coverings

2. Animal foods we get cholesterol from are: milk, cheese, meat, poultry, pork, fish, egg yolks and sea food like shrimps

3. Altogether, we need about 1000 mg of cholesterol daily for the body's functions. If one eats 200 mg in one's diet (e.g egg yoke is 200 mg), one's liver will produce about 800 mg a day to meet the daily requirements to make the important chemicals needed by the body

4. Cholesterol and Triglyceride (TG) in the blood are usually carried together with a protein in a molecule called LIPOPROTEIN. There are many types of cholesterol circulating in the blood, but the important ones are Total, LDL (low density lipoprotein called "lousy" or "bad"), and HDL (high density lipoprotein called "healthy" or "good") cholesterol. About 60–70% of cholesterol is carried in the blood as LDL. When cells need cholesterol or TG, the protein is removed and cholesterol goes into the cells for use

5. When there is excess LDL Cholesterol in the blood, it is deposited in the inside lining of the blood vessels and together with other substances this deposit is

called PLAQUE (plak). The cholesterol is at its core or center, and this leads to a condition referred to as ATHEROSCLEROSIS or hardening of the arteries. The plaques block blood vessels and affect flow of blood, which may also elevate BP. These can be likened to water carrying copper pipes blocked by lime deposits, which therefore affect flow of water

6. Good cholesterol (HDL) on the other hand helps clear the plaque from the lining of the blood vessels and takes it back to the liver
7. High cholesterol is also linked to tendon problems including inflammation
8. High cholesterol can result from diseases like Diabetes, chronic kidney disease, liver disease and Hypothyroidism
9. Chronic use of medicines like steroids and progesterone can lead to high cholesterol
10. High cholesterol has been linked to certain cancers like breast, intestines and brain cancers in animal studies, but currently, according to the American Institute for Cancer Research, there is no link between dietary cholesterol and cancer risk in humans

Triglycerides (TGs)

1. Triglycerides (TGs) are another type of fat or lipids and are chains of fatty acids which we produce in the body or get from fats in our diet. TG is the form of fat that excess calories from carbohydrates we eat are converted to and stored as fatty tissue in cells. Between meals, they are released and used to produce energy
2. Recent research has shown that high TG (hypertriglyceridemia) is associated with hardening of the arteries (artherosclerosis) which is a risk factor for heart disease, stroke and heart attacks. High levels are found in uncontrolled Diabetes Mellitus, Insulin Resistance, Obesity, Metabolic syndrome and sedentary lifestyle
3. There is genetic component to high TG causing young people to have high TGs and this is called Familiar Hypertriglyceridemia. Environment may play a part. It is passed down in families and may cause early heart disease. TG levels range from 200 to 500 mg/dl
4. Foods with a lot of simple sugars raise the TG levels and should be eaten in moderation. These include baked goods, candy, sweetened drinks and cereals, ice cream, cookies etc
5. High TGs may cause acute pancreatitis or inflammation of the pancreas
6. High TGs are associated with uncontrolled Diabetes, Liver disease, Hypothyroid, Kidney disease

Know One's Cholesterol Numbers

It is important to know what one's cholesterol numbers are: Know one's total cholesterol, HDL (good cholesterol) and LDL (bad cholesterol) and TG. The different cholesterol types are together known as "LIPID PANEL" on the blood work, and can be checked by having a fasting (8 to 12 hours of no food or drink except water) blood work drawn. Recently it has been suggested that for Lipid SCREENING non fasting blood work can be used. However, this may not apply to those who are already on cholesterol medicines or have other chronic conditions.

Ideal Numbers for Lipids

Below are for the average individual, however, if someone has had a previous mini stroke, stroke, heart attack or has a history of diabetes, their LDL number should be between 70 to 100mg/dl, with the lower number – 70 being the more acceptable one.

Total cholesterol	less than 200 mg/dl (5.18mmol/l)
LDL cholesterol	Less than 130mg/dl (3.37mmol/l)
HDL cholesterol	More than 40 (1.04mmol/l) in men and 50 (1.3mmol/l) in women
Triglycerides	Less than 150mg/dl (1.7mmol/l)

Research on the effects of Dietary Cholesterol and Other Lipids

1. Lately scientific evidence show that one's body's total cholesterol levels are affected more by the cholesterol one's body produces rather than what one eats in one's diet, and so dietary cholesterol is not the enemy
2. Decreasing saturated fats affects LDL (lousy) cholesterol more than reducing dietary cholesterol
3. Trans Fatty acids (TFAs) are formed mostly from vegetable oils by adding some hydrogen atoms (partial hydrogenated fatty acids) to convert into shortening and margarine (solid fat). They have been found to raise one's TG, total and LDL cholesterol and lower one's (HDL). Many prepared foods like cookies, snacks, cakes, may contain Trans fatty acids
4. Trans Fatty acids increase one's risk for heart attacks, stroke and DM, and so the FDA of America has mandated they be removed from foods by 2020. Some however, occur naturally in small amounts in certain foods like meat and dairy products
5. The interesting fact is that complete hydrogenated fats do not have same harmful effects and do not cause significant cardiovascular risk as the partial hydrogenated ones

Treatment of Hyperlipidemia

It is important that high cholesterol is treated because it can contribute to ASCVD – heart attacks, coronary artery disease, stroke, TIA, and PVD. It is treated by

Therapeutic Lifestyle Changes (TLC) and Medications. Whether on medication or not, the lifestyle changes described elsewhere apply here as well.

Therapeutic Lifestyle Changes (TLC)

Low cholesterol or healthy diet – fruits and vegetables, whole grains, lean meats, fish, and poultry
Exercise and physical activity
Weight loss
Stop smoking
Alcohol in moderation or not at all

Eat Healthy Foods

The following types of foods will help bring cholesterol down.

1. Eat high fiber containing foods like whole grains, citrus fruits, okra, egg plants, apples, strawberries, and other vegetables. Good sources of soluble fiber include oats, oranges, pears, carrots, dried peas and beans. Whole grains have all the edible part of the grain and examples are Brown rice, Wild rice, Whole-grain barley, whole grain wheat, Quinoa, Buckwheat, whole rye, pop-corn, Millet, Sorghum, Bulgur (cracked wheat)
2. Eat fatty fish like salmon, mackerel, and tuna which contain good fats like omega 3. Minimize red meats and choose lean cuts trimming off fat as needed
3. Choose dairy products with low fat content like skim, 1% or 2% milk, low fat cheese, cottage cheese and yogurt. Make choices like baking and grilling instead of frying, cutting down on butter and margarine, and using "good" oils like olive oil, and vegetable oils. Avoid or cut down on Trans fats foods. All the above, help to cut down on cholesterol and saturated fat content of foods
4. Eggs, though high in cholesterol, have not been found to promote or increase cardiovascular disease, however they do in those with Diabetes mellitus

Medications for Treating High Cholesterol

Not everyone with high cholesterol is treated with medications. Every one has to engage in a heart healthy lifestyle (TLC) whether they are on medicines or not. If one has never had a ASCVD, then one's risk for ASCVD can be assessed by their doctor using the American college of Cardiology ASCVD Risk estimator which is used if LDL-C is less than190 and there is no ASCVD. This will give a person's 10 year risk for a heart attack or death from stroke or CAD. One can go online and calculate one's own risk (www.cvriskcalculator.com) by putting in some of one's numbers including race, presence of hypertension, diabetes etc. Ideally, doctors should calculate one's risk and a joint decision can be made about starting medications to treat one's high cholesterol. This risk calculator is for those between 40–79 years of age.

Statins

Examples of these are Atorvastatin, Pravastatin, Rosuvastatin and Lovastatin. These help to lower blood cholesterol and have been shown to decrease death from heart attacks and strokes. Statins have been found to decrease the risk of deaths in breast, prostate, lung, and bowel cancers by 25% to 50%, and may reduce risk of developing colorectal and skin cancer.

Side Effects of Statins

Ways to decrease muscle pain include taking Co enzyme Q10 or reducing the frequency of taking statins to every other day, or to a few days of the week. Reducing the dose or changing to another statin may also be helpful.

Generally, statins are safe and well tolerated by most people, however, a small number of patients on it may develop side effects. There have been a lot of news in the media about side effects of statins and so those who sometimes need to be on them refuse to take them.

They are the only anti-cholesterol medications which have been proven in many studies to reduce stroke, heart attacks and other atherosclerotic conditions.

1. They may cause a slight increase in blood sugar levels, but this can be followed by one's doctor, and exercising and healthy eating can however bring the blood sugar down. Most people think the benefits outweigh the risk of developing prediabetes
2. Statins may cause some muscle aches, joint pain, leg pain, muscle cramps or weakness in some people but these are not common. A very rare side effect is called rhabdomyolysis where muscle cells break down and cause the urine to turn brown. One has to report to a doctor immediately if such symptoms happen, but they are very rare. Less than 10% of people develop any muscle related side effects
3. If a muscle related side effect occurs, inform one's doctor. One may change to another statin, reduce the dose, reduce the number of days one takes the medicines or be put on a different anticholesterol medication. Some patients take statins 3x/week
4. Taking Co enzymeQ10 (CoQ10, Ubiquinone) may decrease the leg cramps or pain, since deficiency of this substance causes muscle aches, and statins tend to reduce the levels in those taking it
5. A few people may have diarrhea, bloating, vomiting, and stomach aches, but these tend to be present initially, and normally resolve within a short time
6. A small proportion – about 2–3% may have elevated liver enzymes on blood work, but this may subside with dose reduction

7. Cognitive impairment (memory issues) have been reported in some individuals who start statins and FDA of the US has changed labelling of inserts with the medications to read that there is concern for cognitive impairment. However, some studies do not support this claim and have found no link between the use of statins, and worse cognitive function (Kwok Leung Ong; Margaret J. Morris et al. Relationship of Lipids and Lipid-Lowering Medications With Cognitive Function. Am J Epidemiol. 2018;187(4):767–776). Recent Australian study found that statins taken for 6 years was not linked to cognitive decline, but rather they may be beneficial to preventing cognitive impairment (No link between statins and cognitive decline Medscape-Nov 22, 2019).

8. At the same time, there are other studies which have shown statins tend to help those who have dementia, and also the association of high midlife high total cholesterol and increased risk of Alzheimer's Disease

9. Avoid grapefruit juice when on statins because it affects the liver's ability to break them down. This is especially true for Atorvastatin, Simvastatin and Lovastatin

10. Take statins at bedtime, since one will not be doing much walking at night, and so less chance of getting leg cramps

11. Low vitamin D may cause muscle cramps like statins do, so ask one's doctor about one's Vitamin D levels. Dark skin lowers vitamin D produced with the sun's help, and so supplements may be needed if one does not obtain enough from foods which include: milk, yogurt, cheese, fatty fish (tuna and sardine), egg yolk, and beef liver.

Other Anticholesterol Medicines

Other medicines are available for treatment but they have not been found to decrease death from heart attacks and strokes, although they lower cholesterol levels.

1. Examples include Ezetimibe, Fibrates, Niacin, Colestipol; one's health professional will decide what to use for one based on one's numbers

2. Ezetimibe when added to statins has been found to reduce coronary events

3. Medicines given to increase HDL-C have unfortunately not been found to lower ASCVD

4. There are new injectable anti-cholesterol medicines but they are very expensive and are not commonly used. They may be suitable for adults with atherosclerotic disease who are on maximum doses of statins but still have high LDL levels or those who cannot tolerate statins or those with familial hypercholesterolemia. They are called PCSK9 inhibitors and examples are Repatha and Praluent, but they are very expensive and cost almost $15,000 a year. They are given as subcutaneous (under the skin) injections one to two times a month by the patient

Dietary Supplements (OTC) for Lowering Cholesterol Levels

OTC supplements used to lower lipids or cholesterol include:

1. Niacin(Vitamin B3), fish oil or omega 3 fatty acids, krill oil, and flax seed oil
2. B vitamins like Vitamin B3, and Vitamin B5 have been used by some people
3. Plant sterols and stanols (phytosterols added to vegetable spreads and cereals or as supplements). Phytosterols are plant steroids found in their cell walls, and are similar to cholesterol. There are over 200 of them, and they can compete with absorption of cholesterol in the bowels and so eventually lead to decrease cholesterol in the blood. The US National Cholesterol Education program advices people with high cholesterol to eat 2 grams of phytosterols every day
4. Fiber supplements like Psyllium, Benefiber, Metamucil or Fibercon may be in pill or powder forms
5. Soy products like soy isoflavone supplements
6. Policosanol from cane sugar has been found in some studies to lower cholesterol
7. On the other hand, garlic, Chromium,Vitamin C, and green tea have not been found to lower cholesterol in reliable studies
8. Red Yeast Rice (RYR) is a chinese medicinal supplement and is often used to treat high cholesterol; however, most of it may contain added chemicals similar to those found in Lovastatin which is one of the statins. It is produced from rice fermented by a yeast that produces a chemical similar to active ingredient found in Lovastatin. One has to be careful where one purchases these, since it may be adulterated by other chemicals or Lovastatin itself

Reminders on Your Radar

Cholesterol and other fat components are called lipids and excessive amounts lead to the condition of hyperlipidemia. When the blood is examined for lipids we concentrate on four main types in the panel: Total, LDL (lousy chol.), HDL (healthy chol.), and Triglycerides. These four affect one's risk for acquiring diseases like coronary heart disease, peripheral vascular disease, strokes and heart attacks collectively known as atherosclerotic cardiovascular diseases (ASCVD). Lifestyle changes are the first line of treatment to lower one's numbers of total cholesterol and LDL, and these are: healthy eating, healthy weight, weight loss and exercise. If these do not reduce one's numbers, then depending on one's calculated risk for ASCVD, one may need to go on medications to lower one's cholesterol.

Heart Diseases

....

What Is the Heart?

The heart is basically a **Muscle Pump** about the size of one's fist and is nestled between the two lungs in the chest cavity. It is made up of four chambers, the two smaller top chambers separated from the larger lower chambers by valves. The heart has blood vessels located on the outside walls which supply oxygen and nutrients to it, and an electrical conduction system which regulates the rate and rhythm of the heart (the number of beats and the type of beat). There are several diseases which affect the heart's vessels, muscle, valves, and its conduction of electric signals and a few common ones will be discussed here.

Coronary Arteries

The arteries around the heart which supply the heart muscle (myocardium) are called CORONARY ARTERIES, and they carry nutrients, glucose and oxygen to it just like arteries do for other organs. The deoxygenated blood (blood which has oxygen removed from it) is carried away by cardiac veins.

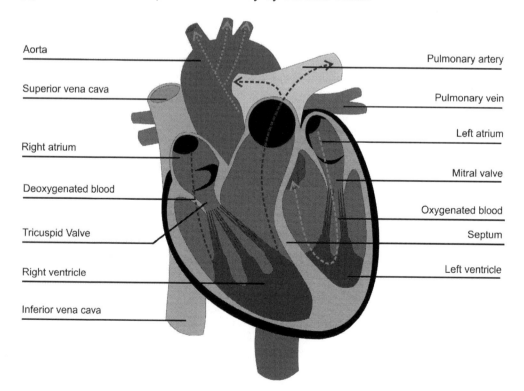

Diagram of the Heart showing how blood flows through it

Atherosclerosis/Arteriosclerosis (Ar-te-rio-skle-rosis)

What is it?

Hardening of the arteries also known as atherosclerosis affects the coronary arteries which supply the heart muscle. When these are blocked by lipids and other substances one has coronary artery disease which can result in chest pain or angina if there is not adequate supply of blood to meet the demands of that part of the heart muscle.

Any artery in the body can become narrowed or clogged over time with fatty substances especially cholesterol and this is termed "hardening of the arteries". The medical term is ATHEROSCLEROSIS (also referred to as ARTERIOSCLEROSIS). The process starts in childhood as FATTY STREAKS in the lining of the walls of the arteries. With age, genetics and the type of diet we eat, the amount increases, gets thicker and hardens in the lining of the vessel. This fatty build up is then called PLAQUE (PLAK). When it occurs in the vessels of the legs, arms or in the neck (carotid arteries) it is known as PERIPHERAL VASCULAR or ARTERY DISEASE (PVD or PAD). I describe CORONARY ARTERY DISEASE (CAD) below, which occurs when the vessels supplying the heart muscle are affected.

Coronary Artery Disease (CAD)

What is it?

When the coronary arteries (blood vessels which supply blood to the heart muscle itself) become narrowed as described above under arteriosclerosis, the condition is known as CORONARY ARTERY DISEASE (CAD). The narrowed artery causes less blood flow and therefore less oxygen or nutrients to that area of the heart muscle it supplies. Some of the names of the coronary arteries are Left Anterior Descending (LAD), Circumflex, (CA), Right Anterior Descending (RAD) and Posterior descending (PDA) arteries. Each coronary artery supplies blood to a specific area of the heart and so if an artery is blocked, then the muscles in that area are affected (due to decreased blood supply and oxgyen), resulting in ischemia (inadequate blood supply) or death of muscle (infarction).

Angina and Heart Attacks

What are They?

Dead or dying heart muscle is what is known as HEART ATTACK or MYOCARDIAL INFARCTION. A similar situation is found in a STROKE which is sometimes referred to as a "BRAIN ATTACK" or CEREBROVASCULAR ACCIDENT (CVA).

Angina (An-gia-na) is when the decreased blood supply to the heart muscles resulting from the narrowed vessels (CAD) causes chest pain or discomfort. One can have CAD without a heart attack but it can result in chest pain or angina when there is increased activity or emotional stress. When the pain goes away with rest, it is known as Stable Angina. When chest pain occurs without activity (at rest) in someone with stable CAD then that signals a worsening situation and its called Unstable Angina.

Heart Attack (Myocardial Infarction)

Heart Attack or myocardial infarction, also known as ACUTE CORONARY SYNDROME occurs when there is the sudden decrease of blood supply through a coronary artery of the heart leading to dead or dying heart muscle (infarction) if process is not reversed quickly. The process starts when the surface of a plaque (see above) is eroded or ruptured. It attracts platelets and other clot-building substances resulting in the formation of a clot. This clot (called thrombus) enlarges and then can block the arteries even more, causing ischemia (lack of blood supply), angina (chest pain) or even a heart attack if artery is partially or completely blocked. Depending on the vessel involved a heart attack can be mild or massive.

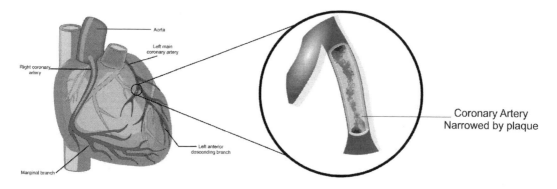

Heart Coronary Vessels – Insert Shows Narrowed Coronary Artery

Widow Maker Heart Attack

This is when the blockage is in one of the main artery called the Left Anterior Descending (LAD). If it is completely blocked it results in a massive heart attack which in most times leads to death. It can also occur in women and the symptoms are similar to heart attacks caused by other blocked vessels, however it is more serious due to the large area of heart muscle it supplies therefore the higher incidence of death.

Other Causes of MI

Most MI occur as a result of a thrombus, however there are other causes which are not common and may involve the coronary vessels or heart muscle. These include trauma to vessels, drug use (cocaine, ephedrine), aneurysm (condition causing ballooning of a vessel), anemia, abnormalities of the vessels, closure of vessel due to variant angina described below, inflammation of the coronary vessels from diseases. Others are enlarged muscles of the ventricle from muscle disease (cardiomyopathy) or from Left ventricle enlargement e.g. from severe hypertension, low blood pressure (hypotension) or severe anemia. Sometimes emboli substances like cholesterol, fat, air, inflammatory cells may travel into the coronary artery and block it. (Myocardial Infarction Cardiology. Medscape.com July 19th, 2018). All these can result in decreased blood flow to heart muscle (ischemia) and or result in death of the heart muscle (infarction).

Prinzmetal Angina
What is it?

This is also called Vasospastic Angina, Variant Angina or Coronary Artery Vasospasm and it is a rare condition resulting in chest pain which is not caused by a blocked coronary artery, but occurs as a result of spasm of muscle within the coronary artery wall. It occurs at rest or even during sleep, or early morning, and is not brought on by exercise or exertion as in normal angina. Pain may be severe and may spread from left chest into arm, shoulder, and jaws lasting from a few minutes to half an hour. Cardiac stress tests and other tests are normal and the coronary arteries do not show blockage. It is rare and one has to do several heart tests in order for this diagnosis to be made. It is common in smokers and those with hypertension and high cholesterol. It has been also found in people who are stressed, those who use cocaine, during alcohol withdrawal and even during environmental changes like cold weather.

Signs and Symptoms of A Heart Attack

Prior to a heart attack – even a few days before – one may have some chest discomfort or feel tired or unwell. However during a heart attack itself the symptoms may include:

1. Pain on the LEFT side or CENTER of the chest, which may move into the left arm, shoulder, neck, jaw, or back. This is also known as ANGINA (an-gia-na)
2. The pain may be sharp, squeezing, pressure like, or intense. It may be accompanied by shortness of breath, rapid heart rate, irregular heartbeat, nausea or vomiting, feeling of indigestion or heart burn, sweating, dizziness and anxiety
3. Pain may last for a few minutes and then go away and come back. As mentioned this is due to decreased blood flow to the heart muscle as blood supply is either decreased or cut off due to blockage or spasm (contraction) of one of the coronary arteries

Atypical Presentation in Women

According to the American Heart Association and US department of Health and Human services, these are more atypical symptoms women should be aware of.

1. Women tend to experience more shortness of breath, nausea and vomiting, and back or jaw pain
2. Chest symptoms described above and pain in upper body, shoulder, either one of both arms, back, neck, upper stomach, light headedness, dizziness, nausea, breaking out in a cold sweat, unusual fatigue and shortness of breath

One has to immediately call for help. In the USA call 911 right away, or in other countries call the phone number for emergency medical services (ambulance) so that one is taken to the hospital.

1. If emergency medical services are not available let someone drive one to a hospital immediately. Women tend to ignore warning signs of a heart attack and this leads to more damage of the heart muscle or even death when treatment is delayed
2. There is a saying "Time is Muscle", so getting help immediately may save some heart muscle from irreversible death or damage

Treatment of Heart Attacks

Time is of an essence in a heart attack, and the expression "time is muscle" is used to signify the importance of getting treatment as soon as possible, otherwise the heart muscle dies from lack of blood supply. Early treatment is the key to saving the heart muscle. In countries with advanced ambulance or emergency medical services, treatment starts before arriving at the hospital. However, it may be wise to take a few ASPIRIN if help is delayed. CHEW and swallow 325 mg or four 75 mg or 81 mg aspirins (low dose Aspirin) while one is waiting for help, or before being driven to the hospital in countries where emergency medical transportation is not readily accessible.

1. Use chewable Aspirin not the enteric coated one which is not absorbed as quickly enough. Aspirin is a blood thinner and prevents more clots from forming by slowing the blood clotting action of platelets. It helps keep the blood flowing in the coronary artery
2. On the way to the hospital, Emergency workers may give Nitroglycerin tablet under the tongue or as a spray in the mouth in the Ambulance. In the hospital a patient will be given aspirin, oxygen, and NITROGLYCERIN as a spray, pill on

tongue or patch on the arm. This medicine dilates or opens up blood vessels so that blood can flow easily through them and it helps with pain as well

3. One may also be given some Morphine Sulphate injection for the pain and anxiety which are usually present

4. Quick arrival to an emergency department prevents further damage to the heart muscle. Death or damage of a large part of the heart muscle results in decreased pumping of the heart and decreased supply of oxygen and nutrients to other parts of the body

5. More than 50% of deaths from heart attacks occur in the first hour and is mostly due to an irregular heartbeat called ventricular fibrillation which frequently develops

6. Other hospital treatments include blood work, EKG, other imaging studies, and if required medications to break up the clot and prevent platelets from sticking together

7. A procedure to open up the blood vessel and restore flow of blood called ANGIOPLASTY or PCI (Percutaneous Coronary Intervention) is also done at times in a Catheterization (CATH) Lab in the hospital. A device is guided into the vessel and at the blocked site a balloon is inflated to open the vessel and then most times a STENT (small pipe-like device) is placed at the site to keep the vessel open and prevent blockage within a short time

8. Sometimes a Coronary artery bypass graft (CABG) (car-bage) surgery is performed, especially if several of the vessels have significant blockage or the sites are not amendable to angioplasty and stenting. These procedures will enable blood flow to the heart muscles and keep the heart working well. During the CABG surgery, an artery or vein from another part of the body is used to bypass the area of blockage of the artery supplying the part of the heart muscle involved. This is major open heart surgery by a highly trained cardiovascular surgeon and is done in specialized centers

Risk Factors for Coronary Artery Disease (CAD)

As with all diseases, certain risk factors have been found to predispose people to develop CAD. When these are lowered, it will lower one's chance of developing CAD and other ASCVD like heart attacks, peripheral vascular disease (blockage of major vessels in the neck and legs) and strokes. We will discuss some of these below.

Certain common risk factors for developing CAD have been identified. These include:

1. Hypertension, Diabetes, high Cholesterol, and Obesity especially in the mid abdomen or commonly called "apple shape" body type

2. Male gender, family history of CAD, and genetics

3. Smoking, excessive alcohol intake, and lack of physical activity
4. Postmenopausal women. Women aged 55 years and over. Before menopause, women have a lower risk for CAD, but after menopause their risk approaches that of males
5. Psychological and social factors also play a part in developing CAD related problems especially in women. These factors include depression, stress, and lack of social support or interaction with others
6. Conclusions from several studies show that long term use of Hormone Replacement Therapy by postmenopausal women increases the risk for heart attack, stroke and even breast cancer. Short term use in early menopause is fine after informed decision by a patient and her doctor

It is important for women to know that both heart disease and stroke kill more women than breast cancer BUT the good news is that most risk factors can be modified by lifestyle changes and medications if needed.

How to Modify Risk Factors FOR CAD

The aim is to modify the risk factors so one does not get CAD, heart attack or stroke. This is done by lifestyle changes and treatment with appropriate medications.
Modifiable Risk factors are:

1. CHOLESTEROL: Reducing the levels of lipids especially bad cholesterol (LDL) and triglyceride in one's blood by diet, exercise or medication, will lower one's cholesterol levels and help prevent coronary artery disease and stroke. Dietary changes which help with cholesterol include increased fruits and vegetables, increased fiber and fish, and less animal proteins like meats. If these do not get the numbers down, medicines are used
2. STATINS can reduce the lipids that are in plaque and may even decrease the thickness of the plaque in the vessels. Other groups of medicines are also available, with recent introduction of an injectable group (PCSK 9 inhibitor) which also has powerful effects on lowering LDL (bad cholesterol) levels in those with established arteriosclerotic disease. One's doctor may recommend that one start medicine if one's cholesterol is high and one has other risk factors
3. HYPERTENSION: Lifestyle changes like eating a healthy diet, low salt intake, DASH diet, exercise with weight loss if needed, together with medications taken to lower blood pressure will help one from getting hypertensive heart disease. Hypertensive heart disease discussed elsewhere is caused by the effect of chronic high blood pressure on the heart's muscle, coronary artery and the conduction system. These will manifest as coronary heart disease, angina, heart attack, enlarged muscles of the heart (Left Ventricular Hypertrophy, or

cardiomyopathy), congestive heart failure (pump failure) and irregular heart beats (cardiac arrhythmia). (Kamran Riaz et al. Hypertensive heart disease. emedicine.medscape.com. Dec 2014.) Sometimes one may need to take 2 or 3 different medicines in order for blood pressure to get to goal

4. DEPRESSION and PSYCHOSOCIAL STRESSORS: Factors like stress at home and work, frequent loneliness, and lack of social support all increase a woman's risk for developing CAD. It is important that if one is suffering from any of the above, ask one's health care provider so one can receive help through counseling. In the case of depression, one may require medicines. Increasing one's circle of friends may help with loneliness, or volunteering and giving back to others, results in happiness and increases one's circle of friends

5. SMOKING: This is a greater risk factor for the development of CAD in women compared to men. Smoking causes over 480,000 deaths a year in the US alone, and according to the US surgeon general's report in 2014, of all the deaths related to smoking, about 28% of them were from ischemic or coronary heart disease. Nicotine causes PLAQUE build up in the lining of the artery. Smoking cessation is important and smokers are encouraged to stop smoking with the aid of medications, counseling, nicotine replacement, or quit cold turkey (stop on their own without any aid)

6. OBESITY: Weight loss is often accompanied by lowering of Blood Pressure and Cholesterol. Healthy diet and exercise, approved weight loss medications and weight loss surgery, are all means which either individually or in combination can help reduce one's risk of developing CAD

Healthy Habits Which Can Prevent CAD in Women

In a recent analysis of data from a big study involving over 60,000 women known as the Nurses' Health Study, the researchers concluded after analyzing data collected for over 20 years on these women, that there are six healthy habits which if adopted by women can prevent up to almost 75% of coronary artery disease in women aged twenty years and over. These include:

1. Exercising about 2 1/2 hours each week (30 minutes 5 days a week)
2. Maintaining a lower body mass index (meaning maintaining a healthy weight)
3. Minimizing television watching to less than 7 hours a week
4. Stop smoking tobacco if one is a smoker
5. Eating healthy – Fruits, vegetables, whole grain, high fiber, fish and less red meat
6. Drinking up to one alcoholic drink a day (see note below on alcohol intake)
    They also found out that about 46% of incidence of Hypertension, Diabetes and high Cholesterol were attributable to poor lifestyle (Journal of American College of Cardiology. January 2015)

The Benefits of Walking in Preventing CAD

The above study emphasizes the importance of, and reasons for lifestyle changes. It is not easy to change behavior, but one can start and encourage a friend or spouse to join one in doing the above and positive changes will result. The important thing is consistency and the life-long goal of incorporating healthy living in one's daily life, and not just a short few months' attempt to change habits one has been used to.

Recent studies have shown that either walking or jogging, for example, can decrease the risk of high blood pressure, diabetes, high cholesterol and cardiovascular disease. (Williams, P., Thompson, P. Arterioscler Thromb Vasc Biol. 2013 May: 331085–1091). One should aim at 10,000 steps a day which also has the ability to decrease what is known as insulin resistance and decrease blood sugar levels, with accompanying weight loss. 5000–7000 may be fine.

How to Get Those Steps In

According to the United States CDC (Centers for Disease Control and Prevention), adults need to get in 150 minutes a week of moderate activity, and this may translate into walking about 7,000 to 8,000 steps a day. Many people invest in a PEDOMETER which can count the number of steps one takes, or a more sophisticated ACTIVITY TRACKER (fitness tracker) Applewatch, etc. which can be used alone, or is synchronized to one's smart phone and so one can keep track of how many steps one is taking in a day, how many calories one eats, as well as one's heart rate.

The activity trackers have become more affordable. Some smart phones also have an Application one can download for counting steps.

Alcohol Intake and Heart Health

The issue about alcohol intake and health can be confusing due to the fact that the risk of CAD as it relates to alcohol, changes with the amount of alcohol consumed.

1. Research shows that lower amounts of consumption like one glass for women and 1–2 glasses for men/day may be beneficial in some ways to one's health. So drinking one glass of red wine (4 oz.) with one's dinner every evening, will have health benefits
2. However; if one was involved mostly with binge or periodic heavy drinking or heavy constant drinking, those are harmful. Heart and brain problems associated with heavy alcohol intake include high blood pressure, strokes, dementia, enlarged size of the heart, heart muscle enlargement, and irregular heart-beats to name a few
3. Such heavy drinking can lead to increased risk of many cancers including breast, mouth, esophagus and liver cancers to name a few

4. So, it is important to interpret news media reports of the benefits of alcohol correctly, and realize that the risks outweigh the so-called benefits of alcohol consumption if it involves excessive amounts

Homocysteine levels

It is thought that high levels of homocysteine which is an amino acid in the blood may contribute to plaque formation in the blood vessels causing increased risk of coronary disease and stroke. Therefore some cardiologists recommend that patients with high risk of these two conditions take Folate, or folic acid, Vitamins B6 (pyridoxine) and B12 which have been found to lower homocysteine levels.

Treating or modifying all the above mentioned risk factors is the key to avoiding any adverse cardiac event or stroke in the first place.

Coronary Microvascular Disease or Small Vessel Disease
What is it?

This is also called "Microvascular Angina" or "Cardiac syndrome X" and like obstructive coronary heart disease, may cause chest pain or angina, but it is not a result of an obstructed large coronary artery but rather of the smaller vessels which branch off the main arteries. It is common in young women, but can occur in older women and men as well.

1. It is thought to be due to spasm of the blood vessels as well as disease of the lining of the small vessels, resulting in their inability to relax or expand to allow blood to flow to the muscles
2. The chest pain is not related to exercises and physical activities, but may come on during normal activities or during stress
3. Apart from chest pain, there may be fatigue, and shortness of breath. The risk factors for developing this are similar to those listed under obstructive coronary artery disease
4. Low estrogen levels around menopause seem to be a risk factor

Treatment

It is quite difficult to diagnose because although a stress test is abnormal, cardiac imaging shows normal large coronary vessels which are not obstructed. After various tests are done similar to those listed under coronary artery disease, a diagnosis is made, and risk factors will have to be controlled, e.g. blood pressure and high cholesterol. It is then treated with other medicines like Aspirin to thin the blood, and Nitroglycerin to cause the vessels to relax.

Sudden Cardiac Arrest or Death
What is it?

This is a term to describe a situation when the heart stops beating suddenly in a person previously healthy or with known cardiac problems. It is due to abnormal electrical conduction through the heart. It is not a heart attack (which has to do with circulation problems), but a heart attack can also cause it as well. In the USA, about 300,000 people die each year of sudden cardiac arrest. As soon as this happens, other organs like respiratory system and brain will also stop functioning with loss in breathing and consciousness because they need blood containing oxygen and energy to function.

The conditions that can lead to sudden cardiac arrest include:

1. Heart attacks, inherited heart diseases, and cardiomyopathy (enlarged muscle of the heart)
2. Severe heart failure, structural abnormalities of the heart and aortic valves, and serious irregular heart rhythms
3. Electrocution – which affects the heart's electrical function
4. It can happen in both young and old, and one commonly hears of young athletes who die of sudden cardiac arrest while practicing with a sports team

Treatment

If this occurs out of the hospital, CPR (Cardiopulmonary Resuscitation) and use of an Automated External Defibrillator (AED) may save a life until patient is taken to the hospital for management. Survival rate is low, but AEDs have saved lives.

Prevention in Living Relatives

It is important that someone whose family member dies of sudden cardiac death lets their doctor know so a careful history and physical exam, and if needed cardiac studies are done to ascertain if there may be a genetic or familial cardiac problem associated with the death. Lowering risk factors for heart attacks may help prevent this, since they can cause irregular heart beats leading to SCD.

Reminders on Your Radar

When a plaque breaks open from the inside wall of the artery a clot (thrombus) forms on the top, and this can block a vessel resulting in a heart attack. There are many risk factors resulting in blockage of vessels and some of the common ones are Diabetes Mellitus, high Cholesterol, tobacco use, Hypertension, lack of exercise and Obesity. Making sure lifestyle changes occur and medical conditions are treated to goal can decrease the risk of Coronary Artery Disease and heart attacks.

Congestive Heart Failure
(Heart Failure, CHF)

....

What Is It?

CHF is due to the heart not being able to pump blood around. It's a "pump failure" and has many causes. These include prolonged uncontrolled hypertension, coronary artery disease and irregular heart rhythm. It causes shortness of breath, difficulty in breathing, fluid retention in the lungs, extremities and abdomen.

Heart failure, also known as CHF, occurs when the heart is not able to contract well and send sufficient blood to the other organs of the body. Heart failure is not the same as heart attack, but in this case there is a weakened pump (heart) due to weakened muscles, and so other organs are deprived of important oxygen and nutrients. Due to the failure of the PUMP, there is fluid buildup (or back up) in the lungs, ankles, legs and abdomen thus the term CONGESTIVE. However, recently, the medical world prefers it to be called "Heart Failure". It is a serious problem, and can be debilitating and cause death. Each year in the USA, more than 3 million people are diagnosed with it. There are many causes which can lead to heart failure.

Common Causes of Heart Failure

- Long-standing or uncontrolled High Blood Pressure
- Coronary Heart Disease (heart artery problems)
- Heart Attack (damaged heart muscle so heart is not pumping well)
- Heart valve diseases (valves separate different chambers of the heart and can be abnormally narrowed, or cause leakage or backflow of blood when diseased)
- Heart muscle (also called myocardium) diseases
- Irregular heart beat (Causes pumping action to be weak)
- Congenital heart diseases (Certain heart conditions that people may be born with)
- Other diseases can affect the heart and cause heart failure. Examples are thyroid diseases and diabetes
- Medications like cancer drugs may cause cancer therapy induced cardiomyopathy

Symptoms of Heart Failure

The excess fluid which results because the pump is not working well, accumulates in the lungs and the lower extremities. Therefore, there are symptoms like:

- Shortness of breath and difficulty in breathing; either at rest or with activity
- Severe shortness of breath with cough at night, not relieved by sitting up
- Cough and wheezing (whistling sound in the chest like in an asthma attack)
- General fatigue or tiredness
- Swelling of the ankles, feet, hands or abdomen (belly)
- Rapid weight gain from accumulated fluid
- Rapid heartbeat (palpitations)
- Difficulty breathing when lying down flat (one uses more pillows or has to sit up in order to be comfortable breathing)
- Sitting up or reclining to sleep or lie down due to difficulty in breathing when lying flat.

What may not be Heart Failure

One needs to seek medical attention when several of the above symptoms are present and point to possible heart failure. Remember, some individuals may get one of the above symptoms in isolation and that does not mean they have heart failure. For example swollen ankles in isolation may not be heart failure. If you sit in a vehicle for a few hours, your ankles or feet may swell, and this does not mean you have heart failure. To prevent swelling in this case, you need to get out of the car, or stand up and walk around for a few minutes when travelling long distances whether in a car or plane. You may also use compression stockings or socks and also keep legs elevated. It is when several of these symptoms are occurring and one also has the risk factors or conditions mentioned under "CAUSES" above; that one needs to be concerned and see a health professional to find out if one has heart failure. However, any one of the symptoms above still needs to be investigated for other conditions.

Treatment of Heart Failure

After taking a history and doing a physical exam, various tests including blood work, chest X-ray, EKG, Ultrasound of the heart (Echocardiogram), and other heart tests may be done to ascertain the diagnosis and the severity of heart failure. The following are used to keep it under control.

An important measurement by an Echo or Stress test is the Ejection Fraction (EF) which tends to decrease in moderate to serve Heart Failure (normal is 55–70%). It tells one the percentage of blood leaving the heart each time it contracts.

- Treatment is aimed at relieving symptoms and helping the heart beat stronger
- Medications can cause the shortness of breath, difficulty in breathing, impaired pumping of the heart, swelling of the feet and fatigue to improve.

- After initial treatment, one has to be on these medications for life unless the cause of the heart failure is reversible or it is curable.
- Some of the medications may be from the classes mentioned under hypertension: It is important to be on a Beta blocker, ACE (Angiotensin converting enzyme) inhibitor or ARB (Angiotensin receptor blocker) and sometimes a Diuretic or digoxin.
- Examples of some of the medicines in the various classes are: Lisinopril, Losartan, Carvedilol, Furosemide, Hydrochlorothiazide, and Spironolactone.
- New Medicines For Heart Failure

    New classes of medicines have also been included to help decrease exacerbations and death. Examples are Sacubitril/Valsartan (Entresto) used together with others and in place of ACEI or ARB mentioned above. It reduces risk of death from cardiovascular disease and hospitalization for HF.

    Dapagliflozin (Jardiance) an oral diabetes medicine has just been approved to be used to reduce hospitalization for heart failure and the risk of cardiovascular death in people with chronic heart failure.
- Sometimes, some people have to be on oxygen on a regular basis if heart failure is severe.
- It has been found that two particular medicines benefit black patients with heart failure and these are Hydralazine, and Isosorbide dinitrate both of which relax arteries

IMPLANTED DEVICES FOR TREATING HEART FAILURE

Some individuals with heart failure need to have a device implanted near the heart to help prevent an irregular heart beat which may result in sudden death, and its called Implantable Cardioverter Defibrillators (ICD). Another device is the Cardiac Resynchronization Therapy device which has electric leads in the left and right ventricles to help the heart beat effectively and supply all the organs with oxygen and nutrients more efficiently. Sometimes a pacemaker is implanted.

Reminders on Your Radar

Congestive Heart Failure or Heart Failure (HF) is a common disease and is caused by the inability of the heart to pump blood to supply the organs in the body. In the acute stage, the patient may be given diuretics (water pill) to flush out the excess fluids. The patient has to be on medications to improve the pumping action, remove fluids and help the patient breath better. Most of the medicines are in certain groups used to treat hypertension. In a person with HF weight gain is a sign of fluid overload and so if one gains more than 2 pounds (or 1 kilo) above normal weight, it is a good idea to go and see the doctor to check for excess fluid retention.

Irregular or Abnormal Heart Beats

....

There are different types of irregular heart rhythms and some are benign like Preventricular contractions (PVCs) while others are more serious like Atrial Fibrillation which can cause strokes if not treated.

When a doctor listens to your heart, he or she is listening to the rhythm or the way the heart beats as well as taking note of the heart rate. Heart rate is measured as BEATS PER MINUTE. Normal heart rate is about 60 to 100 beats/minutes. (60–100/min.)

Slow Heart Rate (Bradycardia) (bra-de-car-diea)
What is it?

Bradycardia is when the heart is beating less than 60 beats per minute. When there are problems with the heart's electrical conduction system or its natural pacemaker called the Sinoatrial node, the result may be a slow heart rate. Some people may naturally have a low heart rate – and this is often seen in runners, especially marathon runners and they do not have any symptoms. Some medicines may also cause slow heart rate e.g. beta blockers, opoids, and even alcohol

Signs and Symptoms

These may include tiredness, fatigue, dizziness or passing out (fainting), because blood is not being pumped fast enough to the brain and other organs. Examination of the heart will reveal a low heart beat and pulse rate.

Treatment

After taking a history and doing a physical exam, the doctor will order various tests which may include a EKG, Chest X-ray, Echocardiogram, and may also let the patient wear a heart monitor called a Holter monitor which may be for 24 to 48 hours. It is like a continuous (EKG)/ECG), monitoring the electrical activity of the heart as person goes about her every day activities. The results will be downloaded and interpreted. If nothing is detected, then a wireless Holter monitor or an event monitor or recorder may be used. They are worn for longer periods (weeks or months); and have a button which is pushed if you have symptoms. This will send the electrical activity to your doctor through the phone. The individual also keeps a diary or log to record any symptoms like chest pain, shortness of breath etc., or irregular heart beat or rhythm they may have felt.

Treatment

One of the ways to treat this is to put in a little electronic device known as a PACEMAKER just under the skin near the collar bone and it has attached electrical leads/wires which go into the right ventricle alone or both right chambers of the heart. This will take over the electrical conduction system of the heart, and initiation of the heart beat when the heart beats too slowly.

Fast Heart Rate (Tachycardia) (tar-ki-kar-di-a)
What Is This?

This is when the heart beats too fast. Some of the common causes include:

Ingesting lots of caffeine (coffee or energy drinks with lots of caffeine)
Fever
Hyperthyroidism (hyperactive thyroid gland)
Obstructive Sleep Apnea
Obesity
Heart electrical conduction system problems

Treatment

If its an acute situation like fever then it will resolve with treatment. After history and physical exam, the heart tests mentioned above (Holter Monitor etc.) are also done together with blood work to identify any abnormal blood chemistry. The heart tests are not always needed, especially if the cause is obvious.

Treatment is correcting the underlying problem, so for example:

If problem is caffeine, decrease or stop it
If it is Hyperthyroidism, treatment will bring down the heart rate
If it is Obstructive sleep apnea, treatment with a CPAP machine or oral device will correct it
If due to irregular or regular fast heart beat as a result of problem with conduction system of heart, there are medications available to treat a fast heart rate and normalize it

Atrial Fibrillation (A FIB) (ay tree-fib-ruh-la-shin)
What is it?

In A FIB, the ineffective pump (heart) cannot support the circulation of blood to all the organs, and can lead to heart failure with its associated symptoms. The same also causes slow movement of blood within the heart, and may lead to formation of blood clots which may break off and travel to the brain to cause a stroke.

A common condition resulting in a rapid heart rate which at the same time is IRREGULAR in rhythm is called ATRIAL FIBRILLATION or A. FIB. Instead of the electric signals originating from one place in the upper right side of the heart (right atrium), irregular electrical signals from different sites disrupt normal signals from atrium to ventricle resulting in fast irregular signals which cause the heart to become an ineffective pump as the upper parts of the heart is out of sync with the lower ventricles. The beats are not strong, and are described like "a bag full of wriggling worms".

Risks for Developing Atrial Fibrillation

Risk increases with age
Heart disease and Hypertension
Diabetes and Hyperthyroidism
Family history of A Fib
Asthma
Following heart surgery
Excessive alcohol use

Signs and Symptoms

Symptoms may include tiredness, fatigue, passing out, chest pain, dizziness, and rapid fluttering of the heart or palpitations.

Investigation of Irregular Heart Beats

After a history and physical exam, tests or studies which may be done include blood work, EKG (Electrocardiogram ECG) and ultrasound of the heart (Echocardiogram). Blood work will check for different electrolytes in the blood, Magnesium, thyroid studies, Anemia etc. since abnormal levels of these may contribute to heart arrthymias (irregular rhythms). However, to have a longer recording of one's heart rate and rhythm, a Holter Monitor or Event Monitor may be worn by the individual. These devices have been described under Bradycardia above.

Sometimes it is difficult to diagnosis the presence of irregular rhythm or rate and because the individual continues to have symptoms of palpitations, fatigue and even chest pain, a device called an implantable loop recorder is placed under the skin near the left chest and it can be used to monitor heart rhythm and rate for up to three years.

Treatment of Atrial Fibrillation

This is treated with

- Medicines which take care of both the fast rate and the abnormal beat or rhythm
- Sometimes the electrical conduction system of the heart is tweaked by "burning" some of the fibers involved in conduction
- The heart may need to be "shocked" with special electrical paddles (defibrillator, de-fib-ril-la-tor) to correct the irregular heartbeat and reset it back to normal rhythm and rate.

- A pacemaker device is sometimes placed under the skin on the chest to regulate the heart rate when it is beating too fast.
- Whatever the form of treatment used to regulate the rate and or rhythm, blood thinners are used to prevent blood clots from forming and leading to strokes.
- Atrial fibrillation increases risk of stroke five times, so it is important to take medications (blood thinners) as ordered by your physician.
- Two common blood thinners used are WARFARIN or ASPIRIN. There are also many other new ones available and these, unlike Warfarin, do not need checking monthly blood levels of how thin the blood is. These include Rivaroxaban, (Xarelto), Dabigitran (Pradaxa, Prazaxa), Edoxaban (Savaysa, Lixiana) to name a few. These new ones, however, are not presently used for treating Atrial fibrillation in people who have heart valve replaced, or have Mitral stenosis (the circumference of the mitral valve area is reduced). These have to use Coumadin or Warfarin to prevent blood clots from forming and going to the brain.

Reminders on Your Radar

The heart may have problems with its rate or rhythm. The heart rate can be either too slow or too fast, and sometimes the cause may be medications or defects in the electrical conduction system. A pacemaker may be implanted to regulate the rate so that it falls within normal range. To detect rhythm problems, a EKG (ECG) may detect an irregular heart rhythm, however, sometimes one has to wear a heart monitor for days to months in order to detect this. Serious irregular rhythms, as may occur following a heart attack, can cause sudden cardiac death. Treatment may include medications and an implanted device in the chest called a defibrillator which can convert a dangerous rhythm back to a normal one if it occurs. A FIB is a serious condition leading to irregular heart beat and rhythm. It is important to treat it since it causes an increased risk for blood clots to form in the heart and can cause stroke.

Varicose Veins

. . . .

What are They?

When superficial veins on the legs (close to the skin) become enlarged and sometimes tortuous they are known as VARICOSE VEINS. They are the result of underlying sluggish or reverse (back flow) flow of venous blood toward the feet instead of to the heart, because the one way valves in these veins are incompetent or ineffective. The veins then swell up with blood. Apart from symptoms and signs mentioned below, cosmetically it can be disfiguring, sometimes affecting one's self-esteem, and looks.

Risk factors for developing these and spider veins (smaller tortuous veins) include:

Family history of Varicose veins
Occupations involving a lot of standing, sales associates, waitresses etc.
Previous injury to the legs
Previous blood clots in legs
Obesity
Pregnancy
Increased pressure in the abdomen and pelvis from obesity
Tumors or masses in the abdomen
Chronic constipation

Signs and Symptoms

Symptoms of Varicose veins include:

Tired or fatigued legs
Swelling of the legs
Discomfort or pain in the involved leg
Night pain in the legs
Itching
Small clots forming in the veins due to the sluggish blood flow
Inflammation, pain, or redness (Thrombophlebitis)
Skin changes which may be red or dark depending on one's skin color
Ulcers around the area where the Varicose vein is located
Some women experience more pain and swelling during their menstrual cycle, when on oral contraceptives or when pregnant

Treatment of Varicose Veins

Treatments include non-surgical or surgical methods.

Nonsurgical methods include support or compression stockings (these compress the veins and cause the blood to flow forward)

Injections into the veins (Sclerotherapy – using special material to shut up or block the vein so blood does not flow through it)

Keeping the legs elevated when seated, or getting up to walk around periodically when seated for long periods of time also help and tend to decrease the pain or discomfort.

Surgical treatments include:

Laser therapy used on the vein
Stripping the involved veins out after tying up some big connecting veins which are part of the problem

14

Brain and Nerve Conditions

Stroke

Stroke occurs in both men and women all over the world, and sometimes even in children with particular medical conditions. It is the second biggest cause of serious long term disability as well. It is a very debilitating disease due to the disabilities it can cause in terms of paralysis or weakness of part of the body, mobility, memory and speech problems. Economically it results in huge medical bills, as well as loss of work with economic consequences.

What is It?

A stroke can be referred to as a BRAIN ATTACK, and can be likened to a Heart Attack. This is because both may involve a blood clot blocking an artery and preventing blood flow and supply to tissues in a particular area.

A stroke is a brain condition due to disruption of blood supply and oxygen to an area of the brain. The lack of blood may be a result of blockage caused by a clot (Ischemic) or to a burst blood vessel in the brain (Hemorrhagic) stroke. According to the CDC, in the USA, each year about 795,000 people suffer from stroke and out of these, 140,000 die of stroke; that is one person every 4 minutes. It is the leading cause of long term disability and costs about $34 billion every year (www.cdc.gov/stroke/facts.htm).

Ischemic Stroke

The commonest type is the Ischemic stroke which makes up about 80% of strokes. The clot (thrombus) may be made up of cholesterol and platelets as in PLAQUE (see under Coronary Artery Disease above) and breaks off from inside a blood vessel and blocks it, thereby depriving the brain area supplied by that artery of blood supply. The clot may also come from elsewhere, like from the heart in cases of Atrial Fibrillation (AF). In AF, the clot forms in the heart and is carried to the brain by the blood (Embolus). A clot may also originate from the carotid arteries in the neck if they have plaque formed due to Arteriosclerosis. This leads to death or dying brain cells resulting in certain long term physical disabilities.

Stroke Characteristics

- An affected individual's symptoms will depend on which part of the brain is affected by the decreased blood supply
- There is a designated side of the brain which controls the function of the oppo-site side of the body when it comes to most areas affected by stroke
- There is a third type of stroke known as Transient Ischemic Attack (TIA) or 'mini stroke' which will be discussed further
- "Cryptogenic Stroke" refers to Ischemic stroke which is transient or complete, but after all the tests and imaging studies the cause of the stroke is not iden-tified (there is no irregular heartbeat observed, the heart echo is normal, and there is no blockage of the vessels in the neck and brain)

About 30% of Ischemic strokes are said to be Cryptogenic, and in that case, long term cardiac monitoring for about one to three months has to be done, since it seems that most Cryptogenic strokes are due to Atrial Fibrillation (irregular heart rhythm) which may be discovered only after continuous heart monitoring for a long time like a month because it can be intermittent, alternating with normal rhythm.

Symptoms of A Stroke

The Acronym FAST has been promoted by the American Stroke Association to help people remember the symptoms of stroke which tend to occur suddenly.

F – FACE DROOPING	When smiling one side of the face droops down
A – ARM WEAKNESS	Cannot raise the affected arm or hand
S – SPEECH DIFFICULTIES	Words are not clear/garbled or speech is incomprehensible
T – TIME TO GET HELP	Call emergency medical services. Get to Emergency room FAST

Other symptoms include:

Loss of vision in one or both eyes
Sudden confusion
Trouble understanding people you are talking to

Difficulty talking
Sudden severe headache
Problems walking
Loss of balance
Loss of sensation of part of the body
Double vision
Difficulty in walking
Loss of consciousness
Most of these may occur together when one is having a stroke.

Risk Factors for Stroke

Stroke is likely to develop in people who have the following medical problems. The risk of a stroke is increased the more risk factors one has. These include:

Previous stroke or mini stroke (TIA)
Atrial Fibrillation (Irregular heart beat and rate)
Hypertension
Diabetes Mellitus
High cholesterol
Coronary heart disease
Certain inherited blood-clotting diseases
Sickle cell disease
Blood vessels malformations in the brain
Use of oral contraceptives for birth control
Use of Leuprolide (Lupron) –medicine used for Prostate cancer
Cocaine or crack Cocaine use
Migraines
Head injury
Stress at work

Stress and Stroke

High level stress plays a role in stroke occurrence. In the 2012 published results (PLOS One Journal 2012) of a 10 year study conducted in women under various degrees of stress at work, the authors Drs. Slopen, Glynn and others, found out that women were almost 40% more likely to have a cardiovascular event over a 10-year period than their counterparts who reported lower job stress. The cardio-vascular events included heart attack, stroke, coronary vascular intervention and death from cardiovascular disease. MACE – Major Adverse Cardiovascular Event.

Stroke in Young People

Stroke can occur in young people as well. The causes are different from that of adults:

Stroke in Sickle Cell Disease

It can occur in children with Sickle cell disease mostly under the age of 15 years and those at high risk can be identified by screening the brain with a test called Transcranial Doppler (TCD). Sickle cell disease affects about 100,000 Americans and stroke occurs in about 10% of all affected children, and it also has a high rate of recurrence. To prevent an initial stroke in these children, as well as a recurrent one, children have to be on blood transfusions for life. In recent studies, researchers found that use of an oral drug call Hydroxyurea did just as well as transfusions.

Arteriovenous Malformation

Another group of children who have been born with malformed blood vessels in the brain known as ARTERIOVENOUS MALFORMATION (AVM) are also at increased risk for stroke. The structures of these vessels are abnormal and make them susceptible to bursting open or tearing. However this is a rare cause of stroke.

How to Prevent A First Ischemic Stroke

There needs to be control of risk factors associated with stroke. Individuals with the risk factors listed above need to keep the controllable ones in check.

- Blood pressure and high cholesterol need to be controlled with medications and lifestyle changes in order to prevent stroke
- Any individual who has Atrial Fibrillation has to be on a blood thinner so that they do not form clots which can block vessels in the brain
- A recent large study in 2015 in China, found that use of 0.8 mg daily of FOLIC ACID (vitamin B9) in individuals being treated for Hypertension (high blood pressure), led to reduced risk for stroke compared to those who were just on the blood pressure medicine. The effect was more significant in those with previous low levels of folic acid in their body (JAMA 2015)

Treatment of Stroke

When symptoms such as those listed above occur, there is need to get medical help as soon as possible. Quick arrival at the hospital is important because early treatment may result in less severe disability and prevents death. Depending on the hospital, an individual may have imaging studies known as CAT scan or MRI to evaluate the brain, CT or MR angiogram (MRA) to look at the blood vessels in brain and neck, Carotid ultrasound, EKG, Holter monitor and Echocardiogram to look at the heart, as well as blood work. A neurologist or doctor trained to treat brain and nerve diseases may be involved in the treatment.

Medications

In developed countries which have advanced medical care, one may receive:

- Medication to burst or "dissolve" the clot which caused the blockage of the blood vessel as soon as one arrives in a hospital
- A "clot buster" cannot be used if arrival at the hospital is more than 4 to 6 hours after symptoms started
- One may be started on blood thinners to prevent more clots from forming in the future
- Aspirin, a common blood thinner may be started as soon as brain studies indicate the stroke is not a bleeding type and if a clot buster was not used
- After the initial stage, other blood thinners called Anticoagulants may be used to prevent blood from clotting and reduce risk of future strokes
- All of the blood thinners carry risk of bleeding and some may interact with other medicines, so make sure one discusses this with their doctor

Warfarin (brand name-Coumadin) is a very common blood thinner but has a lot of interactions with other medicines and with some foods; in addition, one has to have monthly regular blood work to monitor the blood's ability to clot when on Warfarin. The test is called INR/PT and it has to be at a certain level when on Coumadin.

Transient Ischemic Attack (TIA) Mini Stroke

. . . .

What is It?

A mini stroke or TIA is one in which some of the symptoms described above for stroke occur but they last less than 24 hours and then disappear. There is a temporary lack of blood flow to parts of the brain, eyes or spinal cord due to a blood clot and this results in these symptoms. The blood clots may originate from the heart, due to abnormal heart rhythm like Atrial fibrillation described under heart diseases, a hardened blood vessel (Atherosclerosis), or even from inherited diseases which makes a person produce blood clots. The clot can be dissolved or it can move along, causing blood flow to be restored.

Symptoms and Signs

These include changes which are sudden and may typically last from 20 minutes to an hour. They go away as the clot disappears.

They may include disturbances of:

Gait
Speech
Movement
Memory loss
Vision
Behavior

It is important that medical help is received as soon as possible because invariably people who suffer a mini stroke may get a full blown stroke in the future. Some people ignore the symptoms and do not seek help. Seek help immediately.

Treatment of Transient Ischemic Attack (TIA)

After the doctor takes a history and does a physical exam, the following investigations will be done

These include:

Blood work
Heart studies like EKG (ECG) and Echocardiogram (ultrasound of the heart)
Imaging studies like CT brain, MRI and a special MRI which takes images of the blood vessels in the brain and neck called Magnetic resonance angiogram (MRA)
Ultrasound of the blood vessels in the neck (Carotid Ultrasound)
Device worn to detect Atrial fibrillation if that is not detected initially

To detect intermittent Atrial fibrillation one may need to wear an external monitor for 30 days or even have an implantable cardiac monitor also called a Loop recorder placed under the skin. When an irregular rhythm occurs it is recorded, and transmitted to the cardiologist's office.

All these tests are performed just like for full blown stroke to find out the source of the clot which may have caused the brief neurological problems associated with a TIA.

Treatment

The individual is likely to be placed on a blood thinner like Aspirin or Clopidogrel (Plavix) so as to prevent future formation of blood clots.

If there is blockage of blood vessels in the neck (Carotid artery), it is corrected by surgery to remove plaque, or it is ballooned (stretched) open and a stent is placed at the site of the narrowed artery to keep it open.

It is important that any of the risk factors mentioned above, if present, be treated and kept under control. So blood pressure, Cholesterol, blood sugar if diabetic all need to be well controlled with the appropriate medications. Patient is encouraged to engage in healthy eating and exercise.

Post Stroke Care

Post stroke care is needed to minimize the long term complications which may result from the stroke. The earlier it is done, the fewer the permanent disabilities which may result. Post stroke care is essential and caregivers must be advocates to make sure it happens.

It is important to know about post stroke care, which is care one needs apart from medications in the areas of physical and emotional results associated with the stroke. After initial treatment and when the individual is stable, measures are taken to treat the physical and emotional complications of the stroke. Caregivers have to work with medical professionals to motivate the stroke patient to participate in prescribed therapies. These are important since they minimize the complications.

Stroke Complications

These complications may include

Paralysis of one side of the body
Muscle spasm of affected side
Pain in the affected limb(s)
Numbness and tingling
Speech problems
Vision problems
Mobility and balance problems
Memory loss and dementia
Altered thinking process
Depression and anxiety
Anger and frustration

To address these needs one has to have:

- Physical Therapy (PT): To restore muscle function and improve mobility
- Occupational therapy (OT): To help person be independent

- Speech therapy: To help with speech if affected by the stroke
- Psychological Therapy: To help with mood changes like depression

Physical and Occupational Therapy
What are These?

Physical therapy and occupational therapy are important aspects of treatment after a stroke.

Physical Therapy

Physical therapy involves strength training exercises and others to improve the function of either a paralyzed arm or leg. The earlier it is started the better. Walkers, wheelchairs, walking canes, leg or arm splints or braces may be needed.

Occupational Therapy

Occupational therapy involves teaching a post stroke person with deficits and their caregiver ways and tips on how the survivor can be independent as much as possible. For example: Showing them one hand techniques in doing things around the home. Others are tips on how to be safe around the house by recommending devices like raised toilet seat, hand grab bars, bath or shower chair, and other appliances that will make activities of daily living like walking, bathing, moving etc. easier for survivors of stroke. According to the American Occupational Therapy Association, practitioners help stroke victims with physical, cognitive, and emotional challenges enabling them to improve not only movement and physical activities, but memory, concentration and thinking. They also help caregivers assist stroke victims become more independent at home. (www.neurorehabdirectory. com/occupational-therapy-stroke-role-ot).

Speech Therapy

Speech therapists may make sure swallowing is safe and advise on what kind or consistency of food one can eat so as not to choke or aspirate food or liquids. They also help individuals work on regaining their speech through exercises, singing etc.

Music Therapy

This is a therapy that is not often used, but it has been found to help stroke patients. So if you or someone you know has had a stroke, encourage them to listen to music as part of therapy. Writing in the American Journal of Medicine in 2015, Dr. Harvey Simon of the Harvard Medical School in Boston, Massachusetts emphasizes that "music is medicine" and has been found to influence stress, pain, sleep, mood and measurable parameters like blood pressure and heart rate. He cites many studies some of which show that listening to music can affect functions of the brain and may help in stroke recovery. It does this by improving brain function, muscle movements, improve mood, and restoration of speech in some through singing. (Dr. Harvey Simon, "Music as Medicine" The Am. Journal of Med., Feb 2015, vol. 128, No. 2)

Post Stroke Mental Challenges

Some survivors of stroke may be frustrated with their inability to perform functions they used to do, for example, talking or even walking; and so may develop mental challenges like:

Anger and frustration
Depression due to loss of control
Withdrawal and Isolation
Memory loss or forgetfulness
Post stroke dementia

Treatment

Treatment with medications for depression may be needed and so caregivers may need to let the patient's doctor know about their emotional challenges.

Joining a stroke support group or network sometimes helps one face and deal with the many challenges.

Post stroke dementia (problems with memory, concentration and communication) can occur and may be manifested up to 10 years after the event (delayed onset post stroke dementia).

Dementia is more common in those who had Diabetes, Hypertension or Atrial fibrillation prior to the stroke. It seems to also be more frequent in those who have speech problems after a stroke (understanding or expressing themselves verbally).

Post stroke dementia can be reduced by both stroke prevention and early management of stroke and these were discussed above.

Prevention of A Second Stroke

The probability of getting another stroke is higher for someone who has had a previous stroke or TIA. So in order to prevent this, certain risk factors associated with stroke have to be well controlled. These include:

- Smoking cessation
- Controlling high blood pressure (BP)

- Controlling high Cholesterol
- Controlling blood sugar in diabetics
- Use of blood thinners like Aspirin, Warfarin, Clopidogrel (trade names: Coumadin and Plavix respectively)
- Lifestyle changes like healthy diet, weight loss and exercise are also important in order to prevent another stroke. These are the same as one would do for coronary heart disease which was discussed in detail in the previous chapter on cardiovascular diseases

Cognitive Problems
What are These?

These are a number of mental processes of the brain that decline due to many factors. They include deterioration in memory, attention, concentration, thought processes and reasoning. Cognitive decline is a huge problem especially close to and after menopause, and tends to increase with age in both women and men. The problem is being seen in many more people because people are living longer. Decline in cognition is a result of many factors including:

Age
Genetics
Diseases
Environmental factors

Diseases Causing Memory Decline

These include

Cerebrovascular accident (Stroke, CVA)
Parkinson's disease
Alzheimer's disease
Other dementias
Other less known factors influencing memory include:
Sleep problems
Sedentary lifestyle
Decreased brain stimulation

Different degrees and types of memory loss in particular have been identified and we will discuss a few of them. These are the common ones which occur.

Memory Loss Associated With Aging
What is This?

With aging memory that tends to remain stable include: knowledge or certain facts acquired like knowledge about the world. Also the acquisition and later use of a particular skill, for example if one learns how to knit, or build a small toy this is remembered and one continues to do so even as one ages.

This may occur around the age of 50 years in most people and is attributed to structural changes in the brain. Some aspects of memory will naturally decrease with aging while some others remain constant.

Memory Which Decreases With Age

- Remembering personal events and experiences
- The speed at which one processes information
- Ability to perform a future event like taking your medicines
- Recollection
- Remembering new information and combining it with previous long term memory
- Remembering specific information like the ability to recall a specific name, number, or location on demand also declines and many people experience this and get frustrated about it
- Ability to remember names and difficulty remembering and concentrating

Prevention of Age Related Memory Loss

- Eating fish and use of fish oil supplements (Omega 3) has been associated with slowing of age related memory decline. The effect is attributed to their antioxidant properties. Studies in the elderly have shown that these two help with slowing memory decline and imaging studies show that the usual shrinking of brain size seen in people with Dementia (especially Alzheimer's dementia) is not observed in normal elderly individuals who have high levels of Omega 3 in their blood
- Remaining physically, socially, and mentally active may help prevent memory loss associated with aging. According to Dr. Felipe De Brigard who is a memory expert at Duke University USA, things that can help slow memory loss associated with aging include:

  Aerobic exercise
  Healthy living
  An intellectual life
  Sleeping well
  Avoid multitasking by focusing one's attention on the task at hand

(How Memory Works, and How to Preserve It). Medscape.com. Feb 13, 2015).

What About Ginkgo Biloba – Does it Work for Memory Loss?
What is It?

This is a plant which has been attributed to help with several conditions including memory, anxiety, Dementia, insufficient blood flow to brain, and Asthma.

However, according to a big well designed study by NCCIM called Ginkgo Evaluation of Memory (GEM) study in subjects aged 72 to 96 years, the results showed:

- Ginkgo did not decrease cognitive decline compared to "sugar pill" when they looked at memory, attention, language, or executive function (complex function like balancing a check book, organize a trip or an event)
- It did not reduce incidence of Dementia or Alzheimer's disease (JAMA, 2009)
- Generally, there is no strong evidence for its claims

According to Mayo Clinic (A very advanced health care organization in the USA):

- Research does not support its claim to prevent or slow Dementia or memory decline
- It is safe for many adults if taken in recommended doses, however eating raw or roasted Ginkgo seeds can be poisonous or cause a seizure
- It reacts with many medications e.g. aspirin, ibuprofen, statins, Diabetes medicines and anti epileptic drugs.(Mayoclinic.org/drugs-supplements/ginkgo/evidence). Updated 2017

How to Preserve Memory

Based on all the above, one can do the following to preserve memory:

- Use of FISH OIL supplements (DHA omega 3)
- One's diet should include eating fish especially salmon which is rich in omega 3
- Eat diets high in fruits, vegetables, nuts, and legumes. They have antioxidants
- Stimulation of the brain through reading, taking courses or classes (intellectual stimulation)
- Exercise e.g. walking, going to the gym etc. will help your body not just physically but mentally as well
- Recent studies show that "Brain training" by doing puzzles, cross words and computerized programs may not help delay memory loss as was previously thought, however it may stimulate your brain and since it's not harmful, it is recommended

- Group-based computer brain training with a trainer was found to be useful in some studies done

Other Memory Tips include:

- Try to leave usual everyday things in the same place, for example glasses, car keys, cell phone so that one doesn't spend time searching for them or keep losing them
- Try and minimize stress in life
- Get enough sleep every night. If there is difficulty sleeping, discuss this with the doctor. Some sleeping tips called sleep hygiene tips if practiced may help. (See section on sleeping problems)
- Some medications may affect memory (see list below). If an individual is on any of them, they must discuss with their doctor to substitute or replace it with a different medication

Memory loss associated with Menopause

This will be discussed under "Menopause" in a later chapter. It tends to start in women who are about to enter menopause or are in the peri-menopause period of their life. It is believed that hot flashes and sleep disturbances which occur during this time may contribute to this in women.

Memory Loss Associated With Medications

Several medicines have been associated with memory loss and the most common ones are those associated with seizures, sleep and anxiety. Below are a few.

Insomnia Medications

Several drugs prescribed to treat inability to sleep (Insomnia) or are used as OTC products have been associated with memory loss and examples are: Suvorexant, Alprazolam and Diphenhydramine commonly known as Benadryl. Diphenhydramine comes under other names or combined with other drugs like: Acetaminophen (Tylenol) or Ibuprofen (Advil) as Nytol, Excedrin PM, Midol PM, Tylenol PM, and Advil PM. Many people use these to help them sleep. Diphenhydramine has other side effects like drowsiness, dizziness, blurred vision.

Medicines With and Without Anticholinergic Effects

The class of drugs known as Anticholinergics which are used to treat several conditions, as well as common medications that may have anticholinergic effects have been associated with cognitive decline in both older and even younger adults if taken over a long period, or if several are taken together over a short time. (JAMA Intern Med. 2015; 175(3):401–407). Most people may not know this and unfortunately their doctors may not tell them of the memory side effects, or change to other medicines without anticholinergic effects. The more common side effects of these medicines may be mentioned by the doctor, however; the cognitive or memory decline effect is often omitted. Remember Long Term use is the underlying culprit.

These medicines include those used for:

Urine incontinence and overactive bladder: e.g. Oxybutynin, Tolterodine
Insomnia: Diphenhydramine (Benadryl), Chlorpheniramine (Piriton)
Allergies: Diphenhydramine and Chlorpheniramine
Pain or numbness/tingling/depression: tricyclic antidepressants like Amitriptyline
Pain: Codeine, and certain antidepressants called tricyclic antidepressants
Depression, anxiety or sleep: Doxepin, Alpraxolam/Benzodiazepines, tricyclic antidepressants
Diarrhea: Loperamide
Nausea and motion sickness: Dimenhydrinate –Dramamine
Hypertension (BP): Atenolol, Clonidine
Parkinson's Disease: Amantadine
Anticonvulsants/seizures: Phenytoin, Gabapentin, Valproate
Muscle relaxers: Carisoprodol (Soma), Cyclobenzaprine (Flexeril)
Antiemetics Nausea and Vomiting: Prochlorperazine, Metoclopramide
Schizophrenia: Antipsychotics, Chlorpromazine (largactil), Haloperidol, Risperidone (Risperdal), Olanzapine (Zyprexa), Quetiapine (Seroquel)
Bipolar: Lithium
Heart diseases: Atenolol, Digoxin, Amiodarone

In more than 50% of people, stopping the particular medicine improves cognition. Remember this cognitive decline occurs with chronic use, not a week or two use of the medication. Also in the elderly, some of these may increase risk of falls resulting in breaking a bone (fracture).

Medical Conditions Causing Reversible Memory Loss

Other causes of reversible memory loss apart from medications are

Hypothyroid
Hyperparathyroidism
Vitamin B12 Deficiency

Electrolyte imbalance, for example Sodium, Potassium and Calcium
Chronic kidney disease with associated Anemia

Other Conditions Affecting Memory

- LONG TERM USE OF MARIJUANA
  There is a lot of controversy about legalization of Marijuana and what good or harm it can do. Several studies have been done on its effect on the brain. Research shows that long-term Marijuana use results in short term memory loss in the areas controlling sequence of numbers and verbal recall in certain individuals. Its effect on long term memory is still being studied

- OBSTRUCTIVE SLEEP APNEA (OSA)
  OSA can result in excessive daytime sleepiness (EDS), headache, high blood pressure and decreased oxygenation if left untreated. It has been found that as a result of EDS patients with OSA can have impaired memory and decreased daytime functioning. Treatment of OSA is usually with a device called CPAP, or Bipap machine, oral dental device or surgery; all of which help one overcome the obstruction of the airway during sleep. Surgery involves removal of part of the back of the throat and the uvula (long mass hanging from the roof of the throat) to create more space at the back of the throat. Treatment results in day time alertness, sharper memory, less fatigue and tiredness, decrease or better blood pressure control and feeling of being well rested after sleep at night

- ALCOHOL
  Chronic excessive alcohol use can lead to serious effects on the brain, liver, pancreas, high blood pressure, and stroke among other effects. Studies show that men who drink more than two drinks a day on a regular basis may have faster decline of memory. Alcohol impairs memory especially new memory formation. Ironically, limited or mild to moderate consumption of alcohol leads to lower risk of Dementia and other health benefits to the cardiovascular system. Moderate consumption is one drink a day for women and two for men according to the US Food and Drug Administration

- CHEMO "BRAIN"
  This is a term used to describe memory and attention problems that result from Chemotherapy used to treat cancer. For women, breast cancer treatments tend to cause these and lead to some brain fog and memory problems

- CANCER "BRAIN"
  Recent studies indicate that chemicals produced by cancer cells may produce some memory problems prior to Chemotherapy or other treatments. So the

term "Cancer Brain" has been adopted to describe the effects of cancer cells on the brain's cognitive abilities

- OTHER CANCER OR TREATMENT RELATED CAUSES
  According to American Cancer Society, there are many factors causing brain function abnormality like Chemo brain. These include:

  Other medications used in cancer treatment like steroids
  Surgery and Anesthesia
  Infections
  Hormonal treatments used in breast and prostate cancer treatment
  Sleep problems worry, depression, stress and emotional issues
  Patient's age – older patients have more abnormalities

(American Cancer Society www.cancer.org).

So Chemotherapy cannot be solely blamed for the memory problems associated with treatment for breast cancer and other cancers. Radiation to the head and neck areas, brain cancer, brain surgery, metastatic cancers to the brain, and total body irradiation may all cause some cognitive changes as well, mainly memory deficits and speed of processing information.

Symptoms and Signs

It is believed that about 20 to 30% of all **cancer survivors** may experience some amount of memory deficit or problems. These include increased problems with: attention, organizing thoughts, short term memory, finding words, thinking clearly, paying attention focusing or remembering things.

Treatment

There are no specific treatments, but research is ongoing regarding therapies that may help cancer brain. The following may help:

- Computer brain training may be useful
- Treatment of depression and medical conditions like Hypothyroid if present
- Use of occupational therapy helps identify the cognitive dysfunction and then assist individual with problem solving
- Medicines which are "stimulants" e.g. Ritalin (Methylphenidate) may help some cancer survivors
- For those who undergo whole brain radiation therapy, the use of Memantine (Namenda) (used in treating Alzheimer's disease), has been used to reduce possible cognitive impairment

Mild Cognitive Impairment (Memory Loss) (MCI)
What is It?

This condition is characterized by ability to perform activities of daily living, however, there are complaints of memory impairment and changes in memory which is more than expected for the person's age. Not all individuals with MCI develop full blown Dementia and research has shown that the probability of converting from MCI back to normal cognition within a year is twice that of converting from MCI to Alzheimer's disease, so about 40–70% do not progress to Dementia.

Risk Factors

Severe factors have been identified as affecting cognition. These include:

Lack of stimulation of the brain
Presence of medical conditions like Atherosclerosis (hardening of arteries)
Stroke
Sleep disturbances
Lack of exercise
Unhealthy eating

Signs and Symptoms

The symptoms may include memory loss, attention problems, difficulty finding words, problems recognizing or getting disoriented with familiar places or people, BUT there is no social impairment and work is not affected. When SOCIAL INTERACTIONS, BEHAVIOR AND WORK are also affected, then it is termed full blown Dementia.

Prevention Of Mild Cognitive Impairment (MCI)
Avoid Certain Medications

Certain medications described below have been found to be risk factors in developing MCI in adults 65 years and above, especially if used for greater than 60 to 90 days. Unfortunately, a number of older adults are on several of these medicines and so it is important for doctors to minimize the prescription of these. Many older adults also self-medicate with some of these medicines in order to sleep at night. Examples are use of "Tylenol PM and Advil PM" which contain Diphenhydramine or Benadryl.

Avoid medicines that can affect memory in a negative way. They should be substituted with other medicines or therapies. Examples are:

PROBLEM	MEDICATION	SUBSTITUTION
Overactive bladder	Oxybutynin, Tolterodine	Bladder training, Nerve Stimulation Biofeedback Botox
Sleep problems (Insomnia)	Benadryl, Diphenhydramine Tylenol/Advil PM	Sleep hygiene technics, other sleep medicines
Numbness and tingling	Amitriptyline, Nortriptyline	Gabapentin, compound creams
Allergies	Diphenhydramine, Chlorphenramine	Cetirizine, Loratidine

Treatment of MCI (Mild Cognitive Impairment)

....

After a history, including a careful medication history and physical exam by a doctor, the individual will need:

- Imaging Studies: CAT (CT) scan or MRI brain scan
- Blood Work: Electrolytes, Anemia and kidney tests, Syphilis test, Thyroid studies and Vitamin B12, levels have to be checked
- Psychologist: Some psychological and neurological testing need to be done to help doctors determine the severity of the memory loss
- Medications: No specific treatments have been developed but it has been found that using a drug called DONEPEZIL (Aricept) which is used to treat Alzheimer's disease may delay the progression to Alzheimer's in MCI patients with depression
- Therapeutic Lifestyle Changes (TLC): Moderate exercise, healthy diet (fruits, vegetables, whole grains), and intellectually challenging activities may help MCI from progressing
- Mediterranean Diet: Studies show that people who consume the Mediterranean diet have a lower incidence of MCI. This diet incorporates fruits vegetables, nuts, olive oil and fish
- Brain Fitness Program: In a 2015 study presented at Alzheimer's Association International Conference by researchers from USA, one of the lead researchers Dr. Fotuhi suggested that progression can be delayed by doing some of the things in the list below. Their study found that patients with MCI who went through intensive brain training made up of the following improved over 3 months, with participants having an increase in the size of their shrinking brains as well as increase in their cognitive function

Brain fitness program included:

Treatment of any underlying medical conditions
Cognitive skills training
Mindfulness meditation
Advice on exercise and Mediterranean diet
Supplementation with Omega 3 Fish oil

(Fotuhi et al. Alzheimer's Association International Conference (AAIC) 2015. Abstract 4331)

Dementia

What is It?

Dementia is a growing problem with aging being one of the major risk factors. Genetics, environmental and diseases are major risk factors. Alzheimer's Disease (AD) is the leading cause of Dementia, accounting for about 70% of all causes.

Dementia is the term given to conditions resulting in **memory loss accompanied by changes in behavior and socialization.** There are many causes of dementia but the most common is ALZHEIMER'S DISEASE (AD) accounting for about 70% of Dementia cases. Another less common cause of Dementia is VASCULAR DEMENTIA which is due to disease of the blood vessels in the brain resulting in lack of blood supply to certain parts of the brain. Hypertension is one of the leading causes of Vascular dementia. Other causes of Dementia include age related, medications, and medical conditions e.g. stroke, and degenerative brain diseases e.g. Parkinson's, Frontotemporal and Huntington's Disease.

Alzheimer's Disease (AD)

What is it ?

"We remember their love when they can no longer remember."

— Unknown (www.alzheimers.net/quote)

AD is the most common form of Dementia and apart from memory, other cognitive processes are affected. Worldwide, according to WHO reports for 2000, Dementia of any form increases with age but it is not a normal part of aging. The prevalence in those aged 60–69 is about 1%. Interestingly enough, this rises to 39% in those who are 90–95 years. Worldwide, there will be about 106 million individuals affected with AD by the year 2050. The cause is unknown, however, its development is believed to be due to interplay between GENES, ENVIRONMENT, and LIFESTYLE. Most cases are not inherited (sporadic) but 15–25% are familiar with 2–3 relatives affected. It is made up of a number of symptoms as well as changes in the brain. The common symptoms are:

Chronic irreversible memory loss
Changes in personality and behavior

Changes in thinking, reasoning and judgement
Deterioration in socialization

What Happens in the Brain in AD?

In the brain, there is buildup of certain proteins called Amyloid Beta Plaques, (Amyloid) and Tau Protein Tangles (Tangles) which twist and damage nerve cells starting in the areas which deal with memory. There is loss of connection between brain cells, inflammation, as well as shrinking of the brain from brain cell death starting in areas where new memories are formed, resulting in the changes mentioned above. The condition is progressive and eventually results in death.

Prevalence of Alzheimer's Disease

Research into Alzheimer's disease is going on in many parts of the world because many individuals in all countries are affected by the disease. In the USA, according to the Alzheimer's Association, in 2018, it was estimated to be about 5.7 million people suffering from Alzheimer's Disease and this number will increase to about 14 million people by 2050.

Death from AD

The death rate from AD is also increasing and in 2017 it was recorded as the 6th leading cause of death in the USA, killing more people than breast and prostate cancers combined. It is estimated that between 2000 and 2015, deaths from AD increased by 123% and currently, 1 in 3 seniors die with Alzheimer's or other Dementias in the USA (Alzheimer's Association https://www.alz.org/alzheimers-dementia/facts-figures). More women than men are diagnosed with AD after the age of 65 years because women tend to live longer. Blacks or African Americans have a higher prevalence of Dementia of any kind in the USA, with their rate being double that of Caucasians.

Risk Factors

The following are risk factors that may predispose one to Alzheimer's disease, and although one cannot alter one's genes or age, some of the other risk factors can be altered by what one does.

Advanced age
Family history of Alzheimer's disease in parents or close relatives
Hypertension
High cholesterol
Presence of certain genes in your body
Type 2 Diabetes Mellitus

Signs and Symptoms of Alzheimer's Disease

In AD, symptoms initially develop subtly and the individual may try to cover up their memory lapses, but minor symptoms may be noted by relatives or close friends. As the disease progresses it eventually affects the individual's socialization, activities of daily living, and activities which support independent living.

Memory and Behavior problems may be the initial symptoms, however, before discussing these, there are certain definitions one has to be familiar with. These are:

- Activities of daily living (ADL): These include: walking, bathing, dressing, eating, toileting etc
- Instrumental activities of daily living (IADL): These are activities like housekeeping, managing checkbook, using a phone, shopping, cooking, managing medications, driving and using a computer
- Executive function: ability to plan, execute, manage and complete tasks, as well as ability to monitor and control behavior. It is controlled by the frontal part of the brain

Symptoms of AD include:

Memory problems:
  Not remembering newly learned information. Events of the past may be remembered initially
  Confusion
  Losing or misplacing things
  Taking a long time to perform familiar tasks
  Inability to come up with words, so would substitute words, or form new words
  As it gets worse, an individual doesn't recognize familiar people
  Getting lost in familiar surroundings
  Forgetting to pay bills, refusing to participate in an activity they used to love doing

Behavior symptoms:
  Poor judgement
  Behavior changes like suspicious of family and friends occur
  Mood changes
  Changes in behavior or personality (not in early stages, occurs later)
  Sun Downing: Agitation, anxiety, and confusion beginning in the evening
  Sleep disturbances

Late Stages of Alzheimer's Disease

As the disease progresses, there are more symptoms and difficulties encountered by patients. These include:

Difficulties with feeding
Difficulties with walking
Swallowing difficulties
Speech problems and eventually may stop talking
Mood changes like verbal outbursts and anger
Psychiatric symptoms like being paranoid, aggressive, with delusions, and
    *hallucinations
Disinhibition (e.g. taking clothes off)
Being suspicious of caregivers and accusing them of stealing etc
Depression
Wandering out of the house

*seeing and hearing things that are not present

Diagnosis and Treatment of Alzheimer's Disease

Careful history and physical examination can exclude diseases like Parkinson's disease, alcoholism, drug abuse and psychiatric problems all of which can also cause Dementia. Various tests similar to those done in Mild Cognitive Impairment described above are done.

A careful history from a spouse or relatives will help the doctor have a more accurate history of what is happening in the person's life. This is important since patients often play down their memory loss and other symptoms they are exhibiting.

Other common causes of memory problems have to be eliminated by testing the blood for Vitamin B12 deficiency, thyroid problems, Syphilis disease, kidney or liver diseases.

Tests for APOE4 (Apolipoprotein E), a gene tied to higher risk of developing AD may be performed. One's risk is even higher when a person receives this from each parent and so has 2 copies of the gene present.

Special imaging studies may be done and these include CT (CAT scan), PET/CT, and MRI scans of the brain. These help exclude brain tumors, CVA etc.

A series of psychological testing by a psychologist or psychiatrist will have to be done to test the person's ability to recall things, attention span, memory, repetition of words etc.

Once the diagnosis of Alzheimer's disease is made, there are medications used to slow down the progression but they will not reverse the disease. Other non-pharmacological treatments may also help with cognition, functional capacity, and behavior.

Treatment of Alzheimer's Disease

Currently, there is no cure for AD, however, there are medicines and non-drug therapies to help with the symptoms of the disease.

Medications

Cognitive Problems:

- Medications may help lessen the cognitive problems like memory loss, attention, confusion, and reasoning as well as other symptoms like agitation, sleep problems, and depression. They may also help with day to day function like dressing. The dead nerve cells, cannot be restored, but the affected messaging system between nerve cells can be helped by the medications which affect the chemicals involved in message transmission. Their effects may lessen with time, and they may not work for every patient
- Two groups of medicines generally called-Anti Alzheimer Products have been approved to treat the cognitive deficits mentioned above. They are:
  1. Cholinesterase inhibitors (Aricept, Exelon, Razadyne)
  2. NMDA (N-methyl-D-aspartate) receptor antagonists group – Memantine (Namenda – used for moderate to severe cases)

These medicines may also be combined in moderate to severe Alzheimer's Disease. They both give a small improvement in cognition and functional decline.

Treatment for Behavior and Personality changes

Apart from medications, some things can be done which may diminish the behavior changes. These changes and the solutions include:

- Limit changes in the person's surroundings. Solution: Same routine and surroundings as much as possible
- Presence of infections e.g. Urinary tract infection. Solution: Look for and treat infections
- Constipation – Solution: Monitor Bowel movements and give medicines if needed
- Medications – Solution: Change medicines affecting cognition negatively (see below)
- Uncorrected vision and hearing problems – Solution: Use of glasses and hearing aids
- Other simple solutions include making the environment comfortable, e.g. dimming lights, noise reduction, limiting changes in the surroundings, and use of music which can calm a patient and even activate areas of the brain. All these, if done, can help with agitation, and calm down the individual

- If the problem is still present, then medications may be used and these include antidepressants, anti-anxiety, or antipsychotic medicines, all used at minimal doses

Sleep Problems

These are thought to be a result of the impact of AD on the brain, and patients may not sleep at night, nap a lot during the day, and stay awake for many hours. Non-drug approaches include:

Avoiding caffeine and alcohol
Keeping regular sleep times
Making sure they are not in pain

If these don't help, then medications in low doses may be used

Sundowning

This is a term used to describe agitation, confusion etc. which occur in AD patients during late afternoon or evening. Simple solutions include:

Keeping them active during the day
Eating a light meal at night
Daytime light therapy

If no improvement, medicines may be prescribed

Supplements Or OTC Medicines Used for Alzheimer's Disease

Apart from the disease-specific medications, there are others that if used, may probably help or limit some of the symptoms.

- Vitamin E 2000 IU has been found to slightly slow functional decline, especially when combined with the other two groups mentioned above
- Vitamin B complex has been recommended since some believe it may reverse brain degeneration in regions vulnerable to AD process
- Some medicines which have been tried but have not proved beneficial in random controlled scientific trials or have not been subject to such trials include Ginkgo biloba, Huperzine A, coconut oil, Coenzyme Q10, Phosphatidylserine, coral calcium, Omega-3 fatty acids, Statins and NSAIDs (e.g. Ibuprofen). Most have just anecdotal reports, and sometimes the purity is questionable, or there may be adulteration of the products. A healthcare provider has to be notified of any supplements that are being used

Drugs or Medicines To Avoid

- It is also advised to AVOID drugs known as ANTICHOLINERGIC DRUGS or those which have anticholinergic properties because they affect the chemicals involved in transmitting messages from one nerve cell to the other causing more cognitive impairment and confusion
- These are drugs used to treat several conditions including overactive bladder, urinary incontinence, chronic bronchitis, chronic pain, and antihistamines used to treat allergies etc. Examples are Oxybutynin, Ttolterodine, (for overactive bladder) Cyclobenzaprine (Flexeril – which is a muscle relaxant), Ipratropium (for Bronchitis and Asthma), Amitriptyline (depression, pain and migraine prevention), Diphenhydramine (Benadryl – an antihistamine used for allergies and sleep. It is important to avoid these medicines in people with Dementia
- Sometimes over the counter sleep aids may contain Diphenhydramine (Benadryl) and individuals may not be aware of this. These include those combined with a pain medicine like Tylenol or Advil and are known as Tylenol PM and Advil PM

Physical Activity

Recent research suggests that lifestyle of increasing exercise or physical activity improves cerebral blood flow, increasing cognitive function and may even decrease the levels of abnormal proteins associated with Alzheimer's Disease (Amyloid and Tau). It may also decrease the rate of loss of function and slow memory loss.

Ketogenic Diet

Some early research has recently shown that Ketogenic diet helps with the memory impairment in Mild Cognitive Impairment (MCI) and Alzheimer's disease, but this research is in the early stages. The brain in AD loses its ability to use glucose to produce energy like it does in normal people, and scientists believe that may be the reason for some of the decline in brain functions like memory. Ketogenic diets have been found to help the brain use ketones as energy in place of glucose in pilot studies. Ketogenic diets are difficult to adhere to because they have to be low in carbohydrates, so the body utilizes the ketone instead of glucose. The medium chain triglycerides as a supplement may provide this and improve cognitive function as found in one pilot study (Boosting Brain Ketone Metabolism: A New Approach to Alzheimer's-Medscape-Aug 3, 2017). The best source of medium chain triglycerides is coconut oil, although palm kernel oils are also good sources. This research seems to be in line with what has been circulating in the popular media about use of coconut oil to treat symptoms of Alzheimer's disease.

Axona "Medical Food" for AD

Axona, a fractionated coconut oil, which is a medium-chain triglyceride has been touted as a medical food for treating mild to moderate Alzheimer's Disease. It is markcted as an alternate energy source which the brain can use instead of glucose for its function. It's role as a medical food was described as false and misleading in 2013 by the FDA, and it asked the company producing it to stop promoting it as a medical food, because medical foods are usually foods used to treat nutritional deficiencies in certain diseases, and the FDA concluded there are no nutritional deficiencies in Alzheimer's Disease. (www.fda.gov/ICECI/ EnforcementActionsucm381320.htm)

Helpful non drug approaches in AD

Non drug approaches may be helpful in treating some of the symptoms; and these include:

A well-lighted room to prevent or treat sun downing
A quiet environment
Methods to enhance sleep like massage, herbal teas or warm milk
Relaxation music
Decreasing stimuli like noise, and bright light at bedtime
Security in the home to prevent wandering and getting lost
The use of a support group or memory daycare center
Social worker to assist caregivers and families
Exercises to strengthen Muscles and Prevent falls

An Alzheimer's support group will help a caregiver with tips and suggestions which can make caring for a person with the disease a little more manageable.

Mental stimulation in mild to moderate Dementia (e.g. word games, indoor gardening, baking and puzzles) improves cognition and wellbeing.

Occupational therapy training improves cognition. Letting the patient do enjoyable activities seem to help by decreasing the neuropsychiatric symptoms, increase functional abilities and slow memory loss (Ted Epperly et al. Alzheimer Disease American Family Physician Vol 95, Number 12, June 15, 2017).

Prevention of Alzheimer's Disease

Some risk factors like inherited genes related to the disease are not preventable, but others may be controlled, and there are things that one can do to help prevent or delay Alzheimer's disease. In a publication by the Alzheimer's Association, the authors emphasize the fact that there are several risk factors which can be reduced or modified in order to prevent cognitive decline and Dementia. These include:

- Treatment of certain medical conditions like Hypertension, high Cholesterol, Diabetes, and Obesity
- Therapeutic lifestyle changes like smoking cessation, regular physical activity and healthy diet
- Lifelong learning and brain stimulating activities or training

(Matthew Baumgart, Heather M. Snyder et al.). Alzheimer's and Dementia 2015. June 11(6).

Other Factors That May Prevent Or Delay Alzheimer's Disease

Most of these are lifestyle interventions.

- Exercises like walking 5 to 9 miles a week
  Research has shown that of all the lifestyle interventions, physical activity is what helps the most to preserve brain function of memory, attention, focusing and executive functioning. This is definitely a non-expensive way of preserving memory
- Mental activity (reading, cross word puzzles, brain exercises, intellectual stimulation)
- Certain specific diets and foods
  Mediterranean diet consisting of fruits, vegetables, fish, grains, legumes, seeds, nuts, and olive oil. Diets which are high in antioxidants mainly fruits and vegetables are also helpful
- Recent research shows that high intake of trans-fat (as seem in pastries, margarine and candy) was associated with elevated risk of dementia including Alzheimer's disease (Damian McNamara. Medscape, Oct 25th, 2019)
- Reduced stress
- Adequate sleep
- Education
- Possibly Vitamin E 1000 IU 2x daily
- Use of certain blood pressure medications in people with Hypertension

These belong to the category called Angiotensin converting enzyme inhibitors, (ACEI) and Angiotensin receptor blockers (ARB). These may increase blood flow to the brain and also decrease inflammation. Examples of some of these blood pressure medications are: Candesartan, Eprosartan, Irbesartan, Telmisartan, Valsartan, Captopril, Lisinopril, Fosinopril, Ramipril and Periodopril. These in particular cross the barrier between the blood and brain fluid and enter brain cells, having a much greater effect.

Advice from A Well Known Researcher of Alzheimer's Disease

A well-known AD researcher DR. RUDOLPH TANZI does the following to lower his risk.

- Stays intellectually and socially engaged – this activates connection between nerve cells
- He is a vegetarian
- Takes a supplement called ASHWAGANDHA which has anti-Amyloid effects (see above Re: Amyloid)
- Trials have proven that exercise LOWERS RISK OF AD, probably by affecting Amyloid formation
- Sleeping for more than 4 to 5 hours. During deep sleep Amyloid production is turned off and that is when the brain "cleans itself"
- Avoid getting a stroke – Control RISK FACTORS for stroke as discussed previously, because strokes damage the brain and may cause formation of Amyloid and Tau
- Avoid certain medications. These include certain epileptic drugs, (like Phenytoin, Valproate, Phenobarbital), and sleep medicines like Benzodiazepines, Zolpidem and Eszopiclone; and anti-cholinergic drugs like Chlorpheniramine, Diphenhydramine, Promethazine, Dicyclomine. Avoid long term use, or ask your doctor for alternatives
- Maintaining healthy diet in midlife is associated with a larger Hippocampus in later life (this is part of the brain)
- Quit smoking if one is a smoker

Caregivers of Alzheimer Patients

Taking care of a loved one or spouse who has Alzheimer's disease is not an easy task. The primary caregiver has to have support or help from family and friends, the medical community, and paid help so that they do not end up with "caregiver fatigue" or get stressed, depressed or even sick. There is a lot of stress when one is taking care of a Dementia patient and a support group is important to help one feel one is not alone. Some communities have daycare centers for patients and there may be respite care (planned relief for a caregiver) available to give the caregiver a break. When the patient becomes a danger to themselves due to wandering, leaving the home, etc. then they may have to be placed in a long term facility for 24 hour supervision. Many caregivers may feel guilty about this, but sometimes this is the best and safest decision for the patient. Caregivers are heroes and need to be encouraged to use respite care so they do not get "burnout" from the physical and emotional toil of providing care. They need to take care of their own health and mental needs with frequent "Me Time". They must seek help and make use of community resources available for Alzheimer's patients, otherwise both patient and caregiver will suffer tremendously.

Reminders on Your Radar

There is no cure for AD but there are medications which may help so patients can perform some simple activities of daily living, but after a while their effectiveness declines. There are several simple non drug ways to help with some of the symptoms and these should be put into practice. Caregivers are mostly women and they can become exhausted with the increasing demands of the condition, and so it's important they get help from other family members, the community or paid help. Prevention include treatment and control of cardiovascular diseases, physical activity, mental stimulating activities, adequate sleep, healthy eating, and maybe use of Vitamin E supplements.

Headaches

....

There are many different types of headaches and they may be broadly classified as primary and secondary. The primary ones stem from problems with blood vessels, nerves or muscles in the head and neck areas; while the secondary ones are due to conditions or diseases present elsewhere for example Sinusitis, and Meningitis.

Everyone gets an occasional headache which may be associated with another illness e.g. cold, flu, sinus infection, or Malaria. Other causes include, smells, e.g. from perfume or chemicals, dehydration, or lack of adequate sleep. These are usually not chronic but come on when the illness or condition is present. However, some serious diseases may present with headaches and need immediate medical attention.

Headaches are sometimes defined based on broad underlying causes, and these are:

- Vascular: involves blood vessels, e.g. Migraine or as a result of high blood pressure
- Tension or muscle contraction: around head, face and neck which usually goes from back of head to the front
- Traction: headache as a result of brain masses pressing on pain sensitive areas, examples are brain tumors, abscess or blood collected in brain
- Inflammatory: as a result of diseases like Sinusitis, Meningitis, other infections and problems affecting teeth, neck, and ear problems

Headaches That are Concerning

- Headache which is the most severe headache one has ever experienced
- Headache accompanied by vision changes which could signify a Stroke or TIA
- Headache associated with change in a person's mental capabilities or loss of consciousness
- Headache associated with fever, nausea or vomiting, stiff neck or change in consciousness

Such headaches warrant immediate medical attention for proper diagnosis and treatment.

PRIMARY AND SECONDARY HEADACHES

Headaches can be classified as Primary and Secondary:

PRIMARY HEADACHES: These are headaches which are not due to other medical conditions, and they are from nerves, blood vessels and muscles around the head. Two of these are MIGRAINE HEADACHE and TENSION HEADACHE

SECONDARY HEADACHES: The types of headache which result from other medical conditions and include those associated with traction and inflammatory, for example

Head injury which results from an accident involving the head

Meningitis which is a result of infection in the brain or spinal cord

A Stroke or a bleed into the brain

Sinus infections

Obstructive Sleep Apnea

Migraine Headache
What is It?

This is a type of recurrent throbbing headache which is episodic (comes and goes), and has typically existed over several months to years. It typically lasts a few hours to three days, and usually occurs on one side of head often accompanied by sensitivity to light and sound, and sometimes nausea and vomiting. Migraines are more common in women and may run in families, however both men and children can also suffer from migraines. There has been recent research which suggests that people with migraines have a higher risk of getting Strokes and other heart and vascular diseases.

Other Signs and Symptoms

- May be on one side of the head, but can also be on alternate sides or involve both sides

- Headache may be throbbing or pulsating in nature
- The headache may last from 4 to 72 hours typically, and goes away completely
- Physical activity or movement make it worse, and sleeping may help it get better
- Taking pain medicines may help it
- It may occur around one's menses or period (Menstrual Migraine)
- Individual has had this type of headache at least a few times
- May be associated with flashes of light or sounds occurring prior to, during or after the migraine. This is called an "Aura" or warning sign. An aura lasts from a few minutes to an hour for most migraines with aura

Chronic Migraine Headache

This is when an individual experiences a headache greater than two weeks of the month for more than 3 months. This is a very debilitating situation and to avoid that, an episodic or intermittent Migraine has to be treated quickly when an attack occurs.

Atypical Migraine – Hemiplegia Migraine (Stroke like Migraine)

Above describe a classic Migraine but there is another atypical type of Migraine which mimics a stroke called a Hemiplegia Migraine, which presents differently.

What is It?

Occasionally some may experience a serious type of Migraine with symptoms or aura which are similar to a Stroke. They differ from Strokes because Strokes tend to occur suddenly, while these types of symptoms due to Migraine come on gradually. The vision changes in Migraine may be flashes of light or zigzagging lights which are not usually found in Strokes. Those suffering from Hemiplegia migraine may already have a history of Migraine, however any cluster of symptoms like those described below need to be checked out by a doctor. The Hemiplegic migraine may be preceded by aura symptoms like:

Visual problems
Speech problems
Temporary paralysis or weakness of one side of the body
Pins, needles and numbness
Loss of balance on one side of body
Dizziness or Vertigo (spinning sensation)

If someone who has never had a migraine or has migraine gets these symptoms for the first time, it is important to go to the hospital for tests to be done to make sure it's not a Stroke or mini stroke (TIA).

Vestibular Migraines (Migraine related Vestibulopathy)

This is an attack of dizziness and Vertigo, lightheadedness, balance issues, nausea or vomiting in an individual who has a history of Migraines. There may not be any headaches during an attack.

Things or Factors Which May Bring on A Migraine Attack

Certain things may aggravate or on the other hand ease a Migraine attack. Knowing those which will trigger an attack and avoiding them will result in decreased attacks. Triggers include:

- Change in weather: Humidity and temperature change, storms or rainy weather
- Stress: This can cause an attack
- Certain foods: Eating certain foods like chocolate, or aged cheese
- Drinks: Alcohol in red wine which contains Tyramine, and excess Caffeine
- Food additives: Aspartame, nitrates and Mono Sodium Glutamate (MSG)
- Change in sleep pattern: Sleep disruptions, lack of sleep etc. may bring on an attack
- Skipping meals: This or not eating or drinking enough fluids may bring on an attack
- Hormonal changes: Drop in Estrogen levels just before the menses or period time

Things Which May Protect One From A Migraine Attack

- Lowering one's stress level
- Regular meals – no skipping of meals
- Good hydration of the body – drinking adequate fluids especially water
- Postmenopausal state (there is no fluctuations of female hormones)
- Regular exercise

Treatment of Migraine Headache

It is important to let a doctor know when one has a history of Migraine headaches so he or she can take a careful history and examine you. Keeping a headache diary is a good way to keep a record of the headaches. It will help with what kind of treatment one should be given.

Headache Diary

One will document WHEN the headache occurs, the INTENSITY – mild, moderate or severe, WHAT HELPS IT, e.g. what medicine relieved it, if a dark room and sleeping helped it, DURATION, 60 minutes, whole day etc. OTHER symptoms present – nausea, vomiting, vision changes etc. This diary, if given to the doctor, will help determine the appropriate treatment.

Treatment

Initially, after the history and physical exam, a doctor may not order tests or may get a head CT or MRI of the brain, just to rule out conditions like brain tumors or other conditions. Treatment depends on how frequent one gets these headaches. If they are not treated properly, they may transform or change to chronic Migraine headaches. If acute attacks keep reoccurring frequently, then a doctor may have to put the individual on medications that prevent Migraine attacks from occurring in the first place. These have to be taken on a daily basis, just like someone will take a daily medication for high blood pressure. These are called prevention or maintenance medications.

Medications for Treating Acute Episodic Migraines

There are several that can be used, and they have to be started as soon as the headache begins. They abort the Migraine if taken early enough. They include:

- Non-steroidal anti-inflammatory (NSAIDS): e.g. Diclofenac, Naproxen, Ibuprofen
- Combination medications: Excedrin Migraine (Acetaminophen/Aspirin/Caffeine), APC (Acetaminophen, Phenacetin, Caffeine), Fioricet (Butalbital/Acetaminophen/Caffeine) Hydrocodone/Acetaminophen, (the latter is a narcotic and so it is to be avoided since it has addiction tendencies if taken on a regular basis)
- Triptans: e.g. Sumatriptan (Imitrex), Zolmitriptan (Zomig), Rizatriptan (Maxalt)
- Ergotamines : Ergotamine tartrate, Migranal nasal spray
- Antihistamines: Cyproheptadine (Periactin), Promethazine (Phenergan)
- Anti-nausea medications e.g. Promethazine, Ondansetron (Zofran)

Medications for Preventing Episodic Migraines

These are used when the frequency of attacks affects a person's life to such an extent that their work, social and or school work are all affected. Therefore, in order for such an individual to have a "life" besides headaches, they may be put on one of several MIGRAINE PREVENTION MEDICATIONS. These are used on a daily basis and they prevent the development of a Migraine in the first place.

Migraine Prevention Medications

Some of these are blood pressure medicines, antidepressants and anti-seizure medications; however, they do work for Migraine prevention. Examples are:

Propranolol, Metoprolol, Verapamil (BP medicines)
Topiramate, Valproic acid, Gabapentin (anti-seizure medicines)
Amitriptyline, Venlafaxine (antianxiety, antidepressants)

It is important that they are taken DAILY so as to prevent the onset of a Migraine headache.

Medications for Menstrual Migraines

For those who have Migraines associated with periods or menses, they may be put on combined oral contraceptive pills or they may use Estrogen patches or cream a few days before the period to prevent the usual sharp drop in Estrogen level which is thought to cause the headaches.

Injectable Migraine Prevention Medicines

Botox: This has been used for years in those with severe Migraines. One gets several injections around the head and neck for 12 weeks. It blocks pain signals from reaching the nerves in the head and neck area

Monoclonal Antibodies: Newly approved injections given under the skin every month or every three months. Examples are Fremanezumab-vfrm (AJOVY) and Erenumab-aooe (AIMOVIG) which are antibody proteins made in the laboratory that can bind to substances in the body. Currently, only adults can use these

Herbal or OTC Products Used to Prevent Migraine

There are OTC (over the counter or non-prescription) medications which have to be taken on a daily basis to prevent Migraines. One must talk to their health care provider if one has Migraines and would want to try OTC medicines instead of prescription medicines. The American Academy of Neurology and the American Headache Society classify the following as:

Butterbur (Petadolex) effective as per American Academy of Neurology
Riboflavin, Feverfew and Magnesium: probably effective (Feverfew has been used in Germany for years for Migraine)
Coenzyme Q10: possibly effective
Others like ALA, acupuncture, relaxation, biofeedback, spinal manipulation and Melatonin which are sometimes used do not have enough scientific

evidence to prove their effectiveness, however they may be useful. Make sure your doctor knows about any OTC medicines you take (nccih.nih.gov/health/pain/headaches/facts)

Tension Type Headaches
What is It?

This is the second type of headache that tends to affect adult women. It is caused by tense muscles or spasm of the muscles and psychological issues which lead to a headache.

Signs and Symptoms

The headache feels like a band around the head.

Starts from the back at the nape of the neck and comes round to the front or forehead area.

It may be episodic (once in a while) or chronic.

It may be associated with inability to sleep, worry, and anxiety.

May last a few hours or up to a week long.

Unlike Migraine, it is not associated with nausea, vomiting or sensitivity to light and sound.

It is often triggered or brought on by chronic stress or tension.

When it is chronic, it may be present in individuals who also suffer from depression or anxiety.

It may co-exist with Migraines and may lead to Migraine headaches if not treated early when it starts. Other conditions around the head and neck area like tooth ache, sinus infections, or ear infections can trigger this type of headache.

Prevention of Tension Type Headache

Prevention of this type of headache is by minimizing stresses in one's life. There is no need to worry about something that you cannot do anything about or control. One has to find ways of de-stressing and some of these are discussed below. If it is brought on by other conditions around the head and neck, then treating the specific cause will decrease or stop the tension headaches.

Treatment of Tension Type Headaches
Non medication treatment

These include use of cold towel or ice pack, dry heat, or moist heat to areas involved.

Massage, stretching, and relaxation techniques
More complex ones include ultrasound treatment or electrical stimulation.
Injections into muscles or to block nerves that supply the area involved.

For the simpler ones, a chiropractor, massage therapist or physical therapist will be able to do maneuvers which will relax the muscles at the back of the neck and also around the upper back and on the forehead.

Treatment of tension headaches

Medicines: Anti-inflammatories like Ibuprofen, Diclofenac or Analgesics (pain medicine) like Paracetamol/Acetaminophen/Tylenol.

These should not be taken on a daily basis otherwise one would end up with "Analgesic headache" which is a chronic daily headache resulting from overuse of Analgesics.

If the tension headache is triggered by an underlying infection then it gets better when that condition is treated. So for example, if it is triggered by an abscess tooth, treatment with antibiotics, root canal, or extraction of the tooth is important in order to get rid of the headache.

When tension type headache becomes chronic – occurring more than 2 times a week – then prevention medication may have to be used. These include antidepressants and or muscle relaxants which are prescription medications.

Common Headache

Common general forehead headaches which occur once in a while can be triggered by many things. These include:

- Certain foods and drinks like Caffeine, chocolate, cheese, red wine, Monosodium Glutamate (MSG), and processed meats. SOLUTION: Avoid these if they cause headaches
- Sitting in one position for too long especially if one has a phone to the ear or leaning forward (hunched up). SOLUTION: Getting up to change position, walking, and stretching are ways to help with this
- Eye strain by staring at a computer screen or TV monitor for a long time SOLUTION: Reading glasses may be needed to combat eye strain. One can practice the 20-20-20 rule: Every 20 minutes in front of the computer, look away about 20 feet in front for 20 seconds
- Sleep: Too little and even too much sleep can trigger headaches SOLUTION: Keeping a scheduled sleep time may help with this. Some individuals with undiagnosed Sleep Apnea may wake up with headaches in the morning (see below on sleep problems)
- Stress: This can bring on tension and Migraine headaches as discussed above SOLUTION: One has to take time to de-stress and some ways include laughing at oneself, watching comedy, meditation, praying, relaxation breaks and exercising. Talking things over with trusted friends or family may also help

- Dehydration: Everybody needs to drink adequate fluids especially when the weather is hot. The body is very good at signaling that it needs more fluids SOLUTION: Water, fruit flavored water or water with lemon are better than soda, and fruit drinks which may result in consuming lots of empty calories

---

Reminders on Your Radar

Two common headaches which affect women especially are Migraine and Tension headaches, both of which are primary headaches caused by blood vessels and muscles respectively.

Migraines have triggers and these include foods, weather changes, stress, red wine and hormonal changes as seen in some women prior to their periods. Migraines are episodic and when they go away after an attack they do so completely. If recurrence of Migraines is frequent, like once a week, then a sufferer has to be placed on a Migraine prevention medication which has to be taken on a daily basis. Tension headaches involve tensed muscles which start at the back of the head and move to the front like a circular band. It is triggered by stress and psychological issues like anxiety. Unlike Migraines it is not accompanied by sensitivity to light and sound, or nausea or vomiting.

Sleep Problems

Sleep is very important to get us rejuvenated and rested, and many activities to do with our metabolism and other important functions in our cells occur during sleep. However, some people have problems falling asleep (Initiating) or staying (maintaining) sleep, while others find themselves sleeping too much. We will discuss some common sleep problems, their names and treatments.

Insomnia (In-som-nea) Difficulty in Sleeping
What is It?

"That night the king could not sleep. So one was commanded to bring the book of the records of the chronicles; and they were read before the king".

—Bible, Esther 6v1 NKJV

Insomnia is inability to fall asleep, or stay asleep, or waking up early and not being able to go back to sleep. Most healthy adults need 6 to 8 hours of sleep, however with age, some people find it increasingly difficult to sleep. Women have twice the incidence of sleep problems compared to men, and it is higher in older women and in women with changes in hormones like during pregnancy, and peri/postmenopausal period. Adequate sleep has to do with both quantity (amount or duration) and quality (depth, arousals and restfulness) of sleep, and both are important for one to function well during the daytime.

Problems Resulting from Lack of Sleep

Sleep is very important because lack of adequate sleep can cause problems like:

Daytime sleepiness
Motor vehicle accidents
Irritability
Fatigue
Lack of concentration
Not feeling rested in the morning
Work-related accidents
Decreased productivity
Interference with work, and other day time activities
Memory problems

Short Term Sleep Problems

Some people may have short-term sleep problems due, for example, to a temporary stressful situation in their lives like loss of a loved one. However, there are those who have chronic or long-term sleep problems. Factors that contribute to sleep problems range from the mild to the severe and some are addressed below.

Causes of Poor Sleep

- CAFFEINE: Found in coffee, tea, cocoa, soda, and energy drinks can cause people not to fall asleep. Sodas high in Caffeine include Mountain Dew, Red Bull, Pepsi One
- ALCOHOL AND ILLEGAL DRUGS: Alcohol may cause excessive sleep or Insomnia, and illegal drugs like Methamphetamine, Cocaine, Ecstasy, are stimulants and lead to wakefulness and inability to sleep
- MEDICINES: Just as some medicines cause sleepiness, some can cause wakefulness. Sometimes just taking them during the day and not at nighttime may help, but if not, some may need to be discontinued or substituted with another. These include:
- Decongestants: e.g. Pseudoephedrine or Phenylephrine
- Alpha and beta blockers: e.g. Doxazosin, Prazosin, Tamsulosin, Metoprolol, Atenolol
- Steroids: Prednisone, Prednisolone

- Antidepressants: those known as SSRIs and Bupropion (Wellbutrin) Use alternatives or take in the morning
- Antidepressants: TCAs – some of these are activating, e.g. Desipramine, Protriptyline
- Medicines for Alzheimer's Disease: Donepezil, Galantamine
- MEDICAL CONDITIONS: These include some respiratory illnesses like Asthma, chronic cough; Sleep apnea, others like chronic stress, depression, bipolar disease, enlarged tonsils, and heartburn or acid reflux. Treatment resolves the Insomnia
- ACID REFLUX: Stomach acid tends to come up into the throat and mouth and cause burning. Inability to sleep is resolved when the heart burn or acid reflux is treated
- DEPRESSION/ANXIETY: People may stay up at night thinking about issues, and cannot shut their minds off. Depression itself results in sleep problems; either not sleeping or sleeping too much. Once depression or anxiety is treated the problem tends to be resolved, however, if Insomnia continues after the depression has improved, then sometimes a different medication has to be given for the Insomnia. There are particular antidepressants that tend to be used if Insomnia is a big problem. These include Trazodone, Amitriptyline and Mirtazapine (Remeron). The antidepressant called Paroxetine (Paxil an SSRI) may cause Insomnia and so may not be the best choice for someone with that. However some of the SSRIs may cause sleep problems in some, while they will not do so in other people
- PAIN: Pain from Arthritis in the joints, Cancer pain, stomach pain, earache etc. can all cause one not to sleep well. Treating the pain with pain medications will help one get a good night's sleep, but it's important to take care of the underlying problem
- FREQUENCY OF URINATION AT NIGHT: This is known as Nocturia if one is getting up more than once to urinate. It tends to increase with age and there are many reasons causing it. It can disrupt sleep and once the underlying condition is treated, or medication is changed, Insomnia resolves and sleep is restored
  CAUSES OF NOCTURIA:
  Bladder conditions and other conditions. Obstruction to urine flow, overactive bladder, urinary incontinence and infection (UTIs)
- Diseases like congestive heart failure, Diabetes Mellitus with uncontrolled blood sugar also cause Nocturia and sleep disruption
- Medicines include Diuretics, beta blockers, alpha blockers, SSRI antidepressants, weight loss medicines, caffeine containing medicines and Lithium (for bipolar)
- Excessive fluid intake close to bedtime
- Alcohol or drinking too much caffeine which tend to act like diuretics

- UPPER AIR WAY BLOCKAGE: Due to conditions like a small upper airway of the throat area, enlarged tonsils, obesity/overweight, or a large neck, the upper air way may be blocked causing the brain to wake one up when oxygen levels get low

- OBSTRUCTIVE SLEEP APNEA (OSA): This is a condition when airway or throat area is completely or partially closed during breathing while asleep. This cycle occurs many times during sleep and may cause snoring as well. To overcome this, the breathing muscles have to work harder and individual ends up breathing loud or gasping for air. It causes tiredness, day time drowsiness, hypertension, irregular heartbeats and decrease oxygen supply to organs. Once diagnosed by a test known as a sleep study, the individual may be treated with oral mouth devices, weight loss or use of devices like a CPAP (Continuous Positive Airway Pressure) or a BIPAP (Bi-level positive airway pressure) machine. These keep the airway open by increasing pressure in the throat during all phases of breathing, and this results in oxygen being adequately supplied to the lungs, and no waking up which is usually prompted by low oxygen

- PYSCHOPHYSIOLOGICAL (Mind-Body) INSOMNIA: This happens when people are going through stress and so cannot cause their body and mind to relax and fall asleep. Counseling and talking to someone about the problems or stress may help

- RESTLESS LEG SYNDROME: This is a neurological condition in which there is spontaneous leg movement or urge to move the legs when at rest or just before bed. It may feel like something is crawling up the legs. Specific medications help with this

- PERIODIC LEG MOVEMENT DISORDER (PLMD): This is when the desire to move the legs repetitively occurs during sleep and it disrupts sleep, resulting in poor sleep. Sleeping partners or spouses often report the disrupting sleep that occurs from the frequent leg movements

- NEUROLOGICAL DISEASES: Chronic brain diseases like Alzheimer's, Parkinson's disease disrupt sleep patterns causing insomnia. They are discussed in this chapter

- SLEEP PROBLEMS ASSOCIATED WITH MENOPAUSE/PERIMENOPAUSE: When women are in the perimenopause stage of their lives (time when changes signal that menopause is approaching) or have reached menopause (cessation of menstruation for at least 12 months with inability to have children naturally), they may start experiencing hot flashes and night sweats due to the hormonal changes that occur and this may disturb their sleep. There is lack of sleep or frequent awakening which result in tiredness and not feeling rested in the morning. It causes irritability, affects one's moods, decreases desire for sexual intercourse, and socialization with others. When the hot flashes and night sweats are controlled, better sleep is the result. This will be discussed in more detail

Treatment for Insomnia

Where there is a cause or specific reason e.g. side effect of a medicine, a medical problem like depression or Sleep Apnea, then change of medication or specific treatments would be needed. Once the condition is treated, the Insomnia resolves or is at least diminished. We will address sleep problems associated with menopause separately. For some individuals they would need medications to help them sleep if other methods do not work. However, most doctors would like to first try non pharmacological methods to help with sleep.

General Tips to Improve Sleep for People With Insomnia
Sleep Hygiene

Sleep hygiene is the term used to describe the non-drug things one can do to improve sleep and to help get a good night sleep. One can try the following:

- Try to go to bed and also wake up the same time each night
- Don't exercise too close to bedtime (make interval greater than two hours)
- Bed should only be used for sleep, sex, and resting; not reading, watching TV etc
- Avoid Caffeine, alcohol, and Nicotine too close to bedtime
- If one cannot sleep, one should get up and read or do something not too stressful, then go back to lie down when one feels sleepy
- Do not eat a large meal just before bedtime
- Keep the bedroom quiet and the light soft. Use of a bedside lamp helps
- Sometimes soft background music may help one fall sleep
- If something is bothering you, get up and write it down and go back to bed
- Try not to sleep or take a nap in the afternoon. Keep busy during the daytime
- Practice relaxation technics like mindfulness meditation, and deep breathing, prayer
- Make sure one has a good mattress and one can use a body pillow between one's legs
- Aerobic exercise, massage therapy and meditation will release endorphins which relieve pain and stress leading to better sleep
- Break the pain and Insomnia cycle. Pain leads to Insomnia and Insomnia can increase low back pain. Treat pain and use sleep hygiene tips. Focus less on pain, and visualize something peaceful and relaxing

(Some of above are from: Insomnia. www.familydoctor.org).

Herbal Supplements for Sleep

There are several available but there are no real good studies to back most of them, however, if they are safe and do not interfere with other medications they may be okay to take. Let your doctor know of any medicines one is taking.

Melatonin

This is a natural hormone which occurs in the brain and helps with sleep by resetting the body's clock. Studies back it up as a sleep aid. The supplement is used for Insomnia, jet lag and other conditions, with doses ranging from 0.3mg to 10mg. It has to be taken at least half hour before bedtime. There is an immediate release form which can be used if one has trouble falling asleep, while the extended release form is useful if one tends to wake up in the middle of the night. Some experts think effect is better with time release at bedtime and sublingual regular release in middle of night. It appears to be safe but a few people may experience drowsiness, dizziness, and nausea later on.

Valerian Root

This is a plant whose roots are used to make a supplement used for treating sleep problems, anxiety, and depression. Research shows it may help more with anxiety rather than sleep, but some claim it relaxes them.

Chamomile Tea

This herb has been used for calming people and helping with sleep. It usually comes in a tea bag and use 2 or 3 of them to help with sleep. It is safe according to American FDA. It may come in capsules as well.

Tryptophan

It is an amino acid used to build protein, make Niacin (vitamin B3) and Serotonin which is the feel good neurotransmitter which helps with depression, low moods and calming people. Serotonin also helps increase Melatonin levels. Eat Tryptophan rich foods like meats, turkey, eggs, milk, yogurt, nuts, cherries, honey, banana, oats, poultry, peanuts, lentils, tofu, mango, dates close to bedtime. Tryptophan supplements have raised some concerns in terms of side effects and so food sources should be used instead.

Other Herbs

Drink cool or iced herbal teas like Yogi Tea, lemon grass tea, etc. to help one relax and sleep well. Kava has been used for sleep and anxiety, however, it has caused liver damage in some people so talk to one's doctor before using it. Moringa leaves said to be high in Tryptophan have been used for tea and to promote sleep as well.

Aromatherapy

One can use Aromatic essential oils and those that help with sleep include: Roman chamomile oil, Lavender oil, Neroli, and Clary Sage oil. These can be used in a diffuser or vaporizer, or a few drops can be put on a tissue or cotton ball and placed near one's pillow for inhalation at bedtime. Avoid if you have asthma or if it irritates your lungs.

Medications for Treatment for Insomnia

Some individuals cannot sleep despite trying all the non-pharmacologic and herbal treatments suggested above, and so have to go on prescription medications. There are different classes of medications used and some are more appropriate if there are also other medical conditions present like depression, Fibromyalgia or nerve pain. The common ones include:

Antidepressants: Tricyclic ones like Amitriptyline and Doxepin are often used for depression, anxiety, pain, and Insomnia. Antidepressants like Trazodone and Mirtazapine are best used when depression and Insomnia are present. Doxepin is probably the best to use even for the elderly but at lower dose than that used for treating depression, and has been approved by FDA (USA) to treat Insomnia especially if it has to do with maintaining sleep. The main side effects of the tricyclic antidepressants may be dry mouth, excessive sleep, and low blood pressure if dose is too high in older adults

Benzodiazepines: These should be used for only a short time. Examples are Temazepam, and Triazolam. Side effects include addiction potential and drowsiness in the day time

Z drugs: Examples are Zolpidem (Ambien), Zaleplon (Sonata) and Eszopiclone (Lunesta). These are the most prescribed drugs for sleep and they work well. Side effects may include some unusual effects in some people like sleep walking, sleep eating, sleep driving and hallucination. The FDA has, what they call, a black box warning about these side effects

Melatonin like drugs: Ramelteon (Rozerem) acts like Melatonin, but the latter is sold as a supplement and is of course cheaper

Anticonvulsants: Gabapentin (Neurontin) is also used to treat seizures, nerve pain and restless leg syndrome. Side effects may include weight gain and prolonged drowsiness in some people

Tip: If one cannot sleep, try PRAYING, or playing a CD with scriptures or natural sounds. They work for some people.

Tips to Control Perimenopausal and Menopausal Sleep Problems

Sleep problems during the Perimenopause and Postmenopausal periods are very common, and they are mainly due to the hot flashes and night sweats that occur. Another common reason is waking up at night to urinate several times (Nocturia) due to an overactive bladder. Getting the hot flashes and night sweats under control usually helps the sleep problems associated with Menopause. See chapter 23 (p 474).

PARKINSON'S DISEASE (PD)

Parkinson's disease (PD) is a progressive degenerative brain disease and occurs in about 1% of adults greater than 60 years. Worldwide about 6 million suffer from it, and in the USA about one million suffer from PD. It is a result of loss or death of certain nerve cells containing a neurotransmitter and hormone called Dopamine. These cells help with movement. Cause is mostly unknown, but may be due to a combination of age, genetics and environmental factors like toxins, head injury and pesticides. Although known as a movement disorder, it has non motor symptoms and it is important that both types be treated. Symptoms include:

Motor symptoms

Tremors of mostly arms, legs, and body
Rigidity and decreased facial expression
Soft voice
Gait and Posture problems (flexed)
Slowness in walking and decreased swinging of the arms
Restless leg or Periodic leg movement disorder
Late problems include balance and uncontrolled sudden movements called dyskinesia (Dopamine may cause this, that is be a side effect of treatment)

Non-Motor symptoms

Cognitive Problems-memory and thinking problems
Psychiatric-Anxiety, Depression, Hallucinations (latter may be from disease or medication)
Sexual problems like Erectile Dysfunction in men and low libido and vaginal pain in women
Low Blood Pressure with standing up (orthostatic hypotension)
Sleep Problems like Insomnia and increased daytime sleepiness
Overactive Bladder, Urinary Incontinence, Urine Obstruction, or poor stream
Decreased sense of smell, constipation, swallowing difficulties
Dandruff and flaky dry skin (may occur before the diagnosis), or oily skin or excessive sweating
Sensory problems- numbness, tingling, and pain and Vision problems
Fatigue and Apathy
Speech problems- soft or monotone

Treatment

This is for both motor and non-motor symptoms. Currently there is no treatment to slow the loss of neurons, but those currently used are to treat the signs and symptoms. Although a Neurologist is the one in charge of one's treatment, one's primary care doctor may manage you in between neurologist appointments. Other team members may include: physical therapist, occupational, speech therapist, dietitian, psychologist, psychiatrist, nurse, and social worker and even a personal exercise trainer.

Medicines for Motor symptoms (These may be used alone or in combination)

1. Converted to Dopamine in the brain e.g. Levodopa/carbidopa,
2. Mimic effect of Dopamine- e.g. Ropinirole, and Pramipexole
3. Slows down breakdown of Dopamine and Levodopa- MAO-B inhibitors e.g.rasagiline, selegiline, and safinamide.
4. Uncontrolled tremor: Trihexyphenidyl or Benztropine to decrease it if others are not working.

There are others like Amantadine, Entacapone which are added if needed Research is ongoing, e.g. for those with potential for neuroprotection like MAO-B inhibitors, Creatine, and Isradipine a BP drug. (See www.michaeljfox.org).

Like all medicines, all above have side effects which your doctor should discuss with you.

Non drug therapies include: Physical Therapy, Occupational and Speech Therapy, exercise, Rock Steady Boxing (non-contact boxing), Social Networking and support group meetings.

Medicines for non-motor symptoms – this depends on the condition

Constipation – stool softeners(docusate), fluids, high fiber diet, laxative e.g. polyethylene glycol

Drooling – drying agents of saliva include glycopyrrolate and amitriptyline.

Cognitive Problems – memory and thinking-rivastigmine and donepezil (used for Alzheimer's)

Hallucinations – regular drugs used may increase movement symptoms, Pimavanserin is better

Depression and anxiety – Antidepressants like Paroxetine and Venlafaxine

Insomnia – Try sleep hygiene, melatonin or chamomile and medicines discussed under Insomnia

Excess daytime sleepiness – Modafinil

Fatigue – Methylphenidate

Hypostatic Hypotension – fludrocortisone or Midodrine

Pain – e.g. from muscle spasm, need medications ranging from NSAIDs to Narcotics, however, muscle spasm can be treated with massage, exercises, stretching, and water therapy

Sexual Problems – Sildenafil or Tadalafil in men and for women, topical or oral female hormones.

Overactive bladder – Irritation of bladder usually treated with anticholinergic medicines which aggravate symptoms of PD. Behavior therapy discussed under that topic can be used.

Urinary obstruction – may need to use a urinary catheter intermittently to empty bladder

Surgical Treatment – There are two, Deep Brain Stimulation when electrodes are placed in specific areas of the brain to affect electrical impulses and Focused Ultrasound which uses US to destroy brain cells causing the movement problems. Not everyone is suited for either procedures.

Other treatments include Botox injection into salivary gland, speech therapy, Physical Therapy to correct posture, Lip exercises and sucking ice chips.

15

Mouth and Dental Conditions

The Mouth

....

The mouth is one of the port of entries into the body. It is where food is mixed with digestive enzymes found in saliva and digestion begins. It consists of the lips, teeth, gums, tongue, and salivary glands. Apart from initiating digestion, the mouth is also the entry point for foreign objects or organisms to enter our bodies and cause infections or other diseases. We will discuss some important aspects of each part.

"So long as you have food in your mouth, you have solved all questions for the time being".

Franz Kafka, Novelist,
July 3, 1883—June 3, 1924

The Lips

These are the structures which seal the entrance of the mouth and cause things to either enter or be prevented from entering one's body.

Dry lips

The lips can become dry and cracked during the winter, or dry season in some parts of the world; and they can also be dry in individuals who breathe through their mouth while sleeping (mouth breathers) or who snore. Cracked lips can be painful, and so to prevent this, one needs to moisten the lips with any lip moisturizer like Chap Stick, Vaseline, Petroleum jelly, lip gloss, or Shea butter lip balm. Mouth breathing is caused by many factors including sleeping on your back, Allergic Rhinitis, Sleep Apnea, nasal congestion, enlarged adenoids, and septum deviation.

Correction of these can stop or minimize mouth breathing, but untreated, it can lead to inflamed gums (Gingivitis) and bad breath (Halitosis).

Cold Sore (fever blister) Herpes Labialis
What is It?

This occurs on either the upper, lower or corners of the lips, and they are caused by two viruses called Herpes Simplex type I (commonest) and type II. They form painful blisters (contain clear fluid) and after a few days will form ulcers, then get crusted or covered by a scab. When one gets the initial infection with the virus, the ulcer heals in a few days; however, the virus lies dormant in a nearby nerve. When an individual develops fever, stays in the sun for a long time, or is stressed, the virus is reactivated and causes blisters to reappear. Initial infection may result from skin to skin contact like kissing, sharing razors, toothbrushes, cups, utensils, towels with someone who has the virus on the lips or other parts of the body like the eye, anal area, or acquired from the genitals through oral sex.

Signs and Symptoms

The blisters may be preceded by numbness (loss of feeling), tingling, or burning. The carrier or infected person may not have an open sore or ulcer but may still harbor the virus and transmit it to another person. Cold sores on the lips may last for about 5 to 7 days. These two viruses can also cause genital herpes which may present as shallow painful sores on the genitals or anal area. The latter is a sexually transmitted disease (STD) spread through sexual intercourse, which will be discussed in the section about STDs (they are also known as Sexually Transmitted Infections STIs).

Treatment

ANTIVIRAL: They can resolve quickly by the use of anti-viral medicines in the form of creams or oral tablets. Examples of these are ACYCLOVIR, VALACYCLOVIR, and FAMCICLOVIR. When an individual gets more than 6 infections in a year, they may go on suppression therapy. This means they will take an antiviral medication on a daily basis to suppress the virus and prevent an outbreak. Suppression tends to be used more for the genital infection rather than the oral infection, however this therapy may be used for oral infections if they are frequent.

LYSINE: This is an OTC oral supplement which can be taken daily to help prevent recurrent lip herpes or cold sores infections. A dose of 500mg to 1000mg one to two times daily for 6 to 12 months may help prolong infection free periods

10% DOCOSANOL CREAM (Abreva cream): This is an OTC cream which can be used at first sign of lesions or when tingling or pain starts. It cuts down the duration of symptoms

Aphthous Ulcer (Canker Sore)

This is a small round or oval shallow ulcer which develops on the lining of the mouth, gums, tongue, or inner lips. It is called a Canker Sore and tends to recur lasting between 2 to 10 days and heals completely. T usually has a red base with a white creamy covering in the center. The cause is unknown, however, factors like stress, injury to mouth, e.g. hard food, nutritional deficiency, family history and weakened immune state have been implicated.

Treatment include
- Topical steroids (hydrocortisone or Triamcinolone cream)
- Diclofenac paste
- Magic Mouth Wash (e.g. Maalox, 2% lidocaine and diphenhydramine) swish and spit
- Chlorhexidine gluconate mouth rinse
- Doxycycline caps opened and mixed with water as a mouth rinse
- Vitamin B12 sublingually (under tongue) is thought to reduce recurrence
- CAM products: include Aloe Vera, rubbing with Lemon juice and low-level laser Therapy

Teeth and Gums

The teeth are involved in digestion because the chewing process help with softening of the food which mix with digestive juices in saliva before swallowing occurs. The teeth can have cavities (holes), form abscesses, and the surrounding gum around them can develop gum disease. The teeth are also important to give support to the face. If anyone has several teeth extracted or if most of the teeth fall out, one notices that the face or specifically the cheeks appear to sink in, and speech is affected. The tooth consists of more than the eye sees when someone opens their mouth. Below the gum line is the root which is found in the bony part of the jaw. Most people tend to concentrate on the white part (enamel) which is what is above the gum line, however, if for whatever reason the root is not well secured the tooth can get loose and fall out. Serious gum disease causes teeth to be loose.

Tooth Decay (Dental Caries)

Tooth decay also known as Dental Caries or cavities results from infection by bacteria. Using sugar (present in food) in the mouth, the bacteria create chemicals which break down the enamel (hard outer white covering) and that results in a hole or cavity. The break down may start as a white discolored spot on the enamel where minerals are depleted, and if not treated by Fluoride, then the enamel breaks down and a cavity is created. The cavity can be painful and cause severe toothache.

Preventing Cavities in the Teeth

- REGULAR BRUSHING with a Fluoride containing toothpaste two to three times a day after meals
- FLOSSING with FLOSS removes any food particles and bacteria from in between the teeth, because these together may cause cavities. Flossing is when a piece of special waxed string is used to clean the spaces between the teeth and below the gum line
- The use of a FLUORIDE RINSE by swishing one to two teaspoons in the mouth and spitting out after brushing and flossing will help prevent tooth decay. There is a difference between this and a mouthwash. A mouthwash typically does not have Fluoride and it is to freshen one's breath. If it has Fluoride it will say so on the label. Some may have to be diluted and so reading the instructions is very important
- Prolonged continuous use of Fluoride or drinking water high in Fluoride in the first 8 years of life may lead to discoloration of the teeth – turning from white to brown spots known as Dental Fluorosis. It is important to check with one's dentist before using Fluoride rinses
- To further prevent decay, a sealant which is a thin plastic material may be coated on the chewing surfaces of the teeth to prevent plaque and food from going into the ridges and grooves

Gum Disease
What is Gum Disease?

Gum disease is inflammation of the gums and results from bacteria and other substances. Normally, the mouth is full of bacteria and this tends to form a thin sticky film called "PLAQUE" on the surface of the teeth. When plaque is not removed, it can combine with Calcium and Phosphorus from saliva, harden and form a white or blackened substance called 'TARTAR' or Calculus at the gum line. The gum then becomes red and inflamed with easy bleeding. Mild Gum Disease is called Gingivitis, and serious Gum Disease is called Periodontitis.

Mild Gum Disease (Gingivitis)

Gingivitis is mild gum disease, and presents with redness and bleeding of the gums, bad breath (Halitosis), painful gums and receding gum lines making the teeth look longer. Some may also experience pain with chewing food. If it is not treated, then it will lead to periodontal disease.

How to Prevent Gingivitis

Daily brushing at least two times a day – ideally after meals – followed by flossing will remove plaque and prevent its build up. Apart from these, it is necessary to have regular deep cleaning by a dental hygienist or dentist, at least once or twice a year. This will remove plaque, tartar and decrease the accompanying inflammation.

Treatment of Gingivitis

- See one's dentist or dental hygienist for deep cleaning and removal of plaque and tartar
- Another treatment may be an antibiotic rinse called Chlorhexidine gluconate 0.12% solution (Peridex, PerioGard, PerioChip, and Chlorostat). One table-spoon (or as directed) is used by swishing for 30 seconds and spitting, twice a day after brushing for about a week or two to kill bacteria, reduce redness, bleeding and swelling of the gums

Consult a dentist or dental hygienist to find out if this will be appropriate for use. It can cause staining of the teeth and gums if there is a lot of plaque buildup on the teeth, and that is why brushing of the teeth several times a day is important.

Severe Gum Disease (Periodontitis)
What is This?

This is the serious form of gum disease when inflammation and plaque build up around the tooth causes the gum to be pulled away from the tooth creating a "pocket" or space that can become infected by bacteria. There is eventual break down of the tissues that support the teeth and the bone that holds it in place. The tooth can then become loose and must be pulled (extracted) or it falls out.

Treatment

It is treated by dental professionals with deep cleaning and scaling (scraping) every three to four months. The deep cleaning empties the pockets of tartar and bacteria, and causes the inflamed gum to shrink and move closer to the affected teeth. Special antibiotic chips, e.g. PerioChip (Chlorhexidine), Doxycycline or Minocycline may be placed in affected gum pockets every three months after deep cleaning to lower the number of bacteria present and keep the gums healthy. Sometimes laser is used to treat the gum disease and if very serious surgery needs to be done. If the teeth are in very bad shape and the gum is really infected, then extraction of all or most of the teeth would occur.

Who is at Risk for Gum Disease?

It tends to develop more in men, however, there are factors that may predispose a person to gum disease. Saliva protects the mouth, however if it is decreased, bacteria will increase leading to Gingivitis. Risk factors include.

- Smoking
- Dry mouth
- Medical conditions like Diabetes Mellitus, Cancer, and AIDs
- Medications, especially those that make the mouth dry
- Radiation treatment to head and neck

Why it's Important to Avoid or Treat Gum Disease

Some research have associated gum disease with heart disease, Stroke, preterm delivery in women, and uncontrolled Diabetes (DM). For people with Diabetes, the presence of dental cavities, and significant amounts of bacteria in the mouth cause difficulties in blood sugar control. It is advisable to make regular brushing, flossing and visits to the dentist for cleaning part of one's DM care, so that will help keep gums healthy. Good control of blood sugar with medicines, diet and exercise, coupled with healthy teeth and gums will keep one's DM under control and prevent complications of DM.

The process of digestion starts in the mouth and the teeth and tongue assist in this. The teeth is more than what one sees above the gumline. It is important that both the teeth and gums are taken care of by regular brushing at least two times a day, flossing and regular visits to the dentist for professional cleaning. If not, it will result in dental caries or cavities and gum diseases. Gum or periodontal disease may be mild as in Gingivitis or severe as in Periodontitis when the gum is pulled away from the tooth, followed by bone and tooth loss.

16

Digestive System's Diseases and Problems

The Abdomen and the Organs it Contains

....

The abdominal cavity or space covers the area from under the diaphragm to the lower part in the pelvis. In the upper part, the diaphragm separates the chest cavity from the abdominal cavity, and this part contains the liver, stomach, pancreas and spleen and part of the small bowel. The lower part is made up of the small and large bowel, rectum and anal region. Some important organs or structures and their functions include:

"Do you not yet understand that whatever enters the mouth goes into the stomach and is eliminated"?
Jesus Christ (Matthew 15: v17 NKJV).

The Esophagus: Also known as the gullet, this long tube connects the back of the mouth to the stomach, and after swallowing, it moves foods and liquids from the mouth into the stomach

The stomach: Located on the left upper side. The first part is involved in significant digestion of food. It produces acid and other juices involved with digesting foods and there is also absorption of certain Vitamins

The Liver: On the right upper side, just under the diaphragm

The Spleen: On the left upper side just under the diaphragm

Gall bladder: This is a sac which stores a greenish fluid called bile, and this is produced by the liver and helps with the digestion of fat. It is situated below the liver in the right upper part

Pancreas: Produces chemicals called enzymes that aid with digestion and also produces Insulin and Glucagon (hormones) which are involved in controlling the amount of sugar in the blood stream

Small and large intestines: These are the main portions of the digestive system where digestion of food takes place with breaking down of proteins, fats and carbohydrates into simpler substances and absorption of these into the blood stream

The Kidneys: Situated in the posterior aspect just below the rib cage in the back or flank. There are normally 2 kidneys present. They are not involved in digestion but are in the abdominal area right at the back. They deal with removing waste and excess fluid from the body in the form of urine. They will be discussed in a separate chapter. They are strictly not abdominal organs

There are many abdominal conditions that are common and tend to affect women. These include:

- Diseases affecting the Esophagus (gullet)
- Stomach problems
- Small intestine problems
- Large intestine diseases
- Anal and rectal problems
- Liver diseases
- Gallbladder diseases
- Pancreatic diseases

How Digestion Occurs

The digestive system is made up of all the various parts or organs associated with digestion or break down of the food we eat and then the absorption of these nutrients into the blood. The system starts from the mouth which contains the teeth, salivary glands and the tongue.

In the Mouth

Food is chopped into smaller particles by the teeth, moistened, lubricated by saliva, and digested by enzymes in the saliva. It is then moved into the back of the mouth (Pharynx) by the tongue for it to be swallowed and moved into the ESOPHAGUS (Gullet). This is a long muscular tube mostly present above the diaphragm but the lower portion of the Esophagus is below it, and has a sphincter or ring to close it and prevent food from the adjoining STOMACH from moving back up into the esophagus.

In the Stomach and Small Intestines

The stomach contains acid, enzymes, and hormones all of which aid in breaking down food. Digestion continues there for about 2 to 3 hours until food becomes a liquid mixture and moves into the coiled SMALL INTESTINE. This takes up most of the space in the abdominal cavity being about 16 foot long, and it is here that most digestion and absorption of food occurs. The nutrients resulting from digestion are absorbed into the blood stream from the lining of the small intestines, and food and nutrients may spend 4 to 6 hours in the small intestines.

Picture of the Abdomen And its Contents

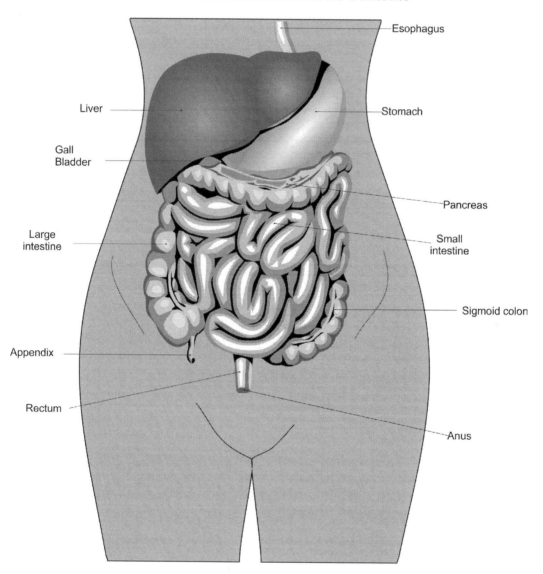

Role of Pancreas, Liver and Gallbladder

The PANCREAS produces enzymes which it discharges into the small intestine to help with digestion, and the LIVER produces bile which is stored in the gallbladder. The GALLBLADDER is situated close to the inferior aspect of the liver and in the presence of fatty food, it releases bile intermittently, to help break fat into smaller particles in the small intestines.

Large Bowel or Intestines

From the small intestine, mostly undigested food is propelled into the LARGE BOWEL OR COLON (large Intestine). The large bowel surrounds the small bowel at its sides and top, and it is about five foot in length. The large bowel starts at the right side and is known as the Cecum with the appendix hanging at its inferior or lower part. From there it lies above the small intestine just below the stomach and is called the Transverse bowel which then becomes the descending colon and sigmoid, on the left side emptying into the rectum.

In the large bowel, water is mostly absorbed into the blood stream leaving a solid fecal material. Some "good" bacteria are present and may remove tiny amounts of nutrients from the feces. Stool or feces is made up of substantial number of bacteria, and indigestible material and water. Stool is kept in the rectum until signals are sent from nerves to evacuate or expel feces. The last part of the colon is the ANUS or opening where stool or feces are discharged from the body.

Diseases of the Esophagus

Food from the mouth is sent down the Esophagus by waves of contractions and at the end of it, there is a sphincter or a circular band of muscle which opens or closes the entrance into the stomach. If functioning normally, the sphincter will close and allow the contents of the stomach to stay inside and undergo further digestion before it is released into the small intestine.

Acid Reflux Disease (GERD)

What is This?

"I can't deal with a lot of spice but I have to eat it. I pay the price — I'm on medication for heartburn, so that's how I deal with it".

— Tom Colicchio (Chef) www.azquotes.com

GASTROESOPHAGEAL REFLUX DISEASE (GERD) is the condition in which acid from the stomach and its liquid contents rise into the Esophagus through the enlarged opening between the two parts caused by a relaxed sphincter. The contents flow back into the esophagus and this is called "REFLUX". It is more than heartburn and has other symptoms.

Signs and Symptoms of GERD

- Heartburn described as pain in front of the chest wall, or pressure in the mid chest area especially after meals (It has nothing to do with the heart; however, since this happens close to where the heart is situated, the symptom is referred to as "heartburn")

- Burning behind the sternum (breast bone)
- Chest pain
- Rushing of fluid into the mouth
- Nausea or vomiting
- Acidic taste in the mouth and throat

When above are present for a while without treatment, complications can occur.

Complications of GERD

- The presence of the acid causes inflammation, irritation and sometimes ulceration of the lining of the Esophagus called Peptic ulcer
- Cough and hoarseness of voice
- Erosion of the enamel of the tooth by acid which backs into the mouth
- Ear infections especially in kids
- Difficulty in swallowing caused by narrowing of the acid damaged Esophagus
- Wheezing or whistling sound in the chest area due to acid in the respiratory tubes as a result of backflow into the voice box
- Bleeding, spitting or vomiting blood when there is ulceration of the lining
- Changes in the lining of the junction between the stomach and Esophagus lead to redness, prolonged inflammation and scarring. If severe or prolonged, it may lead to a pre-cancer state called Barrett's Esophagus
- When the precancerous state is not treated, it can result in cancer of the Esophagus over the long term

Treatment of GERD

Treatment is therefore important if GERD is bothersome and frequent. There are lifestyle changes, medications, devices, and surgery to treat this.

Lifestyle Changes

- If one is overweight or obese, losing weight helps prevent the reflux
- Sleep on more than one pillow thereby lifting the head and neck area up
- Raise the head of the bed by 4 to 6 inches using wooden planks or concrete blocks
- Avoid certain foods like chocolate, onions, tomatoes, coffee, caffeinated drinks, citrus fruits, fermented foods especially before bed, and those high in fat which may aggravate the symptoms
- Eat small meals rather than large amounts at a sitting
- Try not to eat late at night or just before bedtime
- Avoid drinking alcohol late at night
- Stay upright for 3–4 hours after a meal. Don't lie down too soon

- Avoid smoking which can make heartburn worse
- Avoid tight fitting clothes around belly area
- Avoid heavy lifting or bending
- Don't exercise too soon after eating

Medications

- Use of ANTACIDS – Examples are those containing Aluminum, Calcium, and Magnesium. These neutralize the acids produced in the stomach. Magnesium salts may cause Diarrhea, and calcium and or aluminum ones may cause Constipation. Brand names include Alu-Tab, Aludrox, Maalox, Mylanta, Tums, Alka Seltzer and Rolaids
- Use of medications which block production of acid by the stomach – RANITIDINE, CIMETIDINE, NIZATIDINE or FAMOTIDINE. These are non-prescription medicines. The brand names include; Zantac, Tagamet, Pepcid, Peptic relief, Pepcid AC. These should not be used for more than 2–3 weeks at a time without consulting a physician, since heartburn may be a sign of something more serious
- Blocking of acid by another group of drugs called PROTEIN PUMP INHIBITORS (PPIs): These include OMEPRAZOLE, PANTOPRAZOLE, and ESOMEPRAZOLE. Brand names are Nexium, Protonix, Aciphex, Prevacid, Prilosec, Losec, and Pantoloc

EGD (Esophagogastroduodenoscopy)

If using OTC medicines for more than 3 times in a week for several months, it is important to discuss with your doctor so tests can be carried out to further investigate the GERD. A doctor may need to perform upper endoscopy also known as an EGD (Esophagogastroduodenoscopy) with a small lighted tube which has a camera to look into the Esophagus, stomach and first part of small bowel called the duodenum. The state of the lining of the walls of these organs can be visualized, ulcers or masses looked for, biopsies taken to check for cell changes, and to test for the presence of a bacterium called H. Pylori (Helicobacter Pylori).

Surgery

In severe cases of reflux disease when medicines have failed to offer relief, a type of surgery can be performed to tighten the band (sphincter) and the passage way between the stomach and the Esophagus by wrapping upper part of the stomach around the Esophagus. This is known as Fundoplasty, and there are two popular types Nissen and Toupet fundoplication. About 90% of people are symptom free after the surgery.

Other Treatments

ENDOSCOPIC INJECTION: A solution called Enteryx is injected into the lower esophageal sphincter to tighten it and close the space. This prevents acid from flowing backwards

ENDOSCOPIC DEVICES: Magnet device: called a 'LINX' which is a small ring of magnets placed at the lower esophageal sphincter endoscopically and it keeps the sphincter closed so acid does not move back into the esophagus, however it opens to let food and liquid move into the stomach (www.linxforlife.com)

Others strengthen the muscle or make it tighter and the devices involve putting stitches in the Lower Esophageal Sphincter (LES-band) or making tiny cuts which after healing strengthen the LES muscles and prevent reflux. These are the "Bard EndoCinch" system and "Stretta" system respectively.

Common Stomach Diseases

....

Gastritis

What is It?

This is inflammation of the lining of the stomach as a result of various reasons like:

- Stress
- Medications called non – steroidal anti-inflammatory drugs NSAIDs (e.g. Ibuprofen, Aspirin, Diclofenac, and Naproxen) and steroids
- Irritants like spicy foods, and alcohol
- Presence of a bacterium or germ called H. Pylori and viruses

Signs and Symptoms

This may present as stomach pain, fullness, bloating, nausea, vomiting, belching and vomiting of blood.

Treatment

An EGD may be done and it will reveal redness of the lining of the stomach. It is treated with medications which either stop production of acid in the stomach or neutralize the acid. These are similar to those mentioned above for treating GERD. Treating the bacterial infection if present also helps the healing process.

Stomach Ulcer: (Peptic Ulcer Disease)
What is It?

In the past gastric or duodenal ulcers were difficult to treat and ended up in complications from perforations through the wall of the stomach or duodenum. It has now been found that it is mostly a result of an infection with bacteria called H. Pylori. If found in someone with abdominal symptoms, simple treatment with antibiotics and other medications can result in a cure.

Sometimes instead of a general inflammation of the lining of the stomach, an actual ulcer will form and go deeper beyond the lining of the stomach due to erosion of the lining It is due to a combination of many factors like:

Presence of the H. pylori bacterium
Stomach acid
Alcohol
Medicines like NSAIDS

Signs and Symptoms of Gastric Ulcer

The presence of an Ulcer may cause:

Pain in the middle or left part of upper belly just below the breast bone
Nausea and vomiting
Pain after eating a meal
Belching, bloating and feeling gassy
Bleeding with vomiting of blood if a blood vessel under the ulcer is involved
Anemia if there is a lot of blood loss from a bleeding ulcer
TREATMENT: See below

Duodenal Ulcer
What is It?

The duodenum is the first part of the small bowel, right after the stomach. This Ulcer is a type of Peptic Ulcer which develops in the duodenum, as a result of contact with stomach acid, use of NSAIDS and infection with the bacterium Helicobacter Pylori. Other factors like stress, tobacco and alcohol use may increase the occurrence if the initial three are present.

Signs and Symptoms

It may present with constant pain or one that goes and comes, nausea, vomiting or bleeding in which case vomitus will be red in color. Pain may be worse before meals or when one is hungry. Eating may relieve the symptoms.

Complications of Stomach and Duodenal Ulcers

If not identified early, both stomach and duodenal ulcers can have complications some of which can be life threatening. These include:

- Bleeding when ulcer erodes through a blood vessel
- Perforation through the wall of the stomach
- Severe recurrent abdominal pain in the top part of the abdomen or belly
- Anemia (low blood level) as a result of the bleeding ulcer
- Bleeding if it involves a big vessel results in blood loss, and if extensive, can lead to low blood pressure, shock and even death

Treatment of Gastric Or Duodenal Ulcers

These ulcers used to be treated by surgery in earlier times and caused high morbidity (protracted ill health) and mortality (death). However, currently treatment has been very successful with medications. If the ulcers are discovered early, they can be treated with medications, like Omeprazole, Pantoprazole (PPIs) etc. It has been found that Peptic Ulcer disease is mostly a result of infection with the Helicobacter Pylori (H Pylori) bacterium, and so treating this with a combination of antibiotics and an acid reducer, results in healing of the ulcer and resolution of the symptoms. If complicated, e.g. bleeding ulcer, one may need surgery to repair a bleeding ulcer or they can also be cauterized (bleeding vessel is sealed with heat) or clipped.

Hiatal Hernia

What is It?

This is when there is a protrusion or sliding of the upper part of the stomach through a tear or an enlarged opening or defect in the diaphragm into the chest. The diaphragm is the dome-shaped muscle which separates the chest cavity from the abdominal cavity. Hiatal hernia is common and occurs in about 25% of people older than 50 years. Many may be born with it, or it may result from weakness of the muscles around the opening (hiatus) which increases with age, surgery or injury.

Risk Factors for Developing A Hiatal Hernia

There are risk factors associated with getting a Hiatal Hernia. These include:

Being a woman
Pregnancy
Age above 50 years; by 60years, 60% will have a Hiatal Hernia
Obesity

Anything that increases pressure in the abdomen like: chronic cough, lifting weights, straining and excessive vomiting.

Signs and Symptoms

Usually they do not cause any symptoms and it may be discovered when an endoscopy is done or special X-rays or imaging studies are done for other reasons like troubling acid reflux or other abdominal conditions. Symptoms of Hiatal Hernia if present, include:

Heart burn and burning if associated with Acid Reflux
Belching
Fullness in upper abdomen
Chest pain

Treatment

For those with troubling symptoms, the following may help:

- Lifestyle changes like weight loss, eating small frequent meals instead of a large meal at one sitting, and avoiding late night meals
- Delay lying down after eating
- Raise head of bed as discussed under acid reflux treatment
- If symptoms continue to be bothersome despite lifestyle changes, and acid reflux is associated with it, then medications to treat acid reflux may help
- If very large and bothersome, then surgery is done to secure the stomach into the abdomen and prevent it from sliding up into the chest cavity

Diseases of the Small and Large Bowels (Intestines)

There are many diseases which affect the small and large bowels. A few are listed:

Constipation
Hemorrhoids
Diarrhea
Irritable Bowel Disease
Gluten Intolerance and Celiac Disease
Diverticulosis
Inflammatory Bowel Diseases
Colon cancer

Constipation

What is It?

Constipation is a very common condition of the large bowel, when it is difficult to have a bowel movement and the number of bowel movements is reduced to less than three a week.

Signs and Symptoms

The stools are hard, dry and may be little pellet-like, associated with straining, abdominal pain or fullness, and bleeding from the rectum. One may develop hemorrhoids because of excessive straining. In the very elderly, stool may become hard and impacted in the rectum, associated with Diarrhea stools which is from liquid stools passing around the solid impacted stool.

Risk Factors for developing Constipation include:

- Not drinking much fluid, especially water
- Anti-hypertension medicines called Calcium channel blockers e.g. Verapamil
- Pain medicines called Narcotics including Codeine or Hydrocodone
- Some medicines used for treating bladder problems e.g. Oxybutynin
- Irritable Bowel Syndrome (IBS constipation), Parkinson's, Depression, and diverticulosis
- Drinks like coffee, tea and alcohol may cause constipation by acting like diuretics

Treatment

Lifestyle Changes

Increasing fluid especially water in one's diet, increasing fiber in the diet, as well as exercise will help stool move quickly through the bowels. Avoid sorbitol and high fructose corn syrup, try lactose free diet. If severe see doctor, who may do thyroid blood work, colon transit study and colonoscopy

Medications

Over the counter medications available include different types of laxatives and stool softeners.

Lubricants: example is mineral oil which lubricates and retains water in the stool and keeps it moving down can be taken orally with a drink or as an enema.

Bulk forming agents: These fiber containing agents increase volume of stool so it is expelled quickly, e.g. Citrucel, (Methylcellulose), FiberCon, Psyllium like Metamucil, Fiberall

Stool softeners: Gently draw in water. Docusate (Colace), and Kaopectate stool softeners which contain docusate

Osmotic laxatives; These draw water into the bowel so the stool is softened and easily expelled. Examples are Glycerin, Lactulose, Magnesium Citrate, Magnesium Hydroxide (Milk of Magnesia), Sodium Phosphate (Fleet enema)

Stimulant laxative: These stimulate the large bowel to move stool along the bowel quickly. Examples are Bisacodyl (Corrector, Dulcolax), Castor oil, Cascara, Senna (Senokot)

Avoid chronic use of Laxatives, instead, use the other medicines suggested. Chronic use can affect your blood electrolytes, cause your colon to be "Lazy"(reduced bowel movements/ contractions), cause diarrhea, and even risk of colon cancer. On the other hand, fiber types decrease risk of colon cancer by increasing number of "good bowel bacteria" and also diluting any toxins present.

Diarrhea
What is It?

This is defined by excessive or frequent bowel movements of 3 or more watery stools per day.

CAUSES: Diarrhea can be a result of:

Certain medications e.g. some antibiotics

Infection by microbes, including viruses, bacteria, and parasites, (e.g. food poisoning, Cholera, HIV)

Noninfectious causes like Irritable Bowel Syndrome, Bowel Cancer, and two chronic inflammatory diseases of the bowel known as Crohn's Disease and Ulcerative Colitis

Prevention

To prevent Diarrhea it is important that **hand washing** after using the bathroom (toilet) is practiced by all of us. This also prevents the spread of diseases by the oral or respiratory route.

Treatment

Involves replacing fluid and electrolytes (chemicals) that are passed out in large amounts and use of antibiotics if the source is due to bacteria infection.

- The fluid loss has to be replaced with fluids like water, oral rehydration solutions, clear fluids, soups, coconut water and broths
- BRAT Diet: This stands for: Banana, Rice, Applesauce and Toast
- When an infectious source is suspected, antibiotics are used to treat it
- Diarrhea from antibiotics can be minimized by taking Probiotics along with them
- Diarrhea associated with a bug called Clostridium Difficile (C. diff) comes on when people are treated with antibiotics for another reason. It tends to occur in

hospitals and Nursing homes and is spread by orofecal route. May have blood in stool and Colitis. If confirmed, this is treated with antibiotics like metronidazole or vancomycin

- Diarrhea can upset the balance between "good" and "bad" bacteria in the colon, use of probiotics supplements or in foods like some yogurt may help restore the balance
- In non infectious cases – those which do not have blood, or when there is no fever, one can use OTC anti-diarrhea medicines like Bismuth Subsalicylate (Pepto-Bismol, the Pink medicine, Kaopectate), Loperamide (Imodium)
- Prescription medicine like Diphenoxylate and Atropine (Lomotil) tablets
- A supplement from the tree Sangre de grado known as Crofelemer is used for Diarrhea associated with AIDS, traveling Diarrhea, IBS, antibiotic associated Diarrhea and that which is caused by the bacteria Clostridium Difficile, or Cholera

Food Poisoning
What is It?

This is the result of eating food contaminated with bacteria, viruses, parasites (all these are known as microbes) or chemicals. In general, foods usually causing food poisoning include leafy vegetables, and contaminated poultry, meat and dairy products.

Symptoms and Signs

It can cause diarrhea, abdominal pain, bloating, nausea and vomiting, fever and chills depending on the microbe involved.

Treatment

Initially drinking lots of fluids to make up for what has been lost through the stool is the most important thing. Doctors may give antibiotics to eliminate the source of infection, and some other medicines to treat nausea and vomiting, and the abdominal pain.

Prevention

Peeling, washing and cooking foods are the best way to ensure safety of foods.

One has to be careful of sources of food especially if not prepared at home or is from an unknown source.

All employees working in food shops or eating places, have to wash their hands after using the washroom or WC before going back to work.

Everyone has to wash their hands after use of the washroom or toilet.

Children have to be taught handwashing after using the restroom so it becomes a habit.

Cholera

Cholera, an infection resulting in severe Diarrhea and vomiting as a result of eating food contaminated by a germ, called Cholera Vibro, and can lead to serious loss of fluids from the body and death from dehydration and shock. It is common in communities where people live close together without adequate sources of good drinking water and suitable WC or toilets. There are often outbreaks in refugee camps and after disasters like hurricanes etc.

It is treated with fluids, either oral or intravenous and antibiotics. Handwashing is important to prevent transmission of the germ.

Irritable Bowel Syndrome (Spastic Colon) IBS.
What is It?

Irritable Bowel Syndrome (IBS) is a chronic condition of the large bowel, which is characterized by recurrent abdominal pain, bloating (gassy, distended or enlarged belly) accompanied by Diarrhea or Constipation or both off and on. About 3 million Americans suffer from it. It is more common in women and some people may have a predominant Diarrhea type, while others have a Constipation type. There is urgency to defecate or have a bowel movement, and sometimes painful but unsuccessful attempt to defecate (Tenesmus). Note that there is a difference between IBS and Inflammatory Bowel Disease (IBD) which we will discuss later on.

Causes

There is however no underlining infection or inflammation considered to be the cause, with all tests to find the possible cause coming up as negative or normal. Certain risk factors have been identified and these include:

Genetics (family history) runs in the family
Anxiety
An individual's sensitivity to pain
Probably past history of bowel infection
Past use of frequent oral antibiotics
Those with IBS may also suffer from Fibromyalgia and *Celiac Disease

*Celiac disease is a disease in which sufferers are allergic or sensitive to the protein Gluten which is found in wheat, rye and barley

Treatment

After a history and physical exam, accompanied with tests of stool, blood, even studies looking into bowels like a colonoscopy, or imaging studies, the doctor, after coming up with a diagnosis of IBS may prescribe some dietary changes and medicines to help relieve the symptoms. The medicines may be for abdominal pain, flatulence, bloating, Diarrhea or Constipation depending on which symptoms are prevalent. There is general agreement that diet plays a big role in managing the condition and reducing the symptoms.

Dietary Changes Which May Improve IBS Symptoms

- Reducing or eliminating dairy products from one's diet
- If bloating, gas and abdominal pain are frequently present, then fermented carbohydrates should be avoided
- For individuals with constipation type IBS, use of ground linseed or flaxseed seem to help with bowel regularity
- Use of probiotics may be helpful. Probiotics are "good bacteria" or live bacteria that are taken orally and believed to help restore proper balance of the different bacteria normally found in the digestive system. Everyone's digestive tract contains a large amount of "good bacteria" which help with digestion of the food we eat. When the delicate balance between the different types is upset by infection or even antibiotics use, this may result in abdominal symptoms. Many studies show that re introduction of certain micro bacteria (probiotics) back into the intestines can restore this balance and reduce symptoms of Irritable Bowel Syndrome such as abdominal pain and flatulence. Probiotics are either sold in capsules, liquid, chewable gummy bears or are also found in food like yogurt. The ones stored in the fridge seem to be better and retain their potency than those stored in room temperature. Look for ones with one to ten billion cfu (colony forming units)
- Eliminating foods that tend to aggravate the symptoms, e.g. milk, instead use plant based milk like almond or soy.
- If Fibromyalgia is also present, it may be necessary to test for Gluten intolerance. If Gluten intolerance is present, elimination of Gluten from the diet greatly improves both the fibromyalgia and IBS
- Decrease stress in one's life since this seems to aggravate symptoms
- Exercise may help move stool down

Medicines

Prescription medications approved by FDA (USA) for treating IBS-D include, Eluxadoline (Viberzi) which reduces contractions and Rifaximin (Xifaxan) which is an antibiotic that changes the gut bacteria.

For IBS-C the following prescription medications have been approved for use: Linaclotide (Linzess), Lubiprostone (Amitiza), and Plecanatide (Trulance).

Other medications which treat the symptoms and can be used may include:

- Diarrhea:e.g. Loperamide, Kaopectate, Lomotil, Cholestyramine, and Colesevelam
- Abdominal Pain: Dicyclomine, Hyoscyamine or Amitriptyline
- Bloating/distension: Probiotics
- Constipation: OTC laxatives may be used but these can have serious effects if used continuously for a long time, stool softeners may be helpful.

SUPPLEMENTS: These include: Turmeric, Red raspberry leaves, Fenugreek, Zinc, Chia seeds, Apple cider vinegar, garlic, ginger,

Gluten Intolerance and Celiac Disease
What are These?

In the US, about 30% of the population is trying to cut down Gluten from their diet. Gluten free has overtaken fat free and low carbohydrate food fads; it was the second most popular diet in 2012 according to Time magazine. The Gluten free foods market was estimated to increase to $5 billion in 2015.

Gluten intolerance and the more severe form Celiac Disease (umbrella term is Gluten related disorders) are a result of either partial or complete sensitivity to Gluten. Gluten is the protein found in some grains like wheat, rye or barley. A portion of Gluten called Gliadin is not fully broken down in the intestines of all people, and for those who are genetically susceptible, the protein produces an immune response in the intestines (autoimmune reaction). The response leads to reaction against the lining of the small bowel leading to chronic inflammation and damage to the lining. This causes problems with digestion and absorption of nutrients. Most people affected may not have specific symptoms and so may not be diagnosed until adulthood.

Signs and Symptoms

The one specific symptom is an itchy rash which is a reaction to the Gluten and it is found on elbows, knees, scalp and buttocks and occurs mostly in men and in about 25% of individuals with Celiac disease.

However non specific symptoms may occur:

Abdomen: Diarrhea and flatulence/gas, abdominal pain, distention, vomiting, and constipation
Fatigue and weakness
Recurrent streptococcal infections
Iron deficiency anemia
Osteoporosis

Abnormal liver tests

If not treated, serious complications include Lymphoma and Liver Cancers

In children, symptoms may start between the ages of six months and two years and may include the above as well as failure to gain weight, and a short stature

Diagnosis

This is by blood tests, and endoscopy (using a camera to look inside the bowel) associated with biopsy of small bowel lining. Before the endoscopy, diet should not be restricted, otherwise results may be false negative.

Treatment of Celiac Disease

There is need to remove the protein causing the auto immune reaction and the accompanying symptoms. Therefore wheat, rye and barley are eliminated from the diet, or eating less than 50mg of Gluten per day. So instead of wheat flour, rice flour may be used. Gluten free diets are expensive since many American foods are wheat based. Meats, dairy, fruits and vegetables are naturally Gluten free and so can be eaten in any quantities. About 6 to 12 months after a Gluten free diet is started, the blood results will become normal. If there is not a positive response to a Gluten free diet and symptoms persist, then the diagnosis has to be reconsidered. Several intestinal diseases can give similar biopsy results seen in Celiac disease, the commonest ones being intolerance of food like milk, soy, chicken, or tuna.

Hemorrhoids
What are They?

These are swollen veins found in the rectum and may appear at the edge of the anus. The veins tend to have extra pressure on them when there is Constipation, Diarrhea, pregnancy and childbirth or if there is anything that increases pressure or weight in the belly or pelvic area. Some hemorrhoids may appear outside the anus (external) while some may be inside and not be visible (internal hemorrhoids). A large one may appear at the anal opening and become hard, with inability to be pushed back into the anus. It can then become constricted, enlarged inflamed and very painful. This is a PROLAPSED or THROMBOSED HEMORRHOID.

Signs and Symptoms

Some may be without any symptoms, while others may became swollen, itching, painful and may bleed during defecation or bowel movement. Some may become thrombosed as described above causing a painful mass at the anal edge which cannot be pushed back in. If they bleed a lot, then the person may develop Anemia, fatigue and tiredness.

Treatment of Hemorrhoids

- For ordinary hemorrhoids which are not inflamed:
  Prevent them from getting inflamed or from bursting open and bleeding during a bowel movement by doing the following:
  One should avoid getting constipated by drinking lots of fluids
  Eating high fiber in your diet to promote regularity (regular bowel movements)
  Increase consumption of fruits and vegetables which are generally high in fiber
  Use of fiber supplements like Metamucil, Fibercon or Psyllum husk or their generics
  Use stool softeners to help prevent constipation
- If swollen, red, painful and itchy (inflamed):
  Use a Hemorrhoid cream which often contains a steroid like Hydrocortisone, witch hazel creams or pads (Tucks)
  Anti-itch medication in the form of a suppository or cream
  Appy Ice packs to the area
  Sit bath – e.g. sitting in Epson salt lukewarm water in a bath or a large bowl may help the swelling and redness to decrease
- If hemorrhoids bleed a lot, or if there is recurrent occurrence of inflamed hemorrhoids and complications like Anemia, then treatments include:
  Surgical banding or ligation with rubber bands
  Injecting a substance to harden the vein (Sclerotherapy)
  Infra-red treatment and an electrolysis method called Ultroid which is a non-invasive treatment done for a few sessions to destroy the vein
  If these do not work, then surgery to excise or cut out the hemorrhoids is done
- In cases of thrombosed hemorrhoids:
  The blood in that prolapsed part may form a clot and the hemorrhoid may need to be cut open and blood clot removed in order for it to be flattened and help pain to subside

Diverticulosis

What is It?

Diverticulosis is outpocketing of the inner wall of the large bowel through weak spots in the outer walls resulting in pockets or pouches called Diverticula. It is thought to be genetically determined, and is more common in men. It tends to occur in older folks who are 60 years and above. It may result from straining of the muscles in the walls as may occur with chronic constipation but this is not certain. They may be discovered during imaging studies of the abdomen or during colonoscopy.

Signs and Symptoms

They may not cause any symptoms, however some may present with abdominal pain, bloating, Diarrhea or Constipation. They may also be discovered when they present with a complication called Diverticulitis.

Treatment

Keeping stools moving through the bowel may prevent complications discussed below, and therefore avoiding Constipation is important. Drinking fluids, maintaining regularity (regular bowel movements) and increasing fiber in the diet may help. Fiber supplements may be useful.

Complications

- Diverticulitis: They may become inflamed and infected when stool and bacteria lodge in the pockets. This is called diverticulitis (die-ver-q-lye-tis). When diagnosed it has to be treated with bowel rest, (fluids or soft diet only), fluids, pain control and antibiotics
- Complicated Diverticulitis: This is more serious and may cause an abscess, obstruction of the bowel, perforation and bleeding. For example, in an abscess, pus may form around the Diverticula involved and treatment may have to be in a hospital setting because one may be very sick with fever and chills. Treatment may involve draining of the pus, and intravenous antibiotics
- Recurrent Diverticulitis: Some people keep getting attacks and part of the bowel may have to be surgically excised to get rid of the Diverticula to prevent further attacks

Inflammatory Bowel Diseases (IBD)

What are These?

IBDs are not infectious but inflammatory. Crohn's can affect any part of the GI tract, while Ulcerative Colitis is limited to the large bowel and rectal area. They may present with symptoms outside of the bowels including Arthritis, eye, skin, mouth, kidney, Anemia and gallbladder stones.

Inflammatory Bowel Diseases (IBD) are a group of chronic diseases causing inflammation of the gastrointestinal (GI) tract, with the commonest ones being Crohn's Disease (Crohn's) and Ulcerative Colitis (UC). They are usually diagnosed between the ages of 15 to 35 years and they affect men and women equally. They are thought to be due to a combination of genetics, altered immune system and environmental factors, with about 20% of affected individuals having a relative who also has the disease. Initially they were thought to be autoimmune diseases but now they are thought to be due to an overzealous immune system trying to destroy harmless bacteria and viruses in the gut; resulting in inflammation and damage, or probably a mild immune deficiency state.

Signs and Symptoms

Both may present with abdominal symptoms like recurrent abdominal pain, Diarrhea, Constipation, bloody stools or cramps, abscesses and anal tears. There may be nausea and vomiting occurring in Crohn's. Apart from abdominal symptoms, one may present with large joint inflammations, Arthritis, eye, skin, mouth problems, kidney and gallbladder stones, fever, weight loss, fatigue, night sweats, and Anemia. Both diseases may have periods of quietness (remissions) and increased symptoms (flare ups).

Treatment

After blood work, imaging studies and colonoscopy or upper endoscopy with biopsies taken from suspicious areas of the bowel, a diagnosis can be made and treatment can be started.

Treatment include:

Medicines which lower inflammation for example Sulfasalazine and 5-ASA Mesalamine

Those that work on the immune system like Steroids

Biologics which target specific proteins and work on your immune system. Examples of these are Infliximab and Adalimumab

Immunosuppressant drug called Azathioprine

Making sure one has less stress in one's life to prevent flare ups

Eating foods cooked instead of raw vegetables, avoiding spicy foods and high fiber diet especially after a flare up

It is also important to avoid medicines known as Non Steroidal Anti-inflammatory drugs (NSAIDS) examples include Ibuprofen and Naproxen

Make sure one keeps regular appointments with their doctor, and let her/him know if one experiencing any flare ups with GI symptoms or any of the non-GI symptoms like Arthritis, eye problems, skin lesions, etc

Complications

May include abscesses, tears in the anus, bowel obstruction, and Colorectal Cancer. Due to the latter, a person with IBD has to have frequent colonoscopies to make sure any Cancer if present is discovered in the early stages. Patients may also feel depressed at times because of the chronic nature of the disease and its multiple symptoms. One may need to see a therapist/psychologist and also be on antidepressant medications to help one feel better.

Flatulence and Excess Gas

Passing of gas or wind is a regular occurrence and it is due to gas we produce or inhale. It may occur 10–20x in 24 hours. We may swallow more from eating too fast and drinking carbonated drinks, chewing gum and eating foods like beans, cabbage, broccoli, onions, cauliflower, apples, raisins, lactose and Fructose intolerance and constipation. These result in undigested carbs in the colon and they are broken down by the normal bacteria there to produce gas.

SOLUTIONS: Avoid the listed foods, eat slowly, treat constipation and acid reflux, avoid gassy drinks, take a walk after a meal

MEDICINE: Try Gas-X, Simethicone, Beano for bean, Lactaid for milk; if these don't help, see your doctor

Cancer of the Colon or Large Bowel
What is It?

Screening for Colorectal Cancer saves lives and in the US according to the CDC, incidence and mortality have been decreasing due to screening with approved methods. Most develop from polyps; however, most polyps are not cancerous and they tend to increase with age. It may take 10 years for a small polyp to change into a cancer.

Colon cancer is abnormal growth of cells within the last part of the intestines and it is the most common type of Cancer of the digestive system. It is the second leading cause of Cancer related death in the USA after Lung Cancer. It usually starts in the colon or rectal area, and most would start as a polyp (group of non cancer cells), some of which over time develop into precancerous polyps and these may change to become cancer cells later on. The cancer cells usually start in the inner layer of the large bowel and can spread through the muscle to outer layers as well as to nearby blood, lymph vessels, lymph nodes and other distant places like liver, bone and lungs. Most Colon Cancer are of the type called Adenocarcinoma.

Symptoms of Colon Cancer

These depend on whether the condition is early or advance. Symptoms may include fatigue, anemia, abdominal pain, change in bowel habits (e.g. normal to Diarrhea, feeling of incomplete emptying), and blood in the stool. In advance cases there may also be abdominal distension, weight loss, vomiting, or obstruction of the bowel by the Cancer and so Constipation results.

Treatment

Treatment includes surgery to remove the Cancer and part of the bowels, and if needed Chemotherapy and other specific agents which target cancer cells.

Risk Factors for Colon Cancer

Some risk factors are not modifiable, while others are and so altering those risk factors may help decrease one's risk. These include:

Age (those above 45 years)
Family history (only about 25% may have a family history)
Those who have certain bowel diseases called Inflammatory Bowel Disease (Crohn's disease and Ulcerative colitis)
Certain hereditary conditions
Personal history of other cancers like breast, ovarian, and endometrial cancers, or history of colon polyps and colon cancer

Lifestyle risks include tobacco use, heavy alcohol use, obesity, and lack of physical activity. Increased consumption of red meat or processed meats

Grilled and fried meats cooked at high temperatures release chemicals which increase risk

In terms of race, being Black or an Ashkenazi Jew

How to Decrease Risk of Colon Cancer

Apart from modifying some of those mentioned above, one can decrease risk by:
Diets high in fruits, vegetables, whole grain and fiber
Get screened for Colorectal Cancer, and have any suspicious polyps removed

Screening for Colorectal Cancer

There are tests which can screen asymptomatic people for Colorectal Cancer, just like for breast cancer. Early detection as well as removal of precancerous polyps saves lives.

There are about six approved screening tests, and it is recommended for all adults aged from 50 to 75 years who are of average risk (not at increased risk).

Those at increased risk (e.g. one parent had Colon Cancer) may have screening start at a younger age and repeat screening at shorter intervals.

The simplest one is fecal occult blood test (Hemoccult) and the most advanced is Colonoscopy.

In Colonoscopy there is actual viewing of the inside of the colon and its lining by a scope with a camera and any polyps present can be excised and sent for pathological examination. Pictures can be taken of the colon's lining. This exam requires the bowels to be emptied completely before the exam.

Discuss colorectal cancer screening with one's doctor, since early detection and treatment saves lives. The fecal occult test is simple and looks for blood in a sample of stool.

17

Liver Diseases

The liver is a very important organ in the body and it is one of the largest organs in the body. It has many functions including:

Production of protein, cholesterol, hormones, bile, and substances helping with blood clotting

Removing toxins (harmful substances) from the blood

Breakdown of medicines as well as breakdown of red cells

Regulating the amount of glucose, fats and proteins in the blood

Stores glucose, vitamins, and minerals

We will discuss some of the most common liver diseases which people need to be familiar with

Jaundice
What is It?

This is the term used to describe the yellow discoloration of the eyeball, palms and skin (in people of light skin color) due to the accumulation of a substance called BILIRUBIN in the blood. Jaundice is not a disease, but it is a symptom of an underlying disease which must be figured out and treated.

How is Bilirubin Formed

Bilirubin is normally produced in the liver and spleen mostly from the breakdown of old red cells. The red cells contain a nitrogen substance combined with iron called HEME and this is what mostly gives the red cell its color. Through a systematic process the produced bilirubin is incorporated into bile which is yellow greenish liquid stored in the gallbladder. The bilirubin now present in bile is there-after eliminated through the intestine with the stool giving stool its normal color. When there is excessive production of bilirubin or its elimination is slowed down, then bilirubin accumulates in the blood and the level goes up, leading to excess amounts in the urine; causing the color of urine to be deep yellow or orange. The eyes and skin also get affected.

Causes of Jaundice

Some common reasons why an individual will have jaundice are:

- Liver Diseases: e.g. Viral Hepatitis, Cirrhosis of the liver, Cancer of the liver
- Blood Diseases: excessive breakdown of red cells as is seen in sickle cell disease
- Cancer: when cancer from another source spreads to the liver (Metastasis) it can block the elimination of bilirubin from the body and the accumulation in the blood causes Jaundice
- Cancer of organs like the pancreas can block the elimination of bile and lead to Jaundice

Symptoms Accompanying Jaundice

Jaundice may be accompanied by itching, easy bleeding or bruising, nausea and if severe can even affect the brain causing change in a person's mental state, con-fusion, coma and death.

Hepatitis Diseases (Inflammation of the liver)
What is Hepatitis?

Hepatitis means inflammation of the liver cells. There are many things that can cause this, and these include:

Microbes (germs – bacteria, parasites and viruses)
Medications
Autoimmune disease (Body turning against its own cells)
Toxic chemicals
Alcohol

The most common type of Hepatitis is caused by a group of viruses known as Hep-atitis viruses. There are several of these but the most common ones are Hepatitis A, B, and C viruses. (HAV, HBV, HCV)

Spread of Hepatitis Viruses

Spread of Hepatitis B and C:

Contact with infected or contaminated blood

Those who abuse intravenous drugs through sharing needles or using contaminated dirty needles

Sexual contact with semen, or body fluids, of an infected person

Infected mother to a baby in the womb

Infection through contaminated blood transfusion

Unknown causes

Infection Through Contaminated Unscreened Blood Transfusion

Before there was no routine screening of hepatitis in the blood supply by blood transfusion services. Now, many middle aged and older individuals are infected from contaminated blood and blood products given to them while in hospital or for other reasons e.g. during surgery or if anemic. Currently all donated blood is well screened

Spread of Hepatitis A

Hepatitis A (HAV) is spread mainly through food, water, or hands contaminated with an infected person's feces or stool. Less common ways of spread are through blood and body fluids. HAV is common in places with poor sanitation or hygiene.

Infection with Hepatitis Viruses A, B, C

Signs and Symptoms

All three after initial infection, can result in an acute illness characterized by fever, nausea, vomiting, decreased appetite, joint pains, tiredness, itching and skin rash. These symptoms may resemble common illnesses like Flu, Malaria, Typhoid or other viral illnesses.

After a few days, there may be Jaundice of the eyes and skin, pain in the liver area (right upper abdomen), dark urine and pale colored stools.

If severe, liver failure, coma and death will occur.

Hepatitis B can also present with very serious symptoms mainly mental confusion, sleepiness, coma, bleeding from the gut (stomach or intestines) and bleeding from the gums. This is more serious and can lead to death quickly.

Treatment of Acute Infections

Blood tests can be used to find out if one is infected. Certain chemicals called liver enzymes produced by the injured liver cells will rise to very high levels in the blood. Blood tests for hepatitis viruses will show the presence of the antibodies against the particular virus. For all three of them, treatment is supportive, treating the symptoms that are present.

Results of Infection With the Hepatitis Viruses
Hepatitis A

In Hepatitis A infection, the body usually heals itself by attacking and eliminating the virus. The individual then acquires lifelong protection from the disease due to the action of their body's immune system. It does not result in chronic disease, and treatment is mainly supportive treatment, which means that whatever symptoms are present are treated and there is no specific medication for it. Patients may need bed rest, fluids, medicine for nausea and vomiting etc.

Hepatitis B

Most people may recover completely from Hepatitis B in 4 to 6 months after an infection, but about 5 to 10% may continue to carry the virus and are said to have Chronic Hepatitis B which is discussed below.

Hepatitis C

Most individuals with acute Hepatitis C do not even know they are infected, however, treatment of acute infections are symptomatic as for the other two. Most people with Hepatitis C unfortunately do not clear the virus (70–80%) and develop Chronic Hepatitis C, harboring the virus for the rest of their lives and so can spread it to others.

Chronic Hepatitis B and C
What are These?

Some people recover from the initial infections and their immune system can clear the viruses from their bodies. However, others go on to retain the virus and will continue to test positive for the virus after the initial acute illness. The presence of the virus can go unnoticed for several years and infected individuals may not have any symptoms for years. However, eventually they may show symptoms of chronic liver disease.

Symptoms of Chronic Liver Disease

Symptoms of chronic liver disease include liver scarring, Cirrhosis, liver failure, fluid collection and swelling of the abdomen, bleeding from the gut, and eventually Liver Cancer and death. They are also able to pass the virus on to other individuals through the methods mentioned above.

What is Cirrhosis?

Cirrhosis is a disease of the liver resulting from Fibrosis (inflammation followed by body's attempts to repair it), subsequently leading to thick bands (like rubber bands) crisscrossing the liver, giving it an irregular hard surface. It can be caused mainly by Chronic Hepatitis B or C or from excessive alcohol use.

Treatment of Chronic Hepatitis B and C

There are medicines available to treat Chronic Hepatitis B and C. These may take up to a year of therapy, however, recent new oral drugs for treatment of Hepatitis C have been developed which produce cures in about 8 weeks. These newer treatments are very expensive but have shorter treatment duration and less side effects.

Limiting Liver Damage in Chronic Liver Disease

When one has chronic liver disease, It is important to avoid
Other infections or inflammation of the liver,
Medications that affect the liver like Acetaminophen, (Panadol or Tylenol)
Herbal supplement that affects the liver
Alcoholic drinks
One should do regular follow ups with a liver doctor called a Hepatologist
Get vaccinated against Hepatitis A or B viruses if one has Hepatitis C

All these are ways of limiting the damage already done to the liver

Prevention of Hepatitis Infection

Basically, there are three main ways and these are:

Immunization
Practice of safe sex
Testing for the presence of the infections

- IMMUNIZATION AGAINST HEPATITIS (Hep) A AND B
  There are vaccines to protect against Hepatitis A and B, although there is no vaccine yet to protect one against Hepatitis C. Getting vaccinated against Hepatitis A and B will prevent the infections from occurring, and further damaging the liver. In some countries children are immunized against Hepatitis A and B as part of the childhood immunization program. Hep. B vaccine may protect against Hep D
- PRACTICE OF SAFE SEX
  Since hepatitis B and C are transmitted via body fluids like blood and semen, it is important that one practices the A B C of prevention of transmission of

sexually transmitted infections. That is Sexual abstinence (A), Be faithful to one sexual partner, (monogamous relationship) (B) and use of condoms (C), To avoid spreading the viruses to other people, infected individuals should not have unprotected sex, and should always use condoms

- TESTING FOR THE VIRUSES

   Checking for the presence of the viruses through simple blood tests are important, and this is advised if one is at considerable risk due to multiple sexual partners in the past or present. Individuals who have received blood transfusion in the past, or anyone who was born between the years 1946 and 1964 (known as a baby boomer in the US) or donates blood

- OTHER PREVENTIVE MEASURES:

   Not sharing toothbrushes, razor blades, needles for tattoos, body piercing or needles for injections of any kind with other people

   Hepatitis A can be prevented by making sure drinking water is safe, good environmental sanitation, proper hand washing, boiling drinking water if in doubt, not eating raw shellfish, and making sure food is properly cooked before eating

   Employees in eating places and elsewhere should always wash their hands with soap after using the restrooms or toilet

Fatty Liver (Steatosis-stia-to-siz)

What is It?

Fatty liver is caused by alcoholic and non alcoholic factors. Non alcoholic fatty liver (NAFLD) includes simple fatty liver or more serious Steatohepatitis and both have a high prevalence worldwide. They are the commonest causes of chronic liver disease and may result in Fibrosis of the liver, Cirrhosis, and Liver Cancer.

This condition is also known as STEATOSIS, and occurs when there is increased deposit of fatty substances (lipids) mainly in the form of TRIGLYCERIDES (TG) in the liver cells. TG is a type of fat and excess calories not needed by the body is converted to TG and stored in the liver. Inbetween meals or when energy is needed, this is converted to energy to be used by the body. The non alcoholic type of fatty liver (NAFLD) seems to have skyrocketed with the increase of obesity worldwide, and the increased consumption of high fatty foods and foods high in simple carbohydrates. The prevalence worldwide has been estimated at one billion and in the US it affects between 80 and 100 million people. It is the most common cause of chronic liver disease

It can be divided into two main groups:

Alcoholic fatty liver (as a result of excessive alcohol use)
Nonalcoholic fatty liver disease (NAFLD) (not related to alcohol)

Non Alcoholic Fatty Liver Disease (NAFLD)

This is a broad term used to describe both Steatosis (deposition of fatty acids in liver cells) and Non alcoholic Steatohepatitis (STEA-TO-HEPA-TYA-TIS) (NASH), in which there is inflammation damage and or death of the liver cells. About a quarter of those with Fatty liver (Steatosis) will progress to NASH. Both can be present in children and adults, and in the Western world up to 30% of adults and 10% of children are affected. Both genetics and lifestyle play a role in who develops it. Other conditions making one prone to developing fatty liver include:

Medical conditions like Diabetes, Obesity and *Metabolic syndrome
Medications used to treat cancers, for example Tamoxifen for breast cancer and Methotrexate for other cancers and conditions
Nutritional states like starvation and malnutrition
The use of intravenous nutritional feeding in very ill, hospitalized patients

*Metabolic syndrome is used to describe individuals with obesity, high blood sugar, Hypertension and high triglycerides or fatty substances.

Signs and Symptoms

Fatty liver disease is usually without any symptoms, with no pain or tenderness in the liver area, and is usually discovered when blood work for some other purpose shows elevated liver enzymes (due to damaged liver cells). This may be the first clue of the presence of fatty liver. If it is due to other medical conditions, then symptoms and abnormal labs related to those conditions may be present. For example, a woman may be obese or has, increased blood sugar due to Diabetes etc.

Investigations

A liver ultrasound may show a fatty liver, however, at the initial stages, fatty liver changes may not show on ultrasound. A study known as Fibroscan is a special ultrasound study which measures Fibrosis if present. MRI imaging may also be done and eventually, a liver biopsy if done, will give a definite diagnosis. This is when a small sample of liver tissue is removed through the skin during an outpatient procedure and sent for tests. It will tell if there is just accumulation of fat in the liver cells (Steatosis) or if there is inflammation (NASH – non-alcoholic steatohepatitis), or Cirrhosis which is more serious. However, liver biopsies are not routinely done unless there are many abnormal results of tests.

Complications

Fatty liver Steatosis may reverse with lifestyle changes or progress to NASH. NASH can reverse if mild, or stay unchanged. However both can progress and lead to chronic liver disease, Cirrhosis, Liver Cancer and liver failure. There is also increased incidence of coronary atherosclerosis, Atrial fibrillation and heart failure.

Treatment of Fatty Liver

Lifestyle changes are important and need to be used by all people with the condition.

These are Important and include weight loss, healthy diet and exercise.

Medicines for treatment

There is not much success in treatment with medications, but the following have been used:

Cholesterol and diabetes medications like Atorvastatin (Lipitor), and Pioglitazone (Actos) respectively. These have shown varying success in simple fatty liver (Steatosis) and delay development into Steatohepatitis and increased Fibrosis of the liver

CAM Supplements: Not all have been studied in depth. They include vitamin C, vitamin E, Omega 3 fatty acids, Alpha lipoic acid, Milk Thistle (anti inflammatory and antioxidant), Resveratrol (acts like an antioxidant and its found in skin of grapes, peanuts and berries)

If one has a FATTY LIVER, one must ask their doctor if any of these could be used.

Prevention of Fatty Liver

Prevention is important. The measures below may protect against the development or progression of fatty liver:

Lifestyle activities like exercise and healthy eating will prevent this to some extent

Weight Loss by exercise, eating less, Bariatric surgery or medications

Diet plays a key role and many studies have shown that *high fructose intake as found in high fructose corn syrup is associated with fatty liver, and so avoid this. This is found in beverages and baked goods

Healthy diets like the Mediterranean diet as well as complex carbohydrate intake are helpful

High Omega three fatty acids prevent fatty liver

Use oils like olive oil and coconut oil for cooking etc.

Cut back on white simple Carbohydrates like sugar, and flour products

*High fructose corn syrup is made from corn and it is included as a sweetener in many foods, especially in commercial baked goods. Currently, a lot of food manufacturers are excluding it as an ingredient.

Reminders on Your Radar

Fatty liver diseases are the most common liver diseases in the world. They are broadly known as alcoholic and non alcoholic fatty liver diseases. There are no specific medicines to treat them, however, some medicines used to treat Diabetes and Cholesterol have been used. Some CAM herbal products have also been used but studies have been small or not available. Adopting lifestyle changes may help reverse or stop their progression to Cirrhosis, Liver Cancer, liver failure, and heart problems.

Alcoholic Liver Diseases
What are These?

Alcoholic liver diseases are diseases of liver caused by excessive consumption of alcohol. They can be from the simple to more serious or complicated diseases. They include:

Simple alcoholic fatty liver (fatty cells in the liver)
Alcoholic Steatohepatitis (inflammation)
Cirrhosis of the liver (inflammation and scarring)
Cancer of the liver (Hepatoma)

Women tend to develop alcoholic liver disease faster than men. It is important that women do not drink more than ONE alcoholic beverage daily. In individuals with alcohol-related liver disease, cessation of consumption of alcohol can limit the damage or stop progression to serious complications associated with excessive alcohol intake. According to the CDC, the alcohol levels of different standard alcoholic drinks are as follows:

A standard drink is equal to 14.0 grams (0.6 ounces) of pure alcohol. This amount of pure alcohol is found in:
12 ounces of beer (5% alcohol content).
8 ounces of malt liquor (7% alcohol content).
5 ounces of wine (12% alcohol content).

1.5 ounces or a "shot" of 80-proof (40% alcohol content) distilled spirits or liquor e.g., Gin, Rum, Vodka, Whiskey (https://www.cdc.gov/alcohol/faqs.htm).

Elevated Liver Enzymes (LFTs)

....

What is It?

Sometimes blood work will show liver enzymes are high. There are normal amounts of these chemicals or enzymes in the blood; however, excess liver enzymes are released from the liver cells when there is injury or inflammation of the liver. The main ones are called Transaminases and the simple names are abbreviated as ALT and AST.

The causes of elevated liver enzymes are many and include:

Viral hepatitis
Excess alcohol intake
Nonalcoholic fatty liver disease
Metabolic syndrome
Cancer metastasis to the liver
Genetic disease of excessive iron called Hemochromatosis
Celiac disease (Gluten intolerance)
Rapid weight loss
Medications

Medicines Causing Elevated Liver Enzymes

The medicines include: Acetaminophen, cholesterol medications called Statins, Tetracycline, Isoniazid and Rifampin (these two are anti-tuberculosis drugs), some HIV drugs, Lisinopril and Losartan (blood pressure drugs), Methotrexate, antifungal drug like Ketoconazole and Terbinafine, and some nonsteroidal anti-inflammatory drugs like Ibuprofen and Naproxen (these NSAIDs can also affect the kidneys even more).

Treatment of Elevated Liver Enzymes

Most times elevated liver enzymes present in the blood does not cause any symptoms and may be found during routine blood work. If the probable cause is suspected after a careful history, physical exam and blood work; then treatment depends on the cause. Treating the cause would result in the levels going down. For example:

Discontinuation of a causative medication

Cessation of alcohol consumption

If obese, need lifestyle changes and weight loss of 5–10% of body weight

Limiting carbohydrates, high fructose corn syrup and processed foods may help

Usually, the tests will be repeated in a few weeks to see if the levels are trending down. If they persist, an ultrasound of the liver may be needed, which may show a fatty liver. However, it may not show this if less than 30% of the liver cells are affected by the fatty substances. MRI may also be done although it is more expensive. If elevated liver enzymes persist, then sometimes a liver biopsy is done. It is important to treat fatty liver as described above, when tests show that it is present.

Gallbladder Disease

....

What is the Gallbladder?

The gallbladder is a small fluid filled sac which is found on the underside of the liver in the right upper part of the abdomen. It stores BILE in between meals. Bile is a greenish colored fluid produced by the liver and it's made up mainly of water, bilirubin (result of breakdown of red cells in the liver), bile salts and cholesterol. Bile is released periodically from the gallbladder after a fatty meal, and it flows into the small intestine or bowel. The bile aids in digestion of fat and depending on its composition can lead to formation of gall stones in the gall bladder.

Cholecystitis (inflammation of the gallbladder)

Stones can be formed in the gallbladder when there are high concentrations of certain chemicals. The presence of gallstones may not cause any symptoms until one blocks the duct leading from the gallbladder to the intestines. This causes distention of the gall bladder and a condition known as Cholecystitis.

Signs and Symptoms

This includes abdominal pain, especially in the right or middle upper parts just under the ribs, nausea and vomiting, chills and or fever. Examination will reveal tenderness in the location of the gallbladder. The pain may be worse after eating fatty foods and it may be on and off (colicky/cramps) initially, but may later become constant.

Treatment

Treatment is surgical to remove the gallbladder with the stones. Make sure you see a doctor when pain in the upper right side of the belly occurs and does not go away.

Post Cholecystectomy Diarrhea (Diarrhea associated with absence of Gallbladder)

What is It?

After surgery for gall bladder disease, about 20 % of people may experience Diarrhea which may usually last a few weeks to six months. The reason is not exactly clear; however, it is believed it may be due to the presence of excessive amounts of bile salts which move from the liver straight into the bowels without going into the gallbladder, thereby causing a laxative effect resulting in Diarrhea. This will normally stop with time, however, if it does not, talk to a doctor.

Treatment

Avoid certain foods like spicy foods, fatty foods, dairy products, and drinks with high caffeine content like coffee or colas.

To help the Diarrhea, anti-diarrheal medicines like Loperamide (Imodium) can be used.

A doctor may prescribe medicines which affect the absorption of bile like Cholestyramine, Colesevelam (Welchol, Cholestagel, Lodalis) or Aluminum hydroxide.

Pancreatitis (pan-cri-tie-tis)

....

Before discussing Pancreatitis, which is inflammation of the endocrine and digestive gland called the pancreas, a discussion on what this organ is and what it does is important.

The Pancreas

The pancreas is an organ found in the abdomen close to the stomach and it produces two types of chemicals.

- The first group produced are involved with digestion of food and are called AMYLASE and LIPASE. They help the body breakdown protein and fat respectively. They are released into the small intestine as digestion occurs
- The second group of chemicals produced are called HORMONES. The main ones are INSULIN and GLUCAGON and these help with metabolism

(breakdown and use) of glucose in the blood. They were discussed in detail under DIABETES MELLITUS (see endocrine chapter)

Pancreatitis (Pan-cre-thal-tis)

What is It?

Pancreatitis is caused by INJURY and INFLAMMATION of the cells of the pancreas. This can be a result of several factors, however; the main ones are:

GALL STONES which have moved from the gallbladder to block a duct of the pancreas, and these cause about 80% of Pancreatitis

Long term excessive consumption of ALCOHOL

Very high TRIGLYCERIDES (TG – Fatty substances) in the blood (greater than 1000mg/dl)

Any of them eventually cause blockage of the ducts and cell injury within the pancreas leading to inflammation

Signs and Symptoms

An individual with Acute Pancreatitis will present with:

- Pain in the upper abdomen which may be dull or sharp and may go through to the back
- Nausea and vomiting, loss of appetite, and sometimes Diarrhea
- Examination will reveal tenderness in the upper part of the abdomen

Treatment

Pancreatitis is a serious illness and needs to be treated quickly. The individual needs to be admitted into hospital and have blood work, and imaging studies like Ultrasound or CT scans. Treatment involves giving intravenous fluids, pain medications and rest of the bowel and pancreas by not eating any food, until the inflammation subsides and blood work improves. Food is gradually introduced starting with soft bland foods.

Complications

Sometimes a lot of scarring occurs causing the pancreas not to be able to produce enough of the enzymes or hormones. These will then have to be replaced on a regular basis in order for digestion to occur; and for blood sugar levels to be controlled insulin may have to be replaced.

18

Diseases and Conditions Affecting the Urinary System

What is the Urinary System Made Up Of?

....

In simple terms the urinary or renal system is made up of the two kidneys, the bladder, the two tubes (ureters) connecting the kidneys to the bladder; and finally the urethra which is the tube through which urine flows out from the body to the outside.

Urinary or Renal System

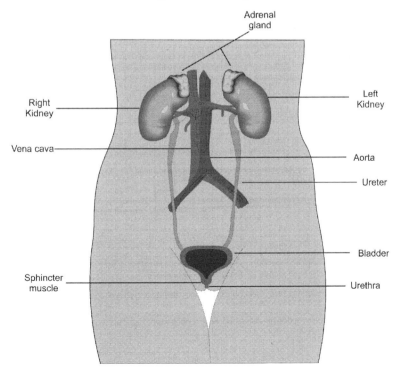

Each of the parts and their functions will be discussed before the discussion of some of the medical conditions that can affect them.

Kidneys

The kidneys are two half-moon shaped brownish organs about 4 × 2.5 inches, in the back of the abdominal cavity of the body. The abdominal cavity is in the mid-section of the body and mainly contains the intestines and other organs associated with digestion. If one places their hands at their sides at the 'waist' or umbilicus (belly button) level, that is approximately where the kidneys are located in the back.
FUNCTIONS: The kidneys have many functions, and these include:

Produce urine which contains fluid and body waste
Help produce red blood cells
Produce an active form of Vitamin D which helps maintain strong bones
Remove drugs/medicines from the body
Keep the amount of fluids in the body well-regulated
Help with regulation of the body's blood pressure
Filter the blood to remove waste products produced by the body's cells
Get rid of excessive fluid from the body

Urine

The removed fluid and waste products form urine which is stored in the bladder and eliminated intermittently through urination. On average, the amount of urine produced per day should be about one and a half (11/2) liters. There is a certain amount of fluid balance that the body needs and if there is too much fluid or increased volume of blood, this affects the pumping ability of the heart, and so the kidney keeps both fluids and electrolytes (salts) well balanced by eliminating the excess fluid. Common table salt contains sodium and too much of it will cause excess fluid retention in the body.

If one is drinking adequate fluids, the urine color may be light yellow or clear, however, when one is dehydrated, urine is concentrated and the color may be dark yellow and smaller in quantity. It is also important to remember that certain foods, or dyes used in foods or medicines can give the urine a yellow or light orange coloration so bear that in mind when considering the color of urine as it relates to adequate fluid intake.

Ureters (u-rea-ters)

These are two tubes which lead from the kidney and get connected to the bladder on either side of the body in the pelvic area. Their function is to carry urine produced in the kidneys to the bladder for storage. The ureters course through the back of the abdomen and enter into the bladder in the pelvis where the reproductive organs are situated.

Bladder

This is the structure for storing urine. The bladder can be compared to an inflated balloon with the mouth held shut. After urine is produced by the kidneys, it is stored in the bladder and urine is kept from leaking out of the bladder by muscles forming a sphincter (a closing mechanism) at the neck or lower part of the bladder. Intermittently, when the bladder is full or partially full, the nerves in the bladder send a message to the bladder neck and there is contraction of the bladder wall, the mouth opens and urine is expelled to the outside.

Urethra

This is a small tube leading from the bladder through which urine from the bladder is expelled to the outside. The urethra is fairly short in women and is situated superior to (top of) the vaginal opening. Both these openings are situated in the VULVA which is the external part of the female genital organs. In men, the urethra is a longer tube and it courses through the penis, with the PROSTATE gland situated below the bladder and surrounding the urethra for a short distance. This is important and will be discussed later.

Urinary Tract Infection (UTI)
What is It?

The close proximity between the urethral opening, vaginal opening and the anal opening through which stool is expelled leads to problems like urinary tract infection (UTI). UTI is infection of any part of the urinary tract and infection of the lower part of the tract is mainly that of the bladder (Cystitis) and urethra (Urethritis), while more serious infection of the kidney is called Pyelonephritis.

Cystitis (sis-tia-tis) Bladder Infection
What is It?

Due to the close proximity of the urethral opening to the vagina and anus, bacteria from the vulva and anal area can go up the urethra into the bladder and cause infection of the bladder or Cystitis. The anus and groin area have a high amount of bacteria which can be transferred to the urethra and into the bladder.

Symptoms

These include:

Burning during urination, pain with urination, and frequency of urination
Smelly urine, cloudy urine, and feeling of incomplete emptying,
Urgency, lower abdominal pain, blood in the urine, and low back pain

Who is Prone to Cystitis or Bladder Infection?

Though all females can get urinary tract infections, there are certain groups that are prone to infections. These include:

- Females who are sexually active (have sexual intercourse): This is because during sex there can be rubbing of the male penis and scrotum on the vulva and this can lead to easy transfer of bacteria from the male skin or the female vulva through the urethra into the bladder
- A newly-wed virgin female or a female having sex for the first time: This woman may end up with HONEYMOON CYSTITIS due to introduction of "new bacteria" from the partner or irritation of the urethral opening by excessive rubbing of the penis
- Young girls or children: Tend to get UTI because they don't clean themselves the right way after bowel movements. Young girls need to be taught the right way of cleaning themselves after a bowel movement. Not wiping properly by cleaning from back to front leads to introduction of bacteria from the anal area to the vagina and urethral area. They have to be taught to wipe from front (vulva) to the back (anus) after a bowel movement (Clean to dirty may be a way of reminding them). Girls like everyone else have to remember to wash their hands after using the toilet
- Peri and Postmenopausal Women: The presence of Estrogen during the reproductive years (when women can have children) keeps the lining of the vagina and vulva area well lubricated with ample blood supply and supple firm tissues. However, during the Peri and Menopause period, the lack of Estrogen causes the tissues around the vulva to become pale, less supple and dry. This leads to easy bruising, pain or burning of vulva and vagina, and coupled with reduced acidity of vaginal fluid make the area more prone to bacteria multiplication and therefore more susceptible to urinary tract infections. Additionally, the urethra gets shorter, and is more susceptible to invasion by bacteria

Treatment of Urinary Tract Infection (UTI)

After seeing a health care provider, urine will be tested. It is important to do a collection known as a "clean catch."

CLEAN CATCH URINE SAMPLE: To do this:

One has to wipe well from front (vulva) to back (anus) with an antiseptic wipe or moist tissue paper, and let the first few drops or urine go into the toilet bowl; next catch a mid-stream portion (middle stream of the flow) into the specimen container, so as to minimize contamination from the vulva area

If urine shows bacteria, one will be treated with antibiotics. Sometimes the urine will be sent for culture and in that case, the specific bacteria causing the infection is grown and identified in the lab, as well as the antibiotic types it is susceptible to

One may need to take medications for three to seven days (take as prescribed) depending on the severity of the infection. Meanwhile:

Drinking lots of water, cranberry juice or cranberry tablets may help with the pain or discomfort. Cranberries have been touted for UTIs but studies are mixed at its effectiveness, in treating infections, because one has to take in a great amount. The juice contains a lot of sugar and not concentrated enough, and so tablets are better to take

Over the counter medicines that help with the pain include Ibuprofen (NSAIDS), AZO, PRODIUM, PYRIDIUM (Phenazopyridine). They are not antibiotics and do not treat the infection, but they help with the pain and discomfort due to bladder contraction until the antibiotics kick in to treat the underlying infection. They may cause the color of the urine to turn orange. NSAIDS eg. Ibuprofen also help

Recurrent Urinary Tract Infections

Some women are prone to recurrent UTIs and may get one every two to three months. It is characterized by two infections in the previous six months or three or more infections proven by positive urine cultures within a 12 month period.

Risk factors for Recurrent UTIs include:

Medicines – Diabetes medicine called SGLT2 Inhibitors cause increased elimination of sugar in urine as well as use of certain antibiotics all lead to recurrent UTIs

Incomplete bladder emptying

Voiding problems, eg constant dribbling or leakage

New sexual partner

Frequent sexual intercourse

Use of spermicidal cream

Pregnancy

Genetically predisposed

Medical problems like Diabetes Mellitus and others that decrease the body's immune system.

Anatomical abnormalities like prolapse of bladder or uterus may result in this.

Signs and Symptoms

These are similar to the ones described above for ordinary UTIs (see above) but occur every few months.

Treatment

After a history and physical exam is done, tests including carefully collecting a "clean catch" or midstream urine which is examined. Urine tests known as urine dip stick, urinalysis, (looking at a urine specimen under a microscope), and urine cultures – when urine is sent for culture to see if it will grow any bacteria – are done. Other urine tests such as how much urine remains in the bladder after voiding, (postvoid residual), and imaging studies like bladder ultrasound may be done as determined by the doctor.

Infections are usually treated with antibiotics the cultured bacteria are sensitive to.

If treated and UTIs continue to occur frequently, one may be put on daily antibiotics for up to six months (Prophylactic antibiotics).

If there is a specific cause like an anatomical problem, then treating that problem will lower recurrence rate.

In postmenopausal women who have low Estrogen levels, it results in thinning of lining of vulva and vagina, as well as reduction in numbers of normal "good bacteria" present, with increase in other bacteria. This leads to frequent vaginitis and increased UTIs. One may be given vaginal Estrogen pill or cream to build up the vaginal and vulva tissue and restore the normal good bacteria numbers. This may help decrease UTIs.

Recent recommendations from American Urological Association (AUA 2019 Annual Meeting) recommends cranberry can be used to prevent infections, but pill form is better, since liquid form may contain a lot of sugar.

Acupuncture, a complementary and alternative medicine procedure has been shown to prevent recurrence of UTIs.

General Measures to Prevent Recurrent UTI

Drink plenty of fluids and urinate often to flush the urinary tract of any bacteria.

Always wipe from front to back after a bowel movement or after urinating.

Empty your bladder before and after sex.

Avoid use of spermicides; they tend to change the normal bacteria, instead use other means for birth control/family planning.

Wash your vulva and urethral area after sex using a water filled squeeze bottle or take a shower.

Take some cranberry tablets before sex.

Take showers instead of lying in the bathtub full of water.

Avoid bubble baths, douching, sprays or soap in vulva as they can alter normal bacteria present.

Taking probiotic capsules or eating yogurt with probiotics may reduce recurrent UTIs.

One may be prescribed an antibiotic to take before sexual intercourse if that is the cause.

One may be prescribed an antibiotic daily or every other day for six months.

If one's sexual partner is uncircumcised ask him to wash his foreskin before and after sex.

Blood in the Urine (Hematuria)
What is It?

Hematuria is when there is blood present in the urine. It is not normal to have blood in the urine, and the urine may be red throughout or red at the end, or urine may look red/brownish in color. It is also known as 'GROSS HEMATURIA'

Causes of Hematuria

Urinary tract infection (see above)

Kidney stones

Kidney infections (Pyelonephritis)

Diseases affecting the kidney itself (the internal tubes and cells)

Tumors and cancer of the bladder

Medications like blood thinners, certain laxatives, cyclophosphamide, and phenolphthalein

In some low resource countries, infection with *Schistosomiasis (also known as Bilharzia)*

SCHISTOSOMIASIS: Caused by stepping in water containing the snails that harbor a parasitic larva resulting in blood in the urine. The larva penetrates the skin and eventually ends up in the bladder causing blood in the urine.

Treatment

Tests and investigations have to be done to find the cause and then treated accordingly, e.g. if infection, appropriate antibiotic medication, if kidney stones – these can pass or be removed, and if diseases affecting the kidneys are the causes, these can be treated with medications.

Microscopic Hematuria

However, sometimes people may have MICROSCOPIC HEMATURIA. Unlike "Gross Hematuria", with Microscopic Hematuria, urine color is normal after urination but laboratory tests will show there is blood in the urine. This is often found incidentally, when a urine test is done for other reasons and blood cells are noticed in the urine. It may be due to several reasons but mainly caused by kidney and bladder problems.

Causes of Microscopic Hematuria

Inflammation of the filtration system of the kidneys (Glomerulonephritis)
Stones in kidneys or bladder
Kidney and bladder infections
Blood diseases like sickle cell disease
Von Willebrand's disease
Hemophilia
Medicines like blood thinners, (Heparin and Warfarin), Aspirin, NSAIDs, Sulfa, Ciprofloxacin, Penicillin, antihypertensive drugs like Furosemide, Triamterene, Captopril, and Omeprazole
Tumors and cancers
Strenuous exercise
In postmenopausal women about 10 to 20% may experience Microscopic Hematuria with no known cause
Idiopathic – no known cause is found

Treatment

Several tests may be done including, special urine tests and blood work.
Ultrasound of the kidneys and bladder.
Cystoscopy is a procedure in which a small camera is used to look inside the bladder and examine the lining of the bladder.
Sometimes after all these tests are done, no obvious cause is found.
However, for those with specific causes, treatment is directed at those.

Urethritis (Ure-thri-tes)
What is It?

This is infection of the urethra, the tube that carries urine outside the body, and is often caused by a sexually transmitted disease, but can be caused by other bacteria, e.g. *E. Coli* coming from the area around the vulva/anus, by viruses e.g. Herpes and non infectious causes like irritation or urethral injury. The common causes are Gonorrhea and Chlamydia. It can affect both women and men.

Signs and Symptoms

It may present with a discharge which is yellow, creamy or greenish from the urethral opening and may have an odor.

There is pain with urination

Urge to urinate

If severe there may be fever or chills but these are not common

There may be pain in the lower part of the abdomen or pelvic area especially if the infection involves the vagina and female organs in the woman

In the male, it may involve the prostate since that surrounds the urethra for a short distance

Treatment

Samples taken with a swab and sent for culture or urine examination will help with the diagnosis. Treatment is with antibiotics if its bacterial related. The individual's sexual partner will also have to be treated to prevent reinfection or even spread to another sexual partner.

Kidney Infection (Pyelonephritis)
(Pye-lo-ne-fri-tis)
What is It?

This is a type of urinary tract infection which occurs in the kidneys. The possible causes include:

Staring in the urethra or bladder and move up to the kidneys

Occurring after a Cystoscope is passed to investigate the bladder (postprocedure infection)

After surgery on any part of the urinary tract

After a urinary catheter has been placed to empty the bladder

All types of UTIs can occur from prolonged use of wet pantie liners

Signs and Symptoms

When infection occurs in the kidneys one may have fever, pain in the back, chills, nausea and or vomiting, and pain with urination. There may be tenderness at the flanks and back when tapped.

Treatment

Urine tests known as urine dip, urinalysis, (looking at a urine specimen under a microscope), and urine cultures may be done. Blood work includes blood cultures and white cell count. The cultures will identify the bacteria causing the infection and the white cell count may show an increase in the number of infection fighting cells. Sometimes if the infection is severe, a CT scan or ultrasound of the kidneys may be done. A strong antibiotic is given for 10 to 14 days, and if severe with high fever, and increased white blood cells in the blood, hospitalization and intravenous antibiotics and fluids will be needed. Pain medications may be needed as well as medicines for nausea and vomiting if present.

Urinary Incontinence
What is It?

"There is a stigma associated with incontinence, so many people never mention it to their doctors or seek treatment. In reality, fecal incontinence is a very common and often very treatable condition."

—Brad Davis. (n.d.). Soccer Player. AZQuotes.com. Retrieved June 21, 2019, from AZQuotes.com

Urinary incontinence is involuntary leakage or expulsion of urine. This can be a bothersome problem for many middle aged and older women. About 25 million women in America have urinary incontinence. There are many women who do not realize that urinary incontinence can be treated and as a result it limits their social activities or interactions. Mentally, for some women, it causes fear of embarrassment in case there is "an accident" so they avoid being with others, and more importantly, there may be fear that they have an odor of urine due to leakage. This can lead to social isolation, depression or anxiety.

Some women may wear pantie liners or pads which when wet can cause odors, and prolong wetness can even lead to urinary tract infections and vulva irritation if they are not changed frequently. Some women may have anxiety about going to places where bathrooms are not easily accessible, and looking out for where a bathroom may be their chief concern when they go out, further increasing anxiety.

There are 3 main types of urinary incontinence:

URGE, STRESS OR COMBINED/MIXED INCONTINENCE

There are other types of incontinence which relate to:

Spinal cord or nerve injury (overflow incontinence)
Functional incontinence which is related to leakage caused by UTI, psychiatric problems, mobility problems etc

Urinary Urge Incontinence (UUI)

This is when "if you have to go, you have to go" (urgency) followed by an "accident" – wetting underwear or clothes (involuntary leakage). In the normal mechanism of elimination of urine from the bladder, there are nerve connections which control how the bladder contracts to eliminate urine.

Causes of UUI

- The nerve connections described above are messed up. This causes irregular contractions of the bladder muscles and results in the urge to urinate even when the bladder is not full
- Medical conditions like chronic cough, smoking and uncontrolled Asthma may contribute to urge incontinence
- Certain medications may lead to incontinence and so they must be taken into consideration. These include:

  Blood pressure medications like Diuretics, (also known as water pills), ACE inhibitors like Lisinopril, Benazepril, Alpha blockers which relax certain muscles (examples are Doxazosin and Prazosin)

  Muscle relaxants

  Sedatives

  Estrogen

  Allergy medicines

  Replacing these with other medicines may help the incontinence

Treatment

There is need to see one's doctor and discuss the problem with him or her. The health provider will take a history of one's medical conditions and medications that one is taking because these can be the cause or contribute to urge incontinence. After examination, one may have some tests done including urine tests, and sometimes more complex ones like ultrasound of the bladder and urine voiding studies.

For those with specific causes, treatment will reduce or eliminate UUI. For example if medication is the cause, replacing that with others may help that. If any infection is present, this is treated with antibiotics. However, if there is no obvious cause then the first line treatment is non-medication. If that alone does not work, then non medication combined with medication is used. Lastly, surgical treatment is also an option, if the first two fail or do not improve the situation.

Non-Medication Treatment

These include:

- Pelvic floor exercises
- Bladder retraining
- Dietary changes
- Weight loss
- Behavior changes to improve urge incontinence

- Exercises to strengthen muscles involved in stopping the expulsion of urine
- Delay of urination
- Timed voiding or urination

Pelvic Floor Exercises

These are exercises which tighten the pelvic muscles and bladder sphincter thereby controlling voiding. One common one is known as KEGEL EXERCISES. These can be done in the comfort of your home. Try these to tighten the pelvic muscles. The more you do them, the better you get at doing them and strengthening your pelvic muscles and other tissues.

Kegel Exercise

To identify the pelvic floor muscles involved in tightening the urethral opening, sit on the toilet, and while urinating, try to squeeze your pelvic muscles to stop the flow of urine. If one's muscles are weak, it will be difficult to stop the flow of urine. Once the muscles involved are identified, one can then do the exercises while standing up or sitting down, by squeezing the pelvic muscles and counting to 5 slowly, and then relax them. This is repeated 5 times per set and one can do three sets a day.

Other Pelvic Floor Exercises

These have been developed by physical therapists which help women strengthen weak pelvic floor muscles and treat urinary incontinence. One such regimen is from the Health Central Hospital rehabilitation services in Ocoee, Central Florida, which is summarized below:

Quick Contractions.

While lying down with a pillow under the knees contract the pelvic floor muscles and hold for 3 seconds. Relax for 3 seconds and repeat these 20 times. Don't stop breathing or hold one's breath.

Endurance Contractions

This is a longer contraction and relaxation routine. Contract pelvic floor muscles and hold for 10 seconds then relax for 10 seconds. Repeat these 10 times. It may help not to stop breathing if one counts one through 10 while contracting and relaxing.

As one does these frequently, one will notice that the muscles get stronger and when one sits on the toilet to urinate and tries to stop the urine flow by squeezing the muscles, it becomes increasingly better for you to hold the urine and not leak.

Pelvic Tilt and Squeeze

Another exercise involves tilting the pelvis and squeezing the pelvic muscles together. While lying down on one's back, draw one's feet toward buttocks while one's arms are at the sides. Then raise one's pelvic area up from the floor while contracting the pelvic muscles; keep it up for a count of 5 and drop down to the floor again. Repeat these 10 times and do it 2–3 times a day. (Health Central Hospital Rehabilitation handout. Ocoee Florida)

Delay of Urination

This is one of the methods used to relearn when to urinate. The urge or sensation to urinate is delayed for about 5 minutes before using the bathroom. If one can do that, then the delay time is increased to 10 minutes. Eventually time is increased until urination is every 3 to 4 hours. Deep relaxation breathing or Kegel exercises can be used to delay urination when the urge is felt. Talking to oneself about not rushing and motivating oneself to do Kegel exercise while walking to the restroom sometimes helps.

Timed Urination or Voiding

This is when urination is on a schedule. One uses the bathroom to urinate, say every one hour whether there is the urge to do so or not. This can be increased to every 2 to 3 hours or a schedule that fits the individual. This is used to train the bladder not to contract irregularly. It takes at least 3 to 12 weeks to master bladder training and so a great deal of patience is needed.

Fluid Management and Dietary Changes

Avoid drinking water or fluids after 6 PM and avoid foods that may irritate the bladder like spices, citrus, tomatoes, chocolate and sodas.

Weight Loss

Studies have shown repeatedly that weight loss helps both urge and stress incontinence to improve in individuals who are overweight or obese. It will also help reduce cardiovascular diseases like Hypertension, coronary heart disease, and elevated cholesterol.

Biofeedback

This can also be used to retrain the pelvic muscles, so there is reduction in the urge to urinate and decrease the number of leakage accidents. A trained therapist usually works with the client who through biofeedback mechanisms trains her mind to strengthen the appropriate muscles using Kegel techniques.

Medicines For Treating Urge Incontinence

When non-medicinal methods are not adequately preventing urge incontinence, then medicines can be used together with the non-medicinal methods.

There are many which may be helpful in decreasing the urge or accidents. The three main categories of drugs used to treat urge incontinence include:

- Antispasmodics: These prevent spasm of the bladder: Hyoscyamine (Anaspaz, Cystospaz, Hyosol, Hyospaz, Levbid, and Levsin) or Dicyclomine (Antispas, Bentyl, Byclomine)
- Tricyclic antidepressants (TCA): They help relax the smooth muscles of the bladder and increase the tone of the urethral sphincter. Examples are Imipramine and Doxepin. Amitriptyline is useful for frequency but not UII.
- Anticholinergic drugs: These help relax the muscles of the bladder by preventing the spasms and are used more frequently than the other two

They include:

Darifenacin (Enablex)
Fesoterodine (Toviaz)
Oxybutynin (Ditropan, Ditropan XL, Gelnique, Oxytrol)
Solifenacin (Vesicare)
Tolterodine (Detrol, Detrol LA)
Trospium (Sanctura)
Oxytrol patch for women is the only drug available over the counter (OTC)

When a single drug treatment does not work, a combination therapy such as Oxybutynin (Ditropan) and Imipramine (Tofranil) may be used. Although their mechanism of action differ, Oxybutynin and Imipramine work together to improve urge incontinence. Each medicine may have side effects which may occur in some women but not in other women. Remember to let one's doctor know if one is started on a medicine and develops side effects. Some of these are drowsiness with the TCAs and dry mouth and Constipation with the Anticholinergics.

Stress Incontinence

This is involuntary leakage of urine when one coughs, sneezes, jumps, runs or lifts heavy objects. In effect, there is leakage when the pressure inside the pelvic or abdominal area is increased. There is weakness of the muscles in the pelvic area causing the urethra to be relaxed and the sphincter or circular muscles around the opening to be weakened. Any increase in pelvic pressure like coughing or laughing causes urine to leak out.

Risk factors for developing stress incontinence include:

Age, especially women who are Postmenopause
Child birth
Overweight and obesity
Previous pelvic surgery like Hysterectomy (removal of uterus)
Pregnancy

Treatment of Stress Incontinence

Behavior: Fluid management and weight loss
Bladder Training: These include Timed Urination, Delayed Urination
Pelvic Floor Muscle Training: As outlined above under urge incontinence

Medicines

There are no effective medicines to treat this, however, some medicines have been used with varying success, although not specifically approved by FDA for this purpose. These include Midodrine, pseudoephedrine, synephrine, and duloxetine. In postmenopausal women, vaginal Estrogen has been found to be helpful especially when combined with any of the first three methods above. When it is combined with urge incontinence (mixed) then medicines used for urge incontinence may help with both types of urinary incontinence.

Devices

Radiofrequency Devices: New devices which tone pelvic muscles are non-surgical treatment options available. The devices use radiofrequency to heat tissues at the bladder base, leading to thicker and firmer collagen which is already present in the tissues. This results in less leakage, and the procedure can be performed in a doctor's office or outpatient setting. Ask a urologist or gynecologist about this if you are interested. An example of this type of device is Renessa.

Home Based Devices

The FDA (Food and Drug Administration) in the USA in 2015 approved a home device to be used for urge and stress incontinence. It is inserted into the vagina and it stimulates the pelvic floor muscles and makes them tight or more toned. It basically does what the Kegel exercises do and strengthens the pelvic muscles. The company has different devices: one for stress urinary incontinence (APEX), one that treats stress and mixed urinary incontinence (APEX M), and one for stress, urge and low sexual function (decreased libido) (INTENSITY). ATTAIN is another one which includes Biofeed back. They even have one that treats fecal or stool incontinence (leakage of stool). Presently only one company has approval from the FDA, but several may soon be approved from other companies. (http://www.incontrolmedical.com).

Surgical Treatment

Several surgical methods are used and these include a sling which is put in to support the urethra (sling support procedure) or a procedure during which special synthetic material is injected near the urethral to cushion it and keep it snug and tight. Newer surgical procedures are being developed.

Mixed or Combined Incontinence

Some individuals have both urge and stress incontinence present. The measures listed above in terms of treatment will apply to mixed incontinence. Medications, surgery or a device will help one or both.

Overactive Bladder (OAB)

What is It?

This is a strong desire to urinate (urgency) often accompanied by frequency. The bladder is not full but it's contracting because of an internal problem which is thought to be caused by over activity of the muscular walls of the urinary bladder. Neurochemicals and nerves associated with bladder muscle function are all thought to be involved in the dysfunction. It increases with age and by

Overactive bladder may occur in children, women and men and is characterized by urgency which may be associated with frequency, nocturia with and without incontinence; and in the absence of infection or other conditions.

70 years 20% of the population may be affected. As with urge incontinence, OAB can be very disturbing and affect an individual's quality of life and her socializing activities in the community and among friends.

Signs and Symptoms

There is urinary **urgency** (strong desire to urinate in spite of small volumes of urine) which may be associated with **frequency** (urinating more than 8 times in 24 hours) and waking up more than 2 times to urinate at night (called **nocturia**). There is no underlying infection e.g. urinary tract infection or inflammation of the bladder.

It may or may not be associated with **urge urinary incontinence** which we discussed above.

It affects both women and men almost equally and tends to increase with age, however, women tend to have urge incontinence associated with it.

Risk Factors Leading to OAB

Those with high risk factors of getting OAB include those who are:

Caucasians

Women aged 75 years and over

Obese individuals

Taking Hormone Replacement medicines for postmenopausal symptoms

Those with diseases like Multiple Sclerosis, Parkinson's Disease, Diabetes mellitus, Stroke, Depression, Arthritis, and enlarged prostate in men (BPH)

Treatment

You must inform your doctor in order to be treated. A careful history, and physical exam will be done by the doctor. Note that certain medications, urinary infections, and severe constipation with stool impacted or stuck in the rectum, may all cause urgency, but these will disappear once the condition is treated or medication is stopped. Tests ordered may include urine examination, ultrasound of the pelvis, bladder and kidneys, and other more complicated tests if needed. Once the diagnosis is made, treatment is initially with three things: Behavioral changes, Pelvic floor Exercises, and Medications. Most treatments control but do not cure overactive bladder.

1. Behavioral Change

This is done to reduce or control intake of dietary irritants, and to retrain the bladder so it releases urine in a controlled way.

- REDUCE DIETARY IRRITANTS
  Dietary irritants are usually "acidic" in nature and need to be used in moderation. Acidic foods are toxic to the bladder and so the bladder will contract to eliminate them. These include: citrus fruits and juices, coffee, cranberries fruit and juices, tea, alcohol, apples, carbonated beverages, pineapple, strawberry, grapes, vinegar, Aspartame, tomato based foods to name a few
- BLADDER RETRAINING
  This is to break the cycle of urgency and frequency, by doing "Timed Voiding" with the goal of ultimately voiding about every 3 hours
  One gradually increases the time between voiding by first identifying the shortest interval between voids, and then voiding only after that time interval passes
  One must try not to urinate in between the time interval as it is increased with time. To make it easier, interval is increased by 15 to 30 minutes every week, until the interval is about every 3 to 4 hours. This works very well, especially

if OAB does not involve incontinence. If incontinence or leakage is a problem, that has to be controlled first before bladder retraining

- LIFESTYLE CHANGES

Other lifestyle changes have been identified as contributing to increasing urinary urgency, frequency or incontinence, and changing these may help decrease OAB as well as urinary incontinence. They include:
  - Obesity: Weight loss has helped some individuals as this takes pressure off pelvic muscles.
  - Excessive intake of fluids: All fluids (include those in foods) should be limited to less than 2400 cc (ml) or 9 cups per day (a cup is about 250 ml) for anyone with OAB, unless they are involved in vigorous exercise, or sweat a lot, etc.
  - Exercises: Regular exercises are needed to strengthen pelvic muscles, and help with weight loss.
  - Constipation: Having regular bowel movement decrease urinary urgency, frequency and incontinence, and so it needs to be prevented and treated. See treatment of constipation (abdomen chapter).

2. Pelvic Floor Exercises

- Pelvic Floor Muscle exercises – These were described above and are known as KEGEL EXERCISES, which are either self directed, or by a physical therapist
- For those who cannot do them on their own, they can use vaginal cones or new devices which help one do the exercises effectively
- The vaginal cones come in a set of identical shapes but have different weights. They are sold on line or in some medical supply shops
- Device known as TENS (electrical stimulator) have an electrode placed in the vagina and it sends a mild electric current to nerves in the lower back. It is thought the stimulation may make the pelvic muscles contract producing "kegel exercises". There are other devices which stimulate other nerves or even cause new nerve cells to grow and cause muscle tone to be increased

3. Biofeedback

This is a type of positive reinforcement of what the body does naturally. A therapist assists the individual to identify muscles involved in contracting pelvic muscles (Kegel muscles) by using electrodes placed on the abdomen and anal area. One then learns to contract them so as to tighten the pelvic muscles that prevent incontinence.

4. Medications

Whe lifestyle changes do not adequately improve overactive bladder (OAB) then medcations may be prescribed. These are either oral or skin patches. Some medicine used to treat it include:

- Anti-cholinergics: OXYBUTYNIN, (Ditropan), TOLTERODINE (Detrol), TROSPIUM (sanctura), PROPIVERINE, SOLIFENACIN (vesicare), DARIFENACIN (Enablex), and oxybutynin patch (Oxytrol patch). The latter is sold as an Over the Counter skin patch in the USA. For older adults Darifenacin and Tolterodine are safer options because they do not cross into the brain and affect thinking process, and have less side effects
- Like all medicines anticholinergics may have side effects but this may not affect everyone. These include dry mouth, constipation, drowsiness and blurred vision. Dose reduction may decrease these side effects
- Vaginal Estrogens: For postmenopausal women, sometimes use of VAGINAL ESTROGEN cream or inserted vaginal tablets may help with symptoms of OAB. Generally women who are on combined oral Estrogen and progestin pills sometimes experience incontinence or worsening of OAB symptoms, but this is not the case with the vaginal Estrogens
- Mirabegron (Myrbetriq) belongs to a different class of drugs and it tends to have lower adverse effects and is better tolerated
- Combination of the above three groups is also possible when one is not effective
- OTC supplements sometimes recommended is VIT D. Some studies have shown that adequate amounts of Vitamin D in the body help maintain urinary continence or stop leakage. Taking between 400 to 1000 IU of VITAMIN D3 may help. It is better absorbed with dietary fats. Magnesium, Yoga and Apple cider vinegar are used but good studies lacking.

Alternate Treatments

For women who have failed the above medications, use of:

1. Botox: this is a protein produced by a bacterium, which is injected into the bladder and it acts as a nerve toxin by blocking muscle contraction
2. Nerve stimulation have been used with success
3. Bulking agents injected around urethra, e.g. collagen (Contigen), Coaptite, Durasphere.

As you may realize, treatment for OAB and urge incontinence do overlap to some extent.

Kidney Failure (Renal Failure)
What is It?

The kidneys are a pair of very important organs in the body and if their funtions deteriorate one ends up with kidney failure also known as Renal Failure. Thee are certain conditions that affect the ability of the kidneys to work at optimal capcity. It is important to know about the risk factors or conditions that may damag the kidneys and therefore affect its function. Reducing these risk factors may helpstop the deterioration of the kidneys. There are different types of renal failure depending on the duration and whether it is reversible.

Acute Kidney Disease

According to the 2010 Global Burden of Disease study, Chronic kidney disease ranged at 18th of total number of deaths worldwide. About 10% of the world's population has chronic kidney disease (CKD) and it increases with age with estimates that in those 65-74 years old, one in five men and one in four women have CKD.

(World Kidney Day: Chronic Kidney Disease. 2015).

Acute Renal Failure occurs over hours and days and once the underlying problem is quickly corrected the kidney function may return to normal.

Chronic Kidney Disease (CKD)

Ongoing renal or kidney disease s referred to as CHRONIC KIDNEY DISEASE when there is kidney damage or reduced function of the kidneys for more than 3 months. This is usually no reversible and it is a slow gradual loss of function. The kidneys have not totally stopped working, but their ability to filter blood, remove toxic substances and regulate water and minerals in your body has diminished. Most people have chronic kidney disease as opposed to acute kidney disease. In the US, about 14% of the populations have CKD, and the main causes are Hypertension and Diabetes according to the National Institute of Health. If CKD continues to get worse, wastes e.g. protein waste, build up in the blood and result in high levels of certain chemicals like creatinine, urea, phosphorus, potassium, low calcium and development of diseases/conditions like anemia, high blood pressure, brittle bones, and nerve problems. Protein wastes can cause nausea and vomiting, change of taste and itching of the skin.

End Stage Renal Disease

This is when the functions of the kidneys are so low, with high accumulation of waste, and it is also referred to as kidney failure. In order for the person to stay alive, the individual must be on DIALYSIS (filtering blood artificially) or get a kidney transplant from a donor.

Risk factors for developing chronic kidney disease (CKD)

- DISEASES: Several diseases or conditions can lead to CKD and these include hypertension, diabetes mellitus, enlarged prostate in men (benign prostatic hypertrophy), history of recurrent kidney infections, kidney stones, and previous kidney disease from diseases like sickle cell disease, and certain inherited kidney diseases
- AUTOIMMUNE conditions: These lead to inflammation of the filtration system as well as the cells of the kidneys. These include conditions like Lupus, Autoimmune kidney disease (IgA nephropathy), and Diabetes Mellitus
- ABNORMAL KIDNEY STRUCTURE: polycystic kidneys – several cysts in the kidneys destroy the cells
- OLDER AGE: Kidney function naturally decreases with age
- FAMILY HISTORY OF CKD: If it occurs in one's parents or close relative
- DISEASES OF KIDNEY BLOOD VESSELS: This may reduce blood flow or circulation to and within the kidneys
- RECURRENT KIDNEY STONES: These or anything that can obstruct the flow of urine in the kidney or tubes (ureters) from the inside or outside
- ENLARGED PROSTATE: In men enlarged prostate can cause obstruction of urine flow
- TUMORS: tumors in the kidneys may block the flow of urine
- MEDICATIONS: Some of these damage the kidney cells or tubes after prolonged use
- HERBAL SUPPLEMENTS: These include; Aristolochia (birthwort, heartwort, and fangji), Some Ayurvedic medications (used in Indian traditional medicine) and some Chinese herbal medications have been found to be contaminated with lead, mercury and arsenic which are toxic to the kidneys. Care also must be taken with use of African herbal medicines as well
- GENETIC: Research shows that about 10% of all CKD is due to genetic causes
- RACE: Being African American, Native American or Asian
- SMOKING: cigarette smoking can cause kidney damage
- HEAVY METALS: Mercury, lead, arsenic
- UNKNOWN CAUSES: Also called 'idiopathic'. In 15% of people with CKD the underlying cause is not known

What to Do to Stop Progression of Chronic Kidney Disease (CKD)

There are certain things you as a patient must do to prevent chronic kidney failure from progressing if you have been diagnosed with CKD. There are degrees of diminished kidney function, and chronic kidney failure is classified from stage 1 to stage 5, with stage 5 being the worse.

To prevent progression, you need to do the following:

- CONTROL BLOOD PRESSURE (BP). BP has to be well controlled. It should be less than 130/80 according to new guidelines by the American College of Cardiology guidelines released in 2017 (2017 Guidelines for high blood pressure in adults www.acc.org/2017-guidelines-for-high-blood-pressure-in-adults). CKD can cause high blood pressure due to fluid retention, and high BP or hypertension can lead to CKD by damaging kidneys blood vessels
- There are two classes of anti-hypertensive medications which are recommended for individuals with CKD and hypertension. These are angiotensin-converting enzyme inhibitors (ACEI) and angiotensin receptor blockers (ARB); both are effective in slowing the progression of kidney disease and lowering mortality
- Another class of drugs which may be added are diuretics (also called water pills) or aldosterone receptor antagonists (e.g. spironolactone and eplerenone) which flush out sodium and water. If you have hypertension and CKD ask your doctor if medications in these classes are right for you
- GOUT or elevated levels of URIC ACID (chemical that leads to gout crystals in joints) can worsen CKD and so it is important that a uric acid lowering medication is used to stop progression
- DECREASE SALT INTAKE: It is recommended that a dietary sodium intake of less than 2.4 g/day (about 2.3 g is in one teaspoon of salt) is appropriate for most adults with CKD and hypertension. The American Heart Association recommends a dietary sodium intake of 1.5 g/day to delay cardiovascular diseases like stroke and heart attacks and so aiming for the lower number is better. One should avoid foods that are pickled, preserved with salt, or are overly salted like salted popcorn, pickles, salted fish, and salted pretzels. Fresh foods are better because you control how much salt you use. Salt can also cause fluid retention and further tax the already damaged kidneys. Be careful of using salt substitutes because they contain potassium salt and this can be retained in the body and cause complications in those with renal disease. Instead use non salt seasonings e.g. mixture of herbs which can help make food palatable without the salt
- DIABETES: If you have diabetes, work with your doctor to make sure your blood sugar is well controlled. Individuals with diabetes who are not well controlled on pills will have to be started on insulin or other injectables to control blood sugar. Being on insulin is not a sign of failure, because it is used for better blood sugar control. Newer groups of DM medicines are now available which may delay insulin initiation
- AVOID CERTAIN MEDICINES: Avoid medicines that may further compromise or affect your kidneys if you already have kidney damage. Such medicines are called "Nephrotoxic" (toxic to the kidneys). They belong to diverse classes of drugs

Some examples include:

- Antibiotics: e.g. ciprofloxacin, vancomycin, sulfonamides, and Aminoglycosides (e.g. gentamicin, tobramycin)
- Anti-inflammatory drugs: e.g. ibuprofen and naproxen, and diclofenac
- Chemotherapy drugs: cisplatin, cyclosporine, and tacrolimus
- Antimalaria drug: Quinine
- Imaging Dyes: Known as contrasts and used for studies like CT and MRI scans
- Others include: amphotericin B, and allopurinol, used to treat gout

What About Aspirin?

Low dose aspirin (75mg to 162mg) is okay to take if you have CKD, but avoid higher doses. Some of the NSAIDs may be bought as brand name medicines like Advil, Motrin, Aleve, and Voltaren etc., and so it's important to read the labels on store bought medications. Although they are good medicines anyone who has kidney disease must stop using them and use other alternative medicines for pain, or inflammation. These may include acetaminophen, low dose tramadol, gabapentin, duloxetine, steroids etc. and use of massage, acupuncture, capsaicin and menthol creams, lidocaine patches etc.

- BE CAREFUL ABOUT CONTRAST GIVEN FOR IMAGING: If you have kidney disease and you have a CT scan ordered with contrast tell them you have kidney disease, because the contrast may make your kidney function worse

Elimination of drugs through the kidneys

Sometimes in kidney disease, the dose of certain prescription medicines eliminated or excreted by the kidney must be reduced so as to avoid accumulation of the drug in the body. Let your doctor know all the medicines you take including herbal medicines, supplements, etc. and find out from him or her if the doses you are taking are okay with kidney disease.

Regular Doctor Check Ups are Important

Go for regular check-ups with your health provider. If you have kidney disease, let any new health provider know when you see her for consultation, so they do not give you any medicines that can further damage your kidneys.

Tests to Check For Chronic Kidney Disease

This may include blood and urine tests, ultrasound or CT scan of the kidneys and bladder, the rate of how the kidney filters urine can be estimated or measured by the lab (Glomerular filtration rate – eGFR). A kidney biopsy may also be done depending on what the suspected cause is. Your health care provider will order these tests and will discuss results with you. Go prepared to ask questions.

Treatment

In the early stages of CKD, one may be placed on certain antihypertensive medications which help with kidney function. As mentioned above, optimal treatment of blood pressure and diabetes, and in some cases a procedure which stretches or dilates a constricted or blocked kidney blood vessel (renal artery stenosis) may result in improved kidney function. There is need for regular follow up with your doctor to do periodic blood work to check your kidneys and to make sure your blood pressure is well controlled. Other medications may be given depending on your blood work results.

Treatment of End Stage Renal Disease (ESRD)

In this case, the kidneys cannot filter the blood well and an artificial kidney has to do that job. This is called DIALYSIS. There are two types:

Hemodialysis

Hemodialysis is a process by which a machine is used to do the normal function of the kidneys by "purifying the blood" through the removal of waste and excess fluid. It is done for about 3 to 4 hours, three times a week.

Peritoneal Dialysis (PD)

In PD a large tissue in the abdominal area (the peritoneum) acts like the filter and together with special fluids introduced into the abdominal cavity, there is removal of the waste and excess fluid from the blood into the fluid that was introduced through a tube placed in the abdomen.

Kidney Transplant

An individual with chronic kidney failure may also have a kidney transplant. This is when the individual receives a kidney from an appropriate or matching donor so that his "new kidney" will perform the functions his damaged kidneys could not do. In humans, one good kidney can do an adequate job of removing the toxins and excess fluids and so two kidneys are not required for this function. A kidney may be donated by a live donor or harvested from an accident victim etc.

Kidney Stones (Nephrolithiasis or renal calculi)
What are Kidney Stones?

Kidney stones are small stones formed from excess chemicals in the urine. Usually when the urine is concentrated or one does not drink enough water, the chemicals precipitate or aggregate to form a small crystal or mass. These can be passed in the urine if very small. However, if the crystals come together and form a bigger stone, it may want to try to pass out of the kidneys through the ureters to the bladder.

What Happens to a Large Kidney Stone?

Due to the large size, it may obstruct the ureter and leads to pain as the ureter tries to get rid of it by contracting. Some stones may form and stay in the kidneys and may not give any symptoms like pain, however if they dislodge and start moving down the ureter they may get stuck and lead to symptoms like colicky pain, and blood in the urine.

Types of Kidney Stones

There are various kinds of kidney stones depending on the chemicals involved in the formation of the stone. Common kidney stones include calcium oxalate, urate, cystine, xanthine, and phosphate.

Risk Factors for Kidney Stone Formation

Hypertension
Diabetes
Obesity
Increased consumption of sugary drinks containing fructose or high fructose
   corn syrup

Symptoms of An Obstructed Kidney Stone (Renal colic).

- Pain – This may be in the back, flank (side), or on either side of the lower abdomen depending on which kidney is involved, or where the obstruction is located. Pain may be felt in the mid lower abdomen, groin, labia of women or the penis in men. Pain tends to come and go initially, (cramping or colicky), but may be sharp or constant
- Nausea and vomiting
- Fever and chills
- Pain during urination
- Blood in the urine
- Frequent urination which is small in amount
- Inability to urinate

Complications

These include bleeding from any part of the urinary system where the stone is.

Large stones can cause obstruction and affect urine flow

Pain which is referred to as renal colic and can be very severe

Infection which needs to be treated with antibiotics

Kidney failure resulting in need for dialysis if not treated early

Treatment

If kidney stones are suspected to be a cause of pain, due to several of the above symptoms, a history and physical examination is done to locate the area of pain. A urine test is the first test done to check for blood, infection and other abnormal cells.

Other studies may include imaging studies of the urinary tract to look for stones. These may include Ultrasound, Intravenous Pyelogram (IVP) of the kidneys, X-rays or CT scan of the abdomen and pelvis.

When confirmed, treatment may include:

Increased fluids by mouth or intravenously (Through the vein)

Medicines to treat pain, and for nausea or vomiting

Medications that may assist the body to pass the stone, e.g. Tamsulosin

Antibiotics may also be given to prevent or treat any infection

If a stone is too big to pass, then special ultrasound sound waves can be used to break it up into smaller bits (Lithotripsy) and they would then be passed out through the urine

A surgical procedure using a special tube and a camera, through a hole in the skin near the kidneys may be used to remove large or irregular shaped stones. Alternatively, the stone may first be crushed with ultrasound sound waves and then the pieces are removed

A small tube called a stent can be placed in the ureter to relieve a blockage.

Prevention of Kidney Stones

There are ways one can prevent or decrease the incidence of recurrent kidney stones. This is through proper diet and use of medications. The most common kidney stone is Calcium Oxalate followed by Uric Acid stones. Preventive measures include:

- Keep oneself well hydrated. If one sweats or exercises, uses sauna, is overheated etc. remember to replace fluids by drinking enough. Dehydration leads to decreased urine production and that can concentrate the chemicals which form kidney stones
- Potassium citrate is often used to prevent formation of kidney stones because the citrate binds to calcium so other stone-forming chemicals cannot bind to it and form stones

- Drink lemonade, limeade and other fruit drinks high in citrate. They perform the same work as Potassium Citrate. Make one's own drink and control the amount of sugar one puts in it
- Appropriate dietary consideration is important. Calcium is not the enemy. Take adequate amounts of calcium in one's diet. Some people think if they avoid calcium, they will have less stones forming, however, research show that this is not the case. Eat calcium and oxalate-rich foods together at the same time, and they will bind together in the intestines before reaching the kidneys where the stones are formed
- Calcium-rich foods are important for women to promote bone health and these include milk, yogurt, cheese, ice cream, soybeans, tofu, and red beans. Others are nuts like almonds, walnuts, Brazil nuts and sesame seeds. Vegetables like broccoli, green beans, okra, spinach, and fish like sardines and salmon with bones are rich in Calcium
- Oxalate-rich foods include peanuts, spinach, beets, tea, chocolate, sweet potatoes, other nuts and green vegetables

Prevention of Uric Acid Stones

- Take medications to prevent uric acid stones from forming. Examples are Allopurinol and Febuxostat which were discussed under prevention of Gout
- Adequate hydration is important as this dilutes the urine preventing stone formation
- Alkalization of urine using Sodium or Potassium Citrate produces a more soluble form of the uric acid molecule
- Dietary wise, one must cut down on animal protein foods, because these are high in purines which form uric acid. These include meats like beef, ham, bacon, deer, veal, and organ meats like liver and tongue. Also cut back on fish like anchovies and codfish
- Increased consumption of Cranberry juice can lead to risk of kidney stones

Remember to regularly take medicines prescribed by one's health care provider and let them know of any non prescribed medicines one takes.

Essential Information About Water and Fluid Intake
Why is Water Important

Water forms about 60% of an individual's body weight and may vary depending on sex, age, which organ, amount of body fat etc. It is very important in keeping the various processes in our cells and organs working, and it forms most of the fluid portion of the blood which transports nutrients and oxygen to cells. It has often been said that everyone has to drink at least eight (8) glasses of water a day, but the experts agree that the amount of water an individual needs depends on:

Age
Weight
Conditions like fever and illness
Climate, e.g. hot weather
How much sweating one is doing
Physical activity and exercise

The Institute of Medicine and other institutions in the USA have determined that on average men need about 3.7 liters or 101 oz of FLUIDS daily (about 13 cups) and women about 2.7 liters or 75 oz (about 9 cups). Now this is total fluid and includes all beverages and foods. One gets on average about 80% of total water intake from water and beverages, and 20% from fruits, vegetables and other foods one eats. Interestingly enough, the body has a way of detecting thirst and that will make an individual drink water or fluids when this occurs.

Too Little or Too Much Water?

"An over-indulgence of anything, even something as pure as water, can intoxicate."

Criss Jami, Venus in Arms (Poetry book)

Drinking too little water or excess loss of water without replacement will cause dehydration and decrease production of urine. If it goes on for a long time, it can cause acute kidney failure due to inadequate blood supply to it and the kidney will stop performing its usual functions.

On the other hand, drinking too much water, can dilute the blood and reduce the concentrations of certain chemicals (electrolytes) like Sodium, Potassium and Chloride leading to serious complications like seizures, confusion, headaches, nausea, vomiting, and muscle cramps.

Bottom Line

If one is thirsty drink fluids. Let thirst be the guide.

If one is losing fluid through sweating, excessive heat or diarrhea; make sure one drinks more to replace that.

19

Diseases of the Pelvic Organs

The Female Genital System

....

The pelvis is just below the abdomen and contains the pelvic organs or reproductive organs, part of the large intestines and the bladder. In the female there is the uterus or womb, the neck of which is formed by the cervix and this opens into the vagina. The fallopian tubes (TUBES) are connected to either sides of the uterus and their wide funnel like ends terminate close to the ovaries. Below is a diagram of the female external genitalia.

Female External Genitalia Area (Perineum)

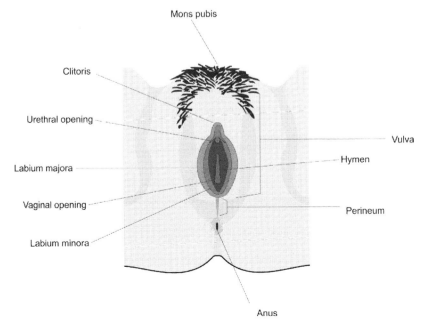

Mons pubis

Clitoris

Urethral opening

Labium majora

Vaginal opening

Labium minora

Vulva

Hymen

Perineum

Anus

There are a number of conditions affecting the female genital organs. Some of these conditions affect either the external or internal female genitalia, however; there is an overlap in some cases. The external parts consist of the vulva, clitoris, external and inner lips (labia) and the vaginal opening. The internal genitalia consists of the "inner parts" like the vagina, cervix, uterus, fallopian tubes and ovaries which are illustrated in a diagram below.

The discussions will focus on the following conditions:

Yeast infection of vagina and vulva (Candidiasis)
Bacterial vaginosis (BV)
Sexually transmitted infections (STIs)
Painful periods (Dysmenorrhea)
Excessive periods or menstruation
Irregular periods or menstruation
Persistent painful sexual intercourse (Dyspareunia)
Other pelvic conditions

Vagina and Vulva Infections

Yeast and Bacterial Vaginosis (BV) are not defined as sexually transmitted infections, but can occur in a woman's vulva and vagina.

Candidiasis – Yeast Infection or "White"
What is It?

This is caused by a yeast (type of fungus) called Candida. It is present normally in small amounts on skin and vulva area, however overgrowth leads to infection. It causes itchy white cottage cheese like discharge (clumps) and irritation of vulva and inside the vagina. Scratching produces redness and or swelling of the vulva and vagina, and sometimes little tears in the lining resulting in irritation and pain made worse during urination.

Risk factors for developing yeast infections

Some women may get frequent yeast infections due to:

Frequent douching
Taking antibiotics for other conditions, e.g for sinus infections or UTIs
Frequent use of scented soaps to wash the vagina and vulva area
Being a diabetic whose blood sugars are not well controlled
Taking chronic steroid medications like Prednisone for medical conditions
Having diseases which decrease one's immune system

These conditions may lead to overgrowth of yeast which is normally present in small amounts. A woman who has a yeast infection can transmit it to her male partner and overgrowth of this can cause him to get the infection as well. Uncircumcised males, those with diabetes or diminished immune system may be more prone to yeast infections.

Treatment

Antifungal medications are used to treat vaginal yeast infections. These include an oral medicine like FLUCONAZOLE (Diflucan), or creams and vaginal suppositories/tablets inserted into the vagina. Examples are Nystatin, Clotrimazole, Miconazole, Terconazole, and a sulfa antibiotic Sulfanilamide 15% (AVC) cream used intravaginally. It is best to avoid sex while undergoing treatment.

Prevention of Yeast Infections

To avoid yeast infections one should:

- Wear cotton underwear or underwear with a cotton lining or gusset. Cotton is ideal because it is a breathable material
- If one has recurrent yeast infections then going to bed without underwear may help
- Wear loose or baggy underwear to bed
- Avoid douching. Douching is attempting to feel "fresh or clean" by using solutions to rinse or wash the vagina area. The liquid used to douche are chemicals mixed with water to "clean" the vagina, however, the process may kill the normal "good" bacteria which are present, and lead to overgrowth of yeast. Some refer to the vagina as a "self-cleaning oven" which does not need soap or anything else to keep it clean
- Avoid using scented soaps or disinfectants to wash/clean the genitalia areas
- Some ladies who have frequent antibiotic associated yeast infections should, along with their antibiotics e.g. Amoxicillin, be given a medicine like one tablet of Fluconazole to prevent a yeast infection
- Using probiotics while on antibiotics tend to prevent elimination of "normal bacteria"
- Some women who have yeast infections around their menses have switched to use of a "menstrual cup" instead of tampons and pads. A menstrual cup is a reusable silicone or rubber cup which is inserted around the cervix to collect menstrual blood. It is rinsed with soap and water and reused

Recurrent Yeast Infections

What is It?

Some women experience recurrent infections with yeast. This means when they are treated the infection recurs and they have about four or more infections within a year. This may be due to treatment resistant yeast species which do not respond to the usual treatment.

Treatment

This requires prolonged treatment with oral or vaginal inserted antifungal medicine. Sometimes treatment may be needed for three to six months. Male partner may need to be treated if he has symptoms to prevent re-infection of the female, if she is the only one treated.

Bacterial Vaginosis (BV)

This is due to overgrowth of normal vaginal bacteria. The vagina contains various bacteria which are normally present and they exist in harmony with each other. When one douches or even takes a lot of bubble baths, the normal balance between the various normal bacteria in the vagina is altered and so there is usually an overgrowth of one type compared to others. This eventually leads to a thin vaginal discharge and an odor, most times a fishy type smell.

Risks Associated with Bacteria Vaginosis

Having recurrent BV can increase the risk of acquiring other infections like Pelvic Inflammatory Disease (PID), sexually transmitted infections and Cervical Cancer (the Cervical Cancer link was seen in a Swedish study). It may also cause difficulty in getting pregnant or increase risk of ending up with an ectopic pregnancy (the embryo does not implant in the uterine cavity).

Treatment

Treatment is to stop douching, no bubble baths and then be treated with either oral or vaginal creams. Examples of such medicines are Metronidazole, Tinidazole, Secnidazole (Solosec, Flagentyl or Tagera Forte) or Clindamycin.

Recurrent Bacterial Vaginosis (BV)

There are a few women who after being treated for Bacterial Vaginosis will get recurrent infections of BV, and in such women, the bacteria persist in the lining of the vagina or may even move down from areas like the mouth or gut. To treat this, women may need to be treated with intravaginal antibiotics twice a week, after the initial seven-day treatment for up to 6 months. DOUCHING SHOULD BE AVOIDED

Alternative Treatment of Recurrent Yeast or BV Infections

Both these two conditions (yeast and BV), if recurrent, as discussed above can also be treated additionally with BORIC ACID 600 mg vaginal capsules which are inserted into the vagina nightly for 7 to 14 days. Boric acid is compounded and may be found at health food or compounding pharmacy shops and is not a prescription medication. One can also make one's own boric acid vaginal capsules by filling an empty capsule (size 0 gelatin) which one can purchase online or in a health food shop with the equivalent of 600mg of the boric acid crystals. It is NOT taken orally. Talk to one's doctor about this treatment if one has recurrent infections of these two conditions and the usual treatments are not working.

Sexually Transmitted Infections (STIs)
What are These?

These were formally referred to as Sexually Transmitted Diseases (STDs), but the name has been changed to "infections" (STIs) because most can be treated and will resolve. These are infections that are transmitted from one individual to another through sexual intercourse either by genital, oral or anal route, or to a new-born from the mother during childbirth as it passes through the birth canal.

General Complications of STIs

Depending on the type, STIs can cause serious health problems like:

Infertility
Chronic pelvic pain (pain in the area of the female organs)
HPV infection leading to precancer, or cervical, anal, vulva and vagina cancers
Genital warts (caused by HPV)
Increased risk of getting HIV/AIDS
Hepatitis and Syphilis
Genital herpes
Death from spread of certain infections into the blood and whole body (Sepsis)
Uncomfortable painful ulcers in the genital and anal areas
Pelvic Inflammatory Disease (PID) and resulting infertility and chronic pain
Low Birth weight or premature infants

There are more than 20 different STIs; however, some are more common than others.

Gonorrhea and Chlamydia

Both are caused by bacteria, and these are called *Neisseria gonorrhoeae and Chlamydia trachomatis* respectively. The infections affect the lining of the vagina, penis, mouth or rectum depending on what type of sex is performed by an infected individual. Infected pregnant women can pass the infections on to their baby at birth as the baby passes through the birth canal. Initially, chlamydia may not cause any symptoms; however, both can cause a pus-like vaginal discharge or penile discharge in the male, back pain, fever, chills, severe abdominal pain, pain with urination, pain during sex, vomiting and nausea.

TREATMENT: Both infections are treated with antibiotics. If not treated, they can progress to Pelvic Inflammatory Disease (PID) which will be discussed below. When an individual is infected with one, health professionals tend to treat for the other as well.

Trichomoniasis (Tric)

This is a common STI caused by Trichomonas Vaginalis, and can present without any symptoms. If symptoms occur they may include bad smelling thin frothy yellow/green discharge from vagina, or penis in the male, itching and pain with urination or sex. It may co exist with other STIs. In pregnant women, it can result in premature delivery of babies or babies who have low birth weight. Other problems include infertility, cervical cells abnormalities.

Treatment

It can be treated with anti-microbes, an example being METRONIDAZOLE tablets or cream or TINIDAZOLE tablets.

Human Papillomavirus (HPV)
What is It?

HPV is the commonest STI in the world, and is spread by skin to skin contact including sexual contact. There are more than 100 HPV types known, however, there are about 40 which affect anal and genital areas. These can be further divided into low and high risk types depending on how they affect or change cells.

The Human Papilloma Virus or HPV is a sexually transmitted virus and is most common STI in humans. There are many types of HPV which affect the genitals, and they can be divided into low risk and high risk types depending on type of long term disease it can cause, for example their ability to change cervical cells to pre-cancer and cancer cells.

Some of the low risk ones cause GENITAL WARTS, which are cauliflower-like growths around the genitals and anal area.

High Risk HPV

On the other hand, high risk HPV can cause abnormal cervical cells which can eventually change to PRE-CANCER cells of the cervix (Cervical Dysplasia) and later lead to CERVICAL CANCER in infected women if not treated. This takes several years to develop. HPV can also cause anal or rectal cancer in men who have anal sex with other men. In females, these pre-cancer or cancer cells may be found on the cervix when a Papanicolaou test, also known as a PAP SMEAR or TEST is done with or without HPV test looking for the specific DNA.

The HPV DNA test can also be done on its own by a healthcare provider.

HPV SELF SAMPLING – As technology has improved, screening for the presence of high risk HPV cells can also be done with a self sampled swab of the vagina by the woman herself in the comfort of her home, or in a healthcare facility. She either gives it to the health center, mails the sample to a lab or takes it to her health provider's office depending on where its done.

VISUALIZATION WITH ACETIC ACID (VIA) – In low resource countries, abnormal cells present on the cervix can also be detected with a simple vinegar solution (Acetic acid), which is used to paint the cervix, and it turns the abnormal cells white, and are referred to as "Acetowhite" cells.

LUGOL IODINE – Another way the abnormal cells are detected in low resource communities is by use of a solution called Lugol Iodine (Iodine solution). It is applied to the cervix during colposcopy. It stains normal cells and the nonstaining areas are abnormal cells like dysplasia or inflammation.

Further Investigations of Abnormal Results

If tests show positive high risk HPV and or abnormal cells present, a biopsy of the cervix and a scrapping of the inside of the cervix (endocervix) using a Colposcope device to view the cervix are done to determine the degree of cell abnormality. A colposcope is a device with light and magnification used to examine the vagina and cervix in detail.

Treatment of precancer cells

Depending on the patient's age, and extent of the abnormality, the cells may be monitored by frequent Pap smears. In women aged 30 years and below, their own immune system can clear the abnormal cells, causing the abnormal Pap smear to revert to normal. It is for this reason that in some countries, Pap smears start at age of 21 years. More definite treatments involve methods that destroy the precancer cells. They include:

Cone biopsy, loop electrosurgical excision procedure (LEEP), cryotherapy (freezing), electrocauterization and laser surgery. More details about pre cancer cervical cells and Cervical Cancer are discussed under CANCER OF THE CERVIX below.

Genital Warts (Condyloma Acuminata)

Genital warts are caused by low risk HPV and the common ones are HPV 6 and 11. They are cauliflower-like growths around the genitals and anal area and may take between 3 weeks and 8 months to show up after an infection. It is spread by skin to skin contact with an infected individual. The lesions may be inside the vagina or at vulva area and may encircle the anus and the space between anus and vulva or around the penis and scrotal area in men. It may present without any symptoms, just the fact that it is present and increasing in size; or may present with burning, itching, pain or bleeding.

Treatment

Diagnosis is usually by visual inspection by one's doctor. They can either resolve without any treatment or they can be destroyed by excision, cauterized with heat, freezing (cryotherapy), or laser. Several topical medicines like Trichloroacetic acid, Imiquimod and Podophyllin which may be applied by a doctor, or by a patient herself in some cases are also available.

Genital Herpes (HSV – Herpes Simplex Virus)
What is It?

Genital Herpes is a sexually transmitted viral infection which causes ulcers in the genitals. There are two types of Genital Herpes; Herpes Simplex 1 and 2. (HSV type 1 and 2). Usually, Type 1 causes the common "cold sore" (fever blister) on the lips, and Type 2 causes genital ulcers. However, they can be interchangeable if oral sex is performed. For example, someone who has a cold core caused by Type 1 can transmit it to a sexual partner's genitals if they have oral sex. Therefore, both can be transferred by sexual contact with someone who has an open herpetic sore, or even without an obvious sore, but who carries the virus on their genitals, in the mouth or lips.

Signs and Symptoms

Initially, for genital infections, there may be general symptoms like fever, swollen lymph nodes in the groin, and muscle aches. This is followed by numbness and tingling around the genitalia or between the buttocks or anal area, followed by small fluid filled vesicles which may burst and become shallow and painful ulcers. If the vagina or vulva is involved there may be vaginal discharge or even pain during urination. The ulcers may crust over in one to two weeks and disappear. However, they may recur sooner or later, or never at all.

Recurrent Herpes Infection

Infection in the genitals with the virus may cause these painful recurrent herpetic ulcers in some individuals. This is known as a "Herpes outbreak". Usually, the body's immune system will try and fight it, however, certain factors may lead to frequent genital outbreaks, and these include stress, illness or around the monthly menses.

Treatment

An outbreak can be treated with anti-viral medications (e.g. Acyclovir or Vancyclovir) for a few days, and people who have frequent outbreaks may be put on prevention or suppression medication which should be taken daily. If outbreaks occur frequently on the lips, antivirals may be taken daily or during an outbreak. An oral supplement called LYSINE has been found to also prevent outbreaks on the lips. These are topical anti-virals-acyclovir,and penciclovir.

Herpes and Pregnancy

An infected pregnant woman may pass on the infection to a baby during vaginal delivery. This can affect the baby's brain or skin, and therefore, if a pregnant woman is known to be a carrier, she will be treated with antiviral medicines and her baby will be delivered by Cesarean section (C-section) instead of vaginally as a precaution.

Human Immunodeficiency Virus Infections (HIV/AIDS)
What is It?

HIV infection is caused by the Human Immunodeficiency Virus, and it is spread by sexual contact with an infected person through exchange of fluids like vaginal fluids, blood, semen, and pre-ejaculate. It can also be transmitted from an infected mother to her baby and through breast milk.

Signs and Symptoms

An HIV infected person may not have any symptoms after initial flu like symptoms, however, after the virus multiples and destroys the immune system, then the individual is susceptible to infection with opportunistic organisms (those which will not otherwise cause infections in people with a healthy immune system) and Cancers. A person is often described as having AIDS (Acquired Immunodeficiency Syndrome) when they are HIV positive and have such low white cell count that they develop an opportunistic infection. Those who have HIV infection are prone to develop other sexually transmitted diseases like Syphilis, Gonorrhea etc. due to their decreased immunity since it's the immune system which helps fight infections.

Treatment

An HIV positive individual may be monitored with frequent blood work to check their white cell count levels and viral load. If they develop a certain low level of white cell count or acquire an opportunistic infection then they will be started on medications. There is no cure for AIDS but treatment is available by several drugs known as Anti retroviral drugs and these decrease the load of the virus in an individual and can cause affected individuals to live long, and have almost undetectable amounts of the virus in the body. These medications have side effects and so patients have to be closely monitored and it is one's responsibility to follow up with health providers frequently for medication refills and blood work. Not all infected persons get the privilege of being treated and so people in low resource countries do die of the disease and its complications.

PREVENTION: Prevention is as for other STIs, Abstinence from sex, Be Faithful to one partner and Condom use. Currently, in some countries a system known as Preexposure Prophylaxis PrEP is used. It is a way for people who are at high risk for HIV infection prevent it by taking a pill every day. The pill is called Truvada and it contains two medicines which are used to treat HIV. It has been found to be highly effective for preventing HIV if used as prescribed. (https://www.cdc.gov/hiv/risk/prep/index.html)

Syphilis
What is It?

This is caused by a bacterium called Treponema pallidum, it is sexually transmitted but it can be passed on to others through other means. These include from an infected mother to her baby during delivery, through contaminated blood transfusion, and infected needles of those who inject intravenous drugs into their veins.

Signs and Symptoms

It may start as an ulcer or sore near the genitals and may produce a rash; or can go on to infect the brain and spinal cord, as well as the blood vessels. It can make one very ill and even cause death if not treated early.

Treatment

It is easily treated with antibiotics e.g. Penicillin; however, it is often very difficult to recognize or identify early enough since it mimics a lot of other illnesses. Early detection and screening of individuals helps with early treatment and prevention of the complications.

Hepatitis A, B and C

These discussed previously, can also be sexually transmitted and were discussed under liver diseases. Chronic Hepatitis B and C can now be treated with antiviral medications if they persist after the initial infection. There are vaccines available against Hepatitis A and B, however, Hepatitis C does not have a vaccine yet. Please see detailed discussion under Liver Diseases.

Pelvic Inflammatory Disease (PID)

What is It?

This is inflammation and infection of the pelvic organs namely uterus, fallopian tubes, and ovaries caused by an untreated STI especially with bacteria like Gonorrhea and Chlamydia. In the case of a pregnant woman, the lives of both the baby and mother may be in danger and lead to Sepsis or blood infection affecting the whole body if infection occurs at that time.

Signs and Symptoms

It may present as pain in the lower abdomen and there may also be fever and chills and vaginal discharge or bleeding from the vagina. Examination of the female pelvic and lower abdomen causes a lot of pain and discomfort.

Treatment

Strong intravenous antibiotics are used to treat this in hospital if it is severe, otherwise mild infections are treated with oral antibiotics. If treatment is delayed it can lead to complications like infertility, ectopic pregnancy, and lots of scar tissue formation, leading to chronic pain in the pelvic area and painful sex (Dyspareunia).

Prevention of Sexually Transmitted Infections (STIs).

As mentioned previously, the prevention of STIs is through the practice of ABC.

ABSTINENCE – not to have sex until one is ready to be in a stable monogamous relationship.
BEING FAITHFUL TO ONE PARTNER – Monogamous relationship
CONDOM USE – Women should make provision for condoms by having them available, men don't usually care much, and in the end it's the women who may acquire an infection.

Though most STIs can be prevented by use of a condom, unfortunately, some of them can be spread despite condom use due to skin to skin contact outside of areas not covered by a condom, or improper use of the condoms. Examples of these are genital warts, HPV and Herpes infections.

Other Pelvic Diseases or Conditions

The Pelvic Area and Contents

The female pelvic area is the area between the lower part of the abdomen and the groin. It contains the reproductive organs made up of the two ovaries, two fallopian tubes (tubes), uterus, cervix, vagina and vulva. There are also other glands that produce fluids for lubrication within the vulva and vagina e.g. Bartholin glands which secrete mucus to lubricate the vagina. Other organs present in pelvic area include part of the urinary system namely the bladder, parts of the ureters and the urethra. There are also parts of the large bowel (colon), pelvic floor muscles, blood vessels, nerves and lymphatic system.

The Female Internal Genitalia

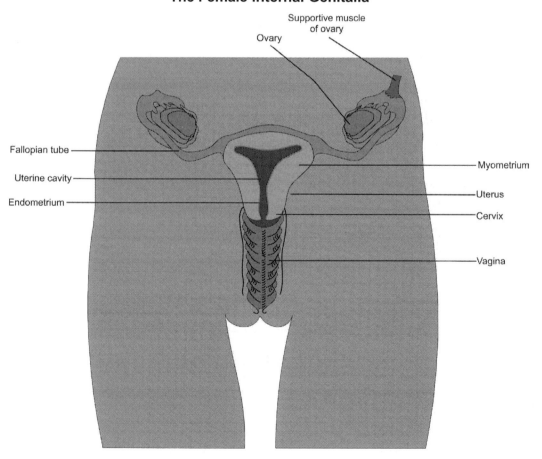

Uterine Fibroids (Leiomyomas)
What are These?

A Fibroid or Leiomyoma is a non-cancerous tumor and is the most common tumor which can grow in a woman's uterus. They are often multiple and are overgrowth of muscle and connective tissues which form a mass in different parts of the uterus. They may grow beneath the lining of the uterus (endometrium), within the muscular wall or in the outside layer of the uterus. They tend to be common in women who are still menstruating or in the reproductive age group. Some are small initially, but may continue to grow during the reproductive years. Fibroid growth is aided by Estrogen, and when this decreases at Menopause the Fibroids tend to shrink in size.

Prevalence of Fibroids

By the age of 50 years, up to 90 % of black women and 80% of Caucasian women may have fibroids, but black women tend to have bigger, multiple and more symptomatic fibroids. Fibroids account for about one third of all hysterectomies performed in the USA, roughly about 100,000 per year.

Signs and Symptoms

Fibroids may present with pelvic pain, irregular bleeding from the uterus, prolonged and or painful periods, pressure in the pelvic area, the need to urinate all the time, Constipation, and pain during intercourse (Dyspareunia). A palpable mass or growth in the pelvis or abdomen may be felt on examination if they are sufficiently large enough. Some women may appear pregnant due to the large size of fibroids in the uterus. Anemia due to excessive bleeding, may occur if they are large and close to the lining of the uterus. They may cause infertility in some women if very large. However others may not present with pain or other symptoms and may be found by chance during an exam or imaging studies like an ultrasound of the pelvic area.

Risk Factors for Developing Fibroids

Black women: maybe due to genes
Black women who use hair perming creams. These contain chemicals called "Hormone Disruptors" which affect hormones of the reproductive organs
Women older than 40 years
Family history of fibroids
History of High Blood Pressure
Obesity
Women who have never been pregnant
Vitamin D deficiency

Treatment

If they do not cause any symptoms, they are just observed and nothing is done. However if a woman is having some of the symptoms mentioned above, and fibroids are discovered through a Pelvic ultrasound or MRI then they have to be treated.

Medical Treatment

- Anti-Inflammatory (NSAIDs): If they cause a lot of pain especially during one's menses, medicines like an anti-inflammatory e.g. Naproxen or Ibuprofen may be used. These have to be taken 2–3x daily for about 5 days.
- Hormones: These include female hormones like Oral Contraceptive Pills which decrease blood flow and pain.
- Some other hormonal drugs may even shrink the size of the fibroids by acting on the pituitary gland in the brain and cause less Estrogens to be produced. These may also be used prior to surgery to shrink them before removal. Examples of these are Leuprorelin (Lupron, Eligard), and another antihormone called Mifepristone RU486 which may also reduce pelvic pain as well.
- Another hormone used is a male hormone (Danazol, Danocrine) which will reduce bleeding in those who suffer from excess menstruation as a result of fibroids.

Surgical Treatment

This is either by destroying the fibroid, removing it or even removing the uterus with the fibroid in it. Your doctor will determine which surgical procedure is best for you after discussing your options with you. The different surgical methods include:

- Myomectomy – This is surgery done to remove fibroids from a woman who still desires to have a future pregnancy or has only one or two small fibroids. The fibroids are removed but the uterus is left intact
- Hysterectomy – This removes the whole uterus and is used to treat women who may have multiple or big fibroids and maybe some other abnormalities of the uterus like Prolapse (uterus drops down)
- Uterine Artery Embolization – The blood supply to the fibroid is cut off by clotting the artery which supplies it. Usually done in the Imaging department under imaging guidance
- MRI guided Ultrasound – In this new procedure under guidance of an MRI imaging, heated ultrasound beams target the fibroids and destroy them

A doctor will recommend the best treatment if one has fibroids that are causing problems.

Painful Periods (Dysmenorrhea) (Dis-meno-reah)
What is It?

Dysmenorrhea or painful monthly menses affects most women during their reproductive years (the child-bearing period of life). There is cramping pain in the lower abdomen during or just before the period starts. It can be primary which tends to start in adolescents when they begin having periods/menses; or secondary (due to another reason) because of a problem in the pelvic organs mainly the uterus. Both types if severe cause loss of work or school time for sufferers.

Primary Dysmenorrhea

Primary Dysmenorrhea is a result of release of certain chemicals at the start of the period which cause the muscle wall of the uterus to contract severely.

Secondary Dysmenorrhea

Secondary Dysmenorrhea tends to occur in older women who previously did not have painful periods, but suddenly have them later on in life. There are several factors which may contribute to secondary Dysmenorrhea, and they include uterine fibroids, Cervical Stenosis (cervical opening is blocked so it is difficult for menstrual blood to flow out), pelvic infections, scar tissue and adhesions from previous infections or surgeries, and Endometriosis (this is discussed below).

Signs and Symptoms

The cramping lower abdominal pain may be associated with nausea and vomiting, back pain, headaches, dizziness, and diarrhea. Pain may last the first 2 or so days of the menses or may be throughout the duration of menses.

Treatment of Dysmenorrhea
Primary Dysmenorrhea

Hot water bottle or heating pad placed over the lower abdomen helps with the pain

Non-steroidal medications (NSAIDS) discussed previously (examples are Ibuprofen, Naproxen, Advil, Motrin etc.) block the action of some of the released chemicals. These need to be started as soon as the period begins. Secondly it is important that they be taken "around the clock" or throughout the day to give effective pain control

Oral contraception pills

IUD (intrauterine device)

Dcpo Provera shots (Progesterone shots)

If nausea and vomiting are present, use an anti-nausea medicine

Other over the counter medicines that have been used and have been found to be helpful by some individuals include Vitamin E, fish oil, Thiamine, Midol (Acetaminophen/Caffeine/Pyrilamine is an Analgesic and Diuretic combination), and other combination OTC medicines containing a Diuretic (water pill) which help with bloating caused by the excess retained fluid. Acupuncture, an alternative medical practice has also helped some sufferers.

Primary Dysmenorrhea gets better with age and after child birth. Teenagers have to be treated so they do not miss many school days.

Secondary Dysmenorrhea

Once the underlying cause is determined, then treatment is geared toward that, and this will help resolve the problem. If either Fibroids or Endometriosis is the cause, then removal of the fibroids or medication like oral contraceptives to treat the Endometriosis will resolve the pain.

Endometriosis (En-do-meat-roses)
What is It?

This is a condition when tissue which lines the uterus forms elsewhere like on the outside of the uterus, fallopian tubes, nearby intestines etc. These also go through the same changes that the lining inside the uterus goes through like getting thick prior to the menses and shedding at time of menstruation.

CAUSE OF ENDOMETRIOSIS: The reason why some women develop it is not certain, but its been suggested that genes, impaired immune system, or possible back up of the tissue though the fallopian tubes into the ovaries and pelvic area has been suggested as well. It tends to occur during the reproductive age (when women can have kids)

Signs and Symptoms

Severe pain and cramps just before and during the menses time, heavy flow, low back pain, and lower abdominal pain. Pain during sex, painful bowel movement or painful urination around the time of the menses. Other women may have difficulty getting pregnant (infertility) if the endometrial tissue is implanted on the ovaries and fallopian tubes.

Treatment

A careful history and physical exam, and tests to rule out other reasons may be done. The definite diagnosis is by laparoscopy, which is direct visualization of pelvic contents. A small tube with a magnifying lens and light is passed into the pelvic area through tiny holes in the abdomen and the whole area can be examined and biopsies taken. Once diagnosis is made, treatment consists of Medicines or surgery, or both can be used depending on one's age, whether one desires pregnancy, and how severe the symptoms are.

Medicines: Include pain pills like NSAIDS, and hormonal based like Birth Control Pills, which will prevent ovulation

Surgery: The implanted tissues can be removed from the organs it is present on. Sometimes surgery to remove all the internal genitals – uterus, ovaries and tubes is done to eliminate all of the pain, if other organs like the intestines are not involved, and there is no desire for pregnancy

Excessive Periods or Menstruation
What is It?

This is also known as "Excessive menstrual bleeding" (EMB) and also called "Menorrhagia", but that term is becoming obsolete. For most women, the number of days of menstruation is between 3 to 7 days. However, when menses or menstrual blood flow is heavy or prolonged enough to interfere with a woman's life – health, sex life, social activities, work etc. then it needs to be investigated and treated. According to the CDC (Centers for Disease Control, Atlanta, USA) menses are excessive if one should change a tampon before 2 hours or passage of several large clots requiring frequent change of pads or tampons.

Results of Excessive Menstrual Bleeding

The excessive blood loss leads to several issues:

- Iron deficiency Anemia: Iron is found in red blood cells and the red blood cells help in transferring oxygen and nutrients to the cells
- Fatigue, weakness, shortness of breath: This is a result of Anemia
- Women may develop PICA: This is the term used to describe the craving for and consumption of substances with no nutrition value by women with iron deficiency Anemia. The substances include ice, clay, or paint. The pica for the most part goes away once the Anemia is treated
- Anxiety: As a result of excessive bleeding some women may refrain from attending social events, or exercise, and may always be afraid they may bleed through their clothes and so are always on edge, anxious or not relaxed. Thus, psychologically it affects them
- Loss of work or school days: Women or school-aged females may lose days of work or school due to excessive menstrual bleeding. In resource poor countries, this sometimes affects the girl child's education, since they may be poor

and not have sanitary wear to keep themselves clean and dry due the excessive bleeding during this time

Causes of Excessive Menstrual Bleeding

The cause may be related to problems in the UTERUS, OTHER DISEASES or HORMONAL ISSUES. In some individuals, the reason is not known or cannot be found.

- UTERUS ASSOCIATED CAUSES
  Uterine fibroids
  Uterine polyps
  Cancer of the Uterus: This is called Endometrial Cancer
  Cancer of the cervix: This is caused mostly by the HPV virus (Cervical Cancer)
  Adenomyosis: This is when the cells lining the uterus grow into the muscle wall. This usually occurs in females who are older than 30 years and have had a previous full-term pregnancy
  With any of the above causes, the bleeding may stop or slow down when the underlying problem is treated
- USE OF AN INTRAUTERINE DEVICE
  An intrauterine device (IUD) also known as the LOOP, is usually used for birth control purposes, and it is inserted into the uterus to prevent pregnancy. Not all IUDs cause long term bleeding. The copper type tends to cause prolonged bleeding, and the Progesterone medicated ones (e.g. Mirena, Skyla, Liletta, Kyleena) may cause diminished or cessation of menstruation
- BLEEDING DISEASES
  These are diseases that may affect the way blood clots because a factor or chemical related to clotting is missing, or platelets found in the blood stream are abnormal and result in blood not clotting well
  Examples of these two conditions are Von Willebrand disease (vW clotting factor defect) and Platelet Function Disorder which relates to abnormal platelets
- Von Willebrand disease:
  Many women may have heavy menstrual flow with heavy clots and may have Von Willebrand disease but not realize it. Other signs include:
  Excessive bleeding after cutting themselves, after dental procedures, nose bleeds, easy bruising, and Anemia

Although vW defect is often inherited due to a defective gene which forms a defective protein in the platelets, some people may get it later on in life (acquired as opposed to inherited). It is not clear why this happens, but autoimmune diseases, use of certain medications, and sluggish or underfunctioning thyroid (Hypothyroid) have all been implicated.

Diagnosis of vW Disease (VWD)

After a careful history and family medical history, special blood tests for VWF antigen which measure the amount of VWF in blood plasma, clotting factors and platelet function may be done. Patients with VWD usually have less than 50% of normal VWF in their blood. The VWF test is often repeated because the levels may fluctuate due to conditions like hyperthyroidism, use of oral contraceptives, pregnancy, stress or exercise.

Treatment of Vw Disease

There are medications for treating this condition, and examples are Desmopressin (DDAVP), recombinant vWF, and vWF/factor VIII (vWF/FVIII) concentrates. In addition, a drug used for treating excessive bleeding – Tranexamic acid – can be used orally or intravenously to treat mild bleeding from gums or skin. The use of oral contraceptive pills and Progesterone containing IUDs are also used to control bleeding.

- OTHER DISEASES
  These include diseases of other organs of the body which affect the uterus leading to excessive bleeding. They include thyroid diseases, liver, kidney diseases and certain cancers
- HORMONAL CAUSES
  Imbalance of the female hormones Estrogen and Progesterone can cause excessive bleeding and is treated as below

Treatment of Excessive Menstrual Bleeding

This depends on the cause of the excessive menstrual bleeding, however one should see a doctor right from the beginning, who will take a history and do a physical exam including a pelvic exam. Tests include blood work, pregnancy test, pelvic ultrasound of the reproductive system (uterus, ovaries cervix and vagina). The doctor may also do a D/C (dilatation and curettage) to scrape the lining of the uterus, or do a biopsy of the lining (endometrial biopsy) and send it for pathology examination for a definitive diagnosis.

- If one is anemic, one may need iron and vitamins like vitamin B12 and folic acid to increase hemoglobin which is what is low in anemia. Some may have such low hemoglobin that they will need intravenous iron or blood transfusion

- The doctor may "burn" the inside lining of the uterus known as Endometrial Ablation
- Sometimes some medicines which decrease blood flow are used during the time of the period, for example Tranexamic acid (Lysteda) is taken for five days
- Use of a specific IUD (intrauterine Device) called the Mirena which is coated with Progesterone hormone can be inserted into the uterus to reduce the bleeding
- If the cause is due to the copper IUD then it has to be removed to stop the bleeding
- If it's a uterus associated cause, treatment of that is required, e.g. if a fibroid or polyp is the cause, removing them will stop the excessive bleeding
- If a large Fibroid is the cause it may require a hysterectomy and not just removing it
- If the cause is based on female hormone problems, then other treatments used include some hormone medications like the birth control pill (this contains Estrogens and Progesterone), Progesterone pills or other appropriate ones prescribed by the doctor
- If due to HYPOTHYOID, one will be placed on thyroid replacement medication and this will stop the excessive bleeding and correct the underactive thyroid

Irregular Periods or Menses
What is It?

This is irregular periods characterized by having two periods in the same month, or continuous spotting, or missing one's menses for a few months. There are many causes but three of the most common causes are related to

Age
Pregnancy
Perimenopause

Age

When a young girl starts having periods at age 10 to 14 years, she may have monthly periods the first 3 months and then not have a period for another 3 to 6 months. This is fairly common and she will need reassurance, that it will resume later on.

Pregnancy

Some women when they become pregnant may have some bleeding or spotting during part of the pregnancy or throughout the entire pregnancy.

Perimenopausal or Premenopausal Stage

This is when a woman is getting close to finally stopping periods. This term means AROUND MENOPAUSE and usually occurs around the late forties.

Other Reasons

These may include Hypothyroid or Hyperthyroid disease, and uterine causes mentioned under excessive bleeding above. Most of these reasons are due to imbalance in the female hormones and blood tests and pelvic ultrasounds may be ordered to pinpoint the reason.

Treatment

One has to see their primary care doctor or gynecologist (doctor who specializes in women's female or reproductive organs problems and diseases) to have the blood work and imaging studies. Treatment is based on the cause. If Anemia is also present that may be treated with iron, folic acid and vitamin B12 as needed. Some of the treatments mentioned above under excessive menstrual bleeding are used to treat irregular menstrual bleeding.

No Menses or Scanty Menses (Amenorrhea) (A-meno-reah)

Amenorrhea is the absence of menses and common causes of Amenorrhea are:

- Pregnancy – this is normal in pregnancy and after delivery may last for a few months especially if breast feeding
- Polycystic Ovarian Syndrome (PCOS) (See below)
- Premature Menopause – When periods cease before the age when it normally stops – which is around 50 years plus or minus a couple of years. Some women may start menopause between 35 to 40 years
- Chemotherapy induced Amenorrhea: Most women who are younger than 50 years and undergo Chemotherapy for breast cancer or other cancers will stop having menses
- Women who are marathon runners/joggers or engage in competitive sports may stop having periods due to hormonal changes associated with the intense exercise
- Hysterectomy – Removal of the uterus for whatever reason will stop periods
- Natural Menopause – At around the age of 50 years most women will cease menstruating
- Tumors in the brain – May affect centers associated with female hormonal control
- Eating disorders like Anorexia and Bulimia affect hormone producing brain centers

- Female athlete triad consists of disordered eating, Amenorrhea or scanty periods and Osteopenia or Osteoporosis (bone loss) and is found in young women who are engaged in serious or competitive sports

If one's period is absent for two to three months see a health provider so they can run some blood work and do other studies as needed. If one is in the reproductive age and is sexually active, one would need to have a pregnancy test done.

Ovary Cysts
What are They?

Ovarian cysts are fluid filled sacs present in the ovary. They are mostly a result of a woman's normal cycle of egg production and release. The two most common ones in this group are called follicular and corpus luteum cysts.

Follicular Cyst

A follicular or functional cyst is formed when the follicle which grows and usually releases an egg does not release it but grows bigger and is usually fluid filled. They may be single or multiple, simple or complex.

Corpus Luteum Cyst

A corpus luteum cyst forms, when a corpus luteum (which is what the follicle becomes after releasing an egg), accumulates fluid inside it, and becomes a cyst.

Signs and Symptoms

Most ovarian cysts will disappear after 2 or 3 menstrual cycles and are not painful. However, some are painful and if large may cause the ovary to twist causing severe pelvic pain which may be accompanied by nausea and vomiting. This is called "torsion of the ovary" and is an emergency. A more common complication is rupture of the cyst which may cause internal bleeding in the cyst and a great deal of pain on the side involved, but pain may also spread to other side of the uterus.

Treatment

An ultrasound exam will usually show ovarian cysts, and if large, a radiologist will ask for a repeat scan after 2 menstrual cycles. A few may be malignant especially if they persist and look complex, and then a surgical removal may be warranted. Some simple ones are treated by oral contraceptive pills, but recent research suggests they are not any better than sugar pills in resolving the cysts. However, use of oral contraceptive pills will help prevent more cysts from forming, so this will help those who tend to form cysts.

Polycystic Ovarian Syndrome (PCOS)
What is It?

Polycystic ovarian syndrome (PCOS) is a common health condition affecting one in ten women (others put it at between 6 to 50%) in the reproductive age group and may start between 20 to 30 years. It is due to female hormonal imbalance resulting in: menstrual irregularities, signs of excessive male hormones (Androgens), changes in the balance of female hormones, no ovulation, and cysts formed in ovaries around immature eggs. It has been found to be more prevalent in women with epilepsy than in the general population.

Symptoms and Signs

Scanty or absent periods
Irregular periods
Infertility or difficulty conceiving
Excessive hair on chin, upper lips, chest, and side burns (due to excessive
    male hormones)
Male pattern baldness with thinning hair at the front and top of the scalp and
    receding hairline
Acne spots on face and chest, and back
Obesity and weight gain

Complications

High cholesterol and triglyceride
Insulin Resistance (impaired response by body to insulin, keeping glucose
    from entering cells)
Infertility
Diabetes or Prediabetes
Hypertension
Risk for Endometrial Cancer

Women may first seek help when they notice their periods are not regular, however, it is important to get help if one notices a cluster of some of the above symptoms. There is a slight increased risk for Endometrial Cancer because the lining of the uterus is not shedding regularly (as in monthly periods), and so it gets thick and the cells can undergo change and become precancerous.

Treatment

After history and physical examination, blood work, and pelvic ultrasound are done, followed by treatments to help every symptom present. Common treatments are:

Birth control pills geared toward treating irregular periods and the excess Androgen in the body

Weight loss is very important and helps insulin resistance, and restoration of regular periods

Treat hirsutism with hair removing creams, laser, etc (See hirsutism treatment under SKIN)

Improving ovulation and fertility by use of medicine or weight loss

Medications frequently used are

1. Metformin (usually used to treat Diabetes and Prediabetes). In this case it helps with weight loss, improve blood sugar and make the periods regular so fertility is improved

2. Spironolactone is used to treat excess facial hair, acne and scalp hair loss

Painful Sexual Intercourse (Dyspareunia) (dis pa-ro-nia)
What is It?

"Beyond the immediate effects of the pain itself, pain during sex (or simply fear or anticipation of pain during sex) can trigger performance anxiety or future arousal problems in some women. Worry over whether pain will come back can diminish lubrication or cause involuntary—and painful—tightening of the vaginal muscles, called vaginismus"

www.menopause.org/for-women/
sexual-health-menopause-online

This is recurrent pain with sexual intercourse, and can be with INITIAL penetration of the entrance of the vagina, or with DEEP penetration which occurs deep within the vagina. This is a frequent problem which can affect intimacy between a woman and a man and causes tremendous relational and psychological problems for those affected. Some women may not have painful sexual intercourse until later on in their sexual life. Causes may be related to the reproductive organs structurally, medical conditions or psychological issues.

Causes of Persistent Painful Sex

1. Related to reproductive organs abnormal structures
   Ovarian cysts, Ovarian tumors, Uterine fibroids or polyps, Endometriosis
   Abnormal position of the uterus – when it is tilted backwards
   Uterine prolapse (uterus dropping down into vagina due to weakened support)
   Abnormal formation of the vagina e.g. presence of double vagina or uterus
   Previous surgery to the pelvic structures leading to scarring

2. Infections or problems of the reproductive and urinary organs
   Problem may resolve when infection or inflammation is resolved
   Pelvic inflammatory disease
   Sexually transmitted infections e.g. Chlamydia, Trichomonas, Gonorrhea

Irritation or inflammation of the cervix (causes redness or erosion of the mouth of the cervix)

Yeast infections

Urinary tract infections

3. Other genital or urinary issues

Bladder and urethral problems or abnormalities

After delivery (postpartum period) there may be tears or cuts made to help with delivery

4. Peri-menopausal and postmenopausal stages of life

The decreased amount of Estrogen produced during the Peri and Post-menopausal phase of life leads to thinning of the vulva and vaginal lining resulting in vaginal dryness, easy bleeding from the lining, a smaller vaginal opening, and shortened length of the vagina. All these can lead to pain during sexual intercourse, causing women in this age group to be uninterested in sex, while their male partners want sex, leading to relationship problems

5. Muscles and skeletal problems

Degenerative disk disease or Arthritis of the vertebrae may lead to back pain and painful sex

6. Psychological factors leading to Dyspareunia

The following lead to psychological problems in a woman, causing intercourse problems

Rape or domestic violence

Previous unpleasant sexual experience

Erroneous ideas about sexual intercourse by a woman

Sexual abuse or molestation as a child

Investigation and Treatment of Dyspareunia

It is important to see a doctor or health care provider, and there is no need to be embarrassed or ashamed about discussing this with a doctor. The doctor will take a careful history including one's sexual history and experiences like rape, sexual assault or domestic violence. After that, a physical examination known as a PELVIC EXAM is usually performed.

Pelvic Examination

During this examination of the female pelvic organs a lubricated SPECULUM (duck beak shaped instrument) is gently introduced into the vagina and it helps with the aid of a light to visualize the vagina and cervix for any abnormalities. It is gently withdrawn and then a bimanual examination with one or two fingers of one hand in the vagina and the second hand on top of the central part of lower abdomen is done to assess the size of the uterus, any tenderness of the cervix, and the sides where the ovaries are usually located.

TESTS: These include

- Swabs taken from the vaginal or cervix areas looking for infections
- Pelvic ultrasound – this will show if there are tumors in the uterus or ovaries etc
- Performing an internal exam of the uterus and organs with the aid of a small lighted tube inserted through the vagina into the uterus (UTEROSCOPY) or through the abdomen (LAPAROSCOPY) may be required. These give direct views of the pelvic and reproductive structures. For example, if a Fibroid or Endometriosis is present it may be visible

Treatment

Treatment depends on the underlying cause. Once a cause for the pain is found, it will be treated and hopefully will result in some relief and make sexual intercourse more enjoyable.

- For Peri and Post-menopausal women, treatment may include vaginal lubricants, moisturizers or local topical Estrogen inserted into the vagina. Estrogen use results in the buildup of the thin vaginal tissues, increased muscle tone, decrease pain during sex and decreased urinary symptoms which also occur during this time in a woman's life cycle
- New devices described under Post menopause problems below (Transitional years), include use of laser therapy at a doctor's office, (Mono Lisa Touch), and INTENSITY (OTC device manufactured by "In Control Medical" and used at home. www.incontrolmedical.com). They are supposed to increase blood flow to the vaginal area resulting in stronger pelvic muscles and greater vaginal lubrication
- Infections like Pelvic Inflammatory Disease (PID), or STIs if present, can be treated with antibiotics
- After a delivery, if the labor process was prolonged, or there was repair of a cut (episiotomy) or surgery was performed, it may take weeks for the new mother to recover from pain. In this case, lubricants or massage of scar tissue may help with the pain. Waiting for at least six weeks before penetrative sexual intercourse after any type of delivery may help reduce pain
- Breastfeeding tends to lower Estrogen levels and so vaginal dryness may occur. Lubricants may be useful in these cases as well as INTENSITY device described above
- Sexual assault or rape victims may have psychological problems accompanied by painful sex (psychosexual problems). The help of a trained SEX THERAPIST or Psychologist may ease the pain as emotions are addressed and healing takes place

20

Sexual Violence and Domestic Violence

Rape and Sexual Assault

....

Rape
What Is It?

Rape is defined by the United States Department of Justice as "an event that occurred without the victim's consent that involved the use or threat of force to penetrate the victim's vagina or anus by penis, tongue, fingers, or object, or the victim's mouth by penis". (Findings from the National Violence against Women Survey Report, November 2000 – ncjrs.gov/pdffiles1/nij/183781. pdf).

Sexual Assault (SA)/Sexual Violence
What is It?

Sexual assault is a term that encompasses sexual contact which involves forced physical or psychological pressure, and it may or may not involve vaginal penetration. The main facts are that:

It is forced and it is of a sexual nature
May involve kissing, holding the victim's breasts or buttocks etc
May not necessarily involve the act of vaginal sex
Sexual assault is an act of violence and is not an act of sexual gratification
It is a crime, which should be punished by law

Societal Views and Response

SA against women is a common occurrence in all societies and developing countries are the worst when it comes to awareness by the public that it is not acceptable. Entrenched warped views of women and their supposed "role" as sexual objects make it hard to change a society's views of sexual assault or abuse. Governments and law enforcement authorities who should be protecting victims and charging perpetrators with crime are insensitive to the plight of unfortunate victims and may not view it as a crime.

It is when women in various societies, social organizations and nations speak out as a group and lobby authorities that will eventually lead to the needed change in societies view of assault on women and young girls. Recent "# Me Too" campaigns to expose sexual assault in all sectors of the workplace has brought it to the limelight and female victims are speaking out and naming abusers. Through this, many rich and famous men have been named by brave women as perpetrators and some of these men have lost their jobs and are facing prosecution. However, there are millions of victims whose voices are silenced, or they are not heard.

Effects of Sexual Assault and Rape on the Victim

Below is an excerpt from a book wrote for victims of child sexual abuse called "*The Dawning of a New Day*", and this part deals with the effects of sexual assault and rape on the victim. It will take you through the journey of RECOVERY from a VICTIM TO A VICTOR as it deals with healing of a survivor's BODY, SOUL, MENTAL, AND SPIRITUAL BEING.

Excerpt from the Dawning of a New Day

There are physical, emotional, psychological and spiritual effects on the victim. If it involves a child, these effects may linger on and be present or be manifested in adulthood.

Sexual Abuse

Intentional physical (e.g. touching breasts) or non-physical (e.g. verbal sexual harassment) contact of a sexual nature between a perpetrator and a victim who has not given her/his consent or who is unable to consent or refuse (e.g. a child).

Effects of Sexual Abuse

Below are some of the recognized results of sexual abuse. Not everyone who is abused or assaulted may exhibit any or all symptoms.

1. Medical/Physical

- There may be injury to the genitals (one's private part)

- Bleeding from the vagina due to tears of the lining or walls
- Urinary tract or bladder infections, pain with urination
- Vaginal discharge due to sexually transmitted infection
- Sexually transmitted diseases like Chlamydia, Gonorrhea, Hepatitis, Human Papillomavirus, Syphilis, Herpes Simplex and HIV/AIDS
- Re-occurring stomach pain, headaches and pain in other parts of your body
- Inability to sleep at night, bad dreams or nightmares
- Eating disorders like Anorexia and Bulimia
- Weight gain or weight loss from over eating or under eating
- Self injury or harm – cutting one's wrists with razor blades
- Not wanting to be touched by other people

Women who have experienced sexual abuse may be reluctant to undergo important pelvic examination or Cervical Cancer screening examination due to the previous encounter involving those areas.

2. Emotional and Mental

The common emotions include:

- Sadness, anger, fear, pain, guilt, moody, shame, violated (feel used), self-blame, flashback (reliving the event), helplessness, confused, hurt, self-hate, argumentative
- Feel your body is unclean or dirty
- Sense of loss of control over your body and yourself
- Inability to express feelings
- Loss of interest in activities once enjoyed
- Suicidal thoughts or plans to kill oneself
  Feeling "jumpy", not at ease, jittery or nervous
- Long term emotional problems including Anxiety, Panic attacks, Depression, Post-Traumatic Stress Disorder (PTSD) numbness (no feelings), low self-esteem, seeing and hearing things which may not be present, bullying others, etc

3. Relational Problems

There may be abnormal social relationships with others, impaired interaction with others, lack of trust of others and inability to form good friendships due to suspicion or fear of betrayal. For adult victims, their relationship with their husbands may even be affected.

4. Social Behavior Problems

Aggression, violent behavior, withdrawal, shyness, not talking much and keeping to oneself, being loud and disrespectful are some of the related social behavior problems. These tend to occur more if the abuse was during childhood or adolescent years.

5. Sexual Behavior Problems

These may be found in up to one third of sexually abused children who may respond to the abuse by becoming sexually reactive. This may result in sexual behaviors ranging from engagement in early sexual activity, promiscuity to prostitution. In addition, whether the abuse occurred in childhood or as an adult, some victims, are unable to enjoy normal sexual relationships with their spouses/husbands and this can affect their marriages. The effects of the abuse may linger on as sexual difficulties or pelvic pain.

(Entsuah, Barbara; The Dawning of a New Day, 2009).

Domestic Violence (DV)
What is It?

Domestic violence (DV) also known as intimate partner violence (IPV), involves physical violence, sexual violence, and threats of physical or sexual violence, verbal or emotional abuse by a current or former spouse or non-marital partner like a boyfriend. It is often committed by a man against a woman, but there are few cases where it is the other way.

Societal Views

Just like sexual abuse discussed above, DV occurs in all countries, and in all educational and socioeconomic strata. Western countries have made great strides to sensitize their societies about the fact that it is a public health issue and it is not okay for an intimate partner to abuse their spouse, wife or girlfriend. It is recognized and accepted as A CRIME, and every year in many countries, women are murdered by their spouses/partners and unfortunately some of the perpetrators get away with this and are not prosecuted by the law. In resource poor countries, people's perspectives and cultural views are slowly changing and women are being empowered to report cases of domestic violence so that their partners can be charged with a crime. Gradually women are accepting the fact that it is not okay for a husband or partner to abuse them physically, sexually, verbally or emotionally.

Ways to Minimize Domestic Violence

To reduce the prevalence a multifaceted approach is used. These include: education, creating awareness, legislation, lobbying, and provision of safe homes or shelters for abused victims. Together they can help combat this "cancer" in societies.

It is important for women organizations in different countries to speak up about intimate partner violence and lobby politicians to make and enforce laws that protect women from this.

Preventing Domestic or Intimate Partner Violence

To prevent this hideous crime, it is important to recognize the signs of abuse. One thing is that the abuser will initially seek to control their partner.

Signs of control include:

If the person belittles or puts one down as a bad spouse or parent
If he lets one stay in the house and does not let one work outside the home
Performs or forces one to engage in sexual acts one is not comfortable with
Threatens he will take one's children away
Prevents one from associating with family and friends
Controls the finances of the house
Makes one feel unsafe or intimidated around him
Controls one's every action and decisions

Some Tips About Domestic Violence

- Women need to know that it is not okay for a partner to abuse them
- It is not a "punishment" they deserve. Women must stop blaming themselves
- One must get help – tell relatives or someone trustworthy and report to relevant authorities
- Leave an abusive relationship. Most of the time there has been ample evidence of previous acts or statements that point to the violence that is occurring even before physical violence occurs
- When an individual hits one, the likelihood that it will happen again is very high
- It is not one's fault and do not rationalize and make excuses for the ongoing abuse
- Sometimes financial security from the partner or the fear of losing one's children are some of the reasons why a woman may stay on and "endure" the violence. One must seek help from appropriate sources who deal with supporting women in intimate partner violence situations
- If one is fearful or have concerns about one's safety in a relationship, seek help from trusted sources
- If one's partner forces one to have sex against your will, it is considered rape

- If one's partner constantly belittles them, makes one have low self-esteem, or bullies them, recognize this as spousal abuse

Some abusive partners after abusing a spouse will turn around and apologize, saying they are sorry for abusing them, and promise they will not do it again, but they do it again and it becomes a cycle. The victim is the one who can break this cycle by moving away and seeking help.

(Some of above information is from the CDC – Centers for Disease Control, Atlanta USA)

21

Cancers of Reproductive Organs
(Reference: American Cancer Society, International Agency for Research on Cancer)

Introduction

....

The Cancers that most often affect women are Breast Cancer, Colorectal Cancer (cancer of the large intestines and rectum), Skin Cancer, Cervical Cancer (the mouth of the womb), Endometrial Cancer (cancer of the womb), and Ovarian Cancer (ovaries). According to the International Agency for Research on Cancer data for 2012:

- Breast cancer was the most common cancer worldwide in women contributing more than 25% of the total number of new cases diagnosed in 2012
- The top three cancers, breast, colorectal and lung, contributed more than 43% of all cancers (excluding non-melanoma skin cancer)
- Cervical Cancer also contributed nearly 8% of all cancers (excluding non-melanoma skin cancer)

(GLOBOCAN 2012 v1.1, Cancer Incidence and Mortality Worldwide: IARC CancerBase No. 11)

Several cancers can occur in the reproductive organs and some of them are discussed below along with any prevention or early detection screening methods available.

Cervical Cancer
What is It?

Cervical Cancer is cancer that affects the cells of the lower part of the uterus (the neck) called the cervix which is connected to the upper part of the vagina. Most Cervical Cancers are caused by the Human Papilloma Virus (HPV). Although there are hundreds of HPV viruses, about forty of them can cause genital infections, and are sexually transmitted or through skin to skin contact during vaginal or anal sex. Fourteen of these are known as "high risk" HPV which may cause cancer of the cervix if they persist in the cells of the cervix. Two main types – 16, and 18 cause about 70% of Cervical Cancer. A high risk HPV is usually present for about 10 years in some cases, before changes in cervical cells occur. GENITAL WARTS, which do not lead to Cervical Cancer, are caused by low risk HPVs.

Persistence of High Risk HPV in a female can lead over time to abnormal cells on the cervix, and progression to Cervical Cancer if not detected early and treated. HPV genital infections are very common and are probably the most common sexually transmitted infections especially in young people.

Incidence

Cervical Cancer is the fourth most common cancer affecting women in the world according to the World Health Organization, and worldwide, there was approximately 530,000 new cases in 2012, representing 7.9% of all **female cancers**. Additionally, about 90% of the 270,000 deaths from Cervical Cancer in 2015 occurred in low – and middle-income countries due to lack of screening and early detection.

Incidence in Resource Poor and Resource Rich Nations

The highest incidence of Cervical Cancer in 2012 was in Africa, Latin America and Caribbean; and the lowest incidence in Northern America and Oceania. In countries where screening occur early and regularly, detection and treatment can result in a cure (GLOBOCAN 2012 v1.1, Cancer Incidence and Mortality Worldwide: IARC CancerBase No. 11). Most resource rich countries who have been screening for Cervical Cancer for over 30–50 years have seen a gradual decrease in incidence of Cervical Cancer, since abnormal cells discovered during screening are quickly treated. This is unfortunately not the case in low resource nations who do not usually have a national screening program in place. Australia in 2018 announced they may be the first country to eradicate Cervical Cancer, due to aggressive preventive measures including screening of women, and immunization of school aged children against the high risk HPV virus. The combination of frequent Cervical Cancer screening and vaccination against the HPV virus can prevent more than 90% of Cervical Cancer.

Detection of Abnormal Cells and High Risk HPV

To detect presence of high risk HPV and abnormal cervical cells the following tests are used:

Detection of HPV in the cervical cells by looking for HPV DNA (nuclear material)
Detection of abnormal cells by means of a Pap smear test
Visual inspection with Acetic acid (VIA) This is used in low resource countries
Visual inspection with Lugol's iodine (VILI). This is used in low resource countries

HPV DNA Test

This is a sophisticated test in which a small device called a cervical brush or other collection device is inserted into the cervix to collect cells for testing. This sample is then sent to the lab for evaluation. It may be collected in the same way as a pap is done or it may be done through "self sampling" when the woman herself inserts the small swab or brush into the vagina, collects the cells and places the brush in a liquid which is sent to the laboratory.

A negative result means that high-risk, cancer-causing types of HPV were not detected and one's risk of having precancer or cancerous lesions in the near future is low.

A positive result means high risk HPV is present and further tests have to be done. This may include further tests to differentiate which type of high risk HPV is present. Depending on the age of the patient and whether a Pap test was also done, and its results, a procedure called a Colposcopy can be done, and details will be discussed below.

PAP Smear

This involves scraping cells from the cervix and looking for abnormal cells (precancer or cancer cells) or signs of HPV in the cells. Pap smears usually start after age 21 years. A positive test means there are abnormal cells present and further investigations are done using a Colposcopy exam. See below for details about a pap smear.

Co-Testing

This refers to the two tests done together at the same time (PAP and HPV DNA). The combined test is usually used in women who are above 30 years because a younger woman's immune system tends to actively destroy the virus and cervical cells may return to normal. In the USA, high risk HPV is recommended to be co tested with a pap smear for women over 30 years. If the two tests are negative, then the testing interval for Cervical Cancer screening can be increased to between 3–5 years depending on a number of factors. In those who are younger than 30 years, if they have an abnormal or unclear Pap result, (when done by itself), then, an HPV test is done to detect if it is present.

Colposcopy

This is a procedure which uses a lighted device with magnification to view the vulva, vagina and cervix and surrounding tissues more closely; and if needed, helps to do a biopsy of abnormal looking tissues. The device is called a Colposcope. Now there are new mobile ones which can be taken out of the office and are being used to screen women for Cervical Cancer or abnormal cells at the community level. They are also being used in emergency rooms to do workup of rape victims.

Visual Inspection With Acetic Acid (VIA)

This involves applying 5% Acetic acid (white vinegar), to the surface of the cervix, waiting a few minutes and looking for change in color from the usual normal pink to areas of white coloration known as "Acetowhite" changes. Acetowhite indicates that abnormal cells are present. Such areas would either need to be biopsied or treated right away since they are suspicious for cell changes which could be pre-cancer or cancer.

Challenges and Solutions in Low Resource Countries

In low resource countries where there are challenges to accessing well equipped clinics or hospitals, and staffing problems (especially availability of trained doctors), creative ways have been developed to screen women in their communities using mobile devices which have a magnifying lens and smart phones with ability to take pictures. These devices are referred to as "Mobile Colposcopes" and they are able to send real time images via the internet to gynecology consultants in their offices many miles away to review and give advice. The woman is also able to see how her cervix looks like on the smart phone.

Community health nurses, midwives and other trained nurses can use a technique known as "see and treat" to screen with VIA, and if they observe an Acetowhite area they will treat with Cryotherapy or other methods to destroy the cells. With more serious looking lesions, the pictures are relayed to the specialists and the woman is sent to a health facility to have a biopsy for definitive diagnosis and treatment using an appropriate method.

Risk Factors for Developing Cervical Cancer

Apart from the presence of high risk HPV, there are other factors that contribute to the development of Cervical Cancer in someone with high risk HPV. These include:

Weak immune system brought about by HIV/AIDS and some medicines
Smoking tobacco
Infection with other sexually transmitted infections
A woman with a history of any cancer

Papanicolaou (PAP) Test or Smear
What is This?

This is a simple test which has been in existence for over 50 years and was developed to detect Cervical Cancer or abnormal pre-cancer cells of the cervix in women. It is often referred to as a "PAP" test. When a woman has a pap test, the doctor inserts a speculum which is a small duck beak-shaped instrument into the vagina. Under the guidance of light, she will lightly scrap some cells from the surface of the cervix, and just inside the cervix (endocervix) and sometimes from the vagina and these are sent to a lab to look for abnormal cells. At the same time, a test to detect the presence of the HPV virus may be done (Co-testing). After the speculum is removed from the vagina, the health care provider may also do a PELVIC EXAM. This was described above under conditions affecting the reproductive organs. This whole exam is often referred to as a "well woman examination", because its not a sick visit and it is to detect Cervical Cancer as well as any reproductive organ abnormalities which may be present.

Picture of A PAP Smear Procedure

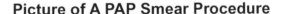

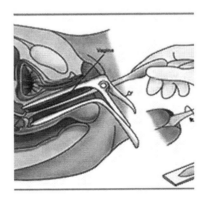

(Image credit: University of California – www.soc.ucsb.edu/sexinfo/article/pap-smear)

Treatment of Abnormal Cervical Cells or Positive HPV Test

There are different grades of abnormal cells of the cervix (Cervical Dysplasia) and treatment may depend on whether the abnormality is severe or mild and the age of the woman. Both abnormal cells and the presence of what type of HPV virus (low risk or high risk) is present are used to determine the treatment. If one has both HPV and Pap smear done, and the Pap (cervical cells) is normal, but there is presence of high risk HPV, then one may have a repeat Pap smear and HPV test in a few months to a year. If the repeat shows both are negative, then one will continue with annual screening Pap. If at repeat, either one is positive, one will have a Colposcopy (see above) and biopsy of suspicious areas. If there is Cervical Cancer or severe abnormality of cells present (moderate or severe cervical dysplasia) then usually the treatment may range from a simple to a complicated procedure to get rid of the abnormal cells.

Treatment of Abnormal Cells

These include:

Cone Biopsy: An extensive removal of tissue from the cervix, which removes the abnormal along with some normal cells in a wedge shape, and specimen is sent to the lab. The procedure is used for both diagnosis and treatment

Thermal Coagulation: Sometimes abnormal cells may be treated by either "burning" or coagulation of the cells at the surface of the cervix by heat or carbon dioxide

Loop electrosurgical excision procedure (LEEP): If the inner cervix (endocervix) is involved, then a procedure called a LEEP, which uses a loop with low electrical current to cut away the affected cells or Cone biopsy are used

Hysterectomy: (surgical removal of the uterus and cervix): In cases of severe Dysplasia or Cervical Cancer this is used for treatment

Prevention of Cervical Cancer

This involves not getting infected with the HPV virus in the first place. Now since it's difficult to know if one's sexual partner has the infection with HPV (as with all other sexually transmitted infections), one must be smart.

Practicing the ABC rule is prudent; although use of condom does not necessarily prevent skin to skin contact around the genital area.

Sexual Abstinence, Being faithful to one partner and Condom use, are the methods which help stop STIs transmission. (ABC of STIs prevention).

Vaccines Against HPV

HPV can cause not just Cervical Cancer but can cause cancers of the mouth, throat, vulva, vagina, penis, and anus. So there are vaccines which have been developed to prevent HPV infections. Initially it was approved for those who are 11 to 26 years old for both female and male, however, in 2018 it was approved for men and women up to 45 years old by the FDA (USA). Vaccination against the high risk HPV is the best protection, because one has a 85% reduction of life time Cervical Cancer risk, making the vaccines very effective ones.

There are three vaccines available Gardasil 4, Cervarix, and Gardasil 9 and each protects again 4, 2 and 9 different types of HPV respectively. In the USA, since 2017, Gardasil 9 (9vHPV) which is a 2 series shot for girls and boys aged 9 through 14 years is what is available and the other two have been phased out. The 9vHPV also protects against genital warts.

Safety of Vaccines

Immunization starts at age 11 years in most countries where it is available, but even 9-year-old kids may receive it. The first two vaccines have been around for more than 10 years and have been found to be safe; and they do not cause auto-immune diseases or venous blood clots as has been speculated by some individuals. More parents need to get their children vaccinated, to prevent HPV related cancers in the future. In the USA, adolescents aged 9 to 14 years receive 2 doses, and those 15 to 26 years receive 3 doses. The WHO requires the vaccination as part of routine vaccinations in all countries and recommend 2 or 3 doses depending on age and immune status. Vaccination is very important since it not only prevents pre cervical or Cervical Cancer, but also anal, vulva, vaginal, penis, mouth, throat and tonsils cancers caused by HPV.

Endometrial Cancer (En do me trial) (Cancer of the Uterus or Womb)
What is It?

Endometrial Cancer is a type of cancer affecting the endometrium or lining of the uterus. There is another type of cancer which affects the muscle of uterus called Uterine Sarcoma but it is less common. Endometrial cancer is usually present in post-menopausal women or in women after the age of fifty years. According to the American Cancer Society, risk factors for developing this cancer include:

- Women who have never had children
- Using Estrogen treatment without Progesterone for a woman who has a uterus
- Beginning menses at an early age, e.g. 10 years and cessation at a late age, e.g. after 51 years (long menstruation history)

- Taking certain anti-cancer drugs like Tamoxifen acts like estrogen on the uterus but as an anti-estrogen on the breasts
- Obesity
- History of Polycystic Ovary Disease (PCOS)
- Women whose close relatives have Uterine cancer, e.g. Mother, Sister, or Daughter
- Women with increased thickness of the lining of uterus as seen on imaging studies like ultrasound
- Women with infertility problems

Symptoms of Endometrial Cancer

- New vaginal bleeding in a post-menopausal woman
- Blood tinged discharge from the vagina
- Persistent or recurrent bleeding between periods for women still menstruating
- Persistent Pain in the pelvic area (lower part of the abdomen)
- Persistent pain when urinating, despite treatment for urinary tract infection
- Pain during sex

It is important that women should realize that vaginal bleeding after one has already stopped menstruation (referred to as post-menopausal bleeding) is not normal and is a serious condition which needs immediate consultation with a doctor. Never think you have reverted to the reproductive period after not having a period for 12 or more months and you are in the post-menopausal age range.

Treatment of Endometrial Cancer

After a history and physical examination which included a pelvic exam, tests which may be ordered include a pelvic ultrasound, CT scan, and blood work. A dilatation and curretage (D&C – scraping the inside lining of the uterus and sending specimen to the lab), and hysteroscopy are done to confirm the cause of the symptoms. The most successful treatment is by total hysterectomy (removal of the uterus) with chemotherapy or radiation treatments, if needed.

Cancer of the Ovary (Ovarian Cancer)
What is It?

Cancer of the ovary can be very subtle and present with non-specific symptoms. It occurs mostly in post-menopausal women. Due to its non-specific presentation, one should consider a constellation or pattern of symptoms to be suspicious of its presence. These include:

- Abdominal lump, bloating, or swelling
- Early feeling of fullness or satiety

- Abdominal pain especially in lower belly, back, and legs
- Urinary symptoms like urinating often (frequency) and urgency (intense desire to urinate)

It is important to consult a health provider if you have several of the symptoms mentioned above.

Risk Factors for Developing Ovarian Cancer

According to the American Cancer Society, it tends to occur in:

- Older women
- Those who have infertility problems
- Women who have not had any natural birth children
- Women who have used Estrogen alone for hormone replacement therapy (to treat menopausal symptoms)
- Women with a history of Breast Cancer or previous Ovarian Cancer
- Those who have inherited Colon Cancer Genes (special genes associated with colon cancer)
- Defects in BRCA 1 and BRCA 2 genes (abnormal genes associated with some breast cancers)
- Those who eat high animal fat diet like, beef, veal, or pork etc

Treatment of Ovarian Cancer

A health provider will take a history and will do a pelvic examination to feel abnormal masses or tenderness in the pelvis. Ultrasound or CT (CAT Scan) of the pelvic may be recommended together with blood test. Treatment depends on the size and position of Tumor; whether it's localized or spread beyond the ovary. Surgery to remove the ovaries or all the genital organs and Chemotherapy are the usual treatments; however, Radiation therapy may be added depending on extend of Cancer to shrink the tumor or destroy the Cancer cells. Ovarian cancer is usually discovered late and so most of the time it does not carry a good prognosis and survival is usually short.

Vulva and Vagina Cancer
The Vulva

The vulva is the external part of the female genitals and it consists of the outer large vaginal lips (labia majora) and smaller inner lips (labia minora), clitoris (sensitive orgasm arousing tissue), vaginal opening, urethral opening (leads into the bladder), and the mons pubis which is the hair covered fat pad area at the superior or upper part of the vulva. The inferior part of the vulva is formed by the perineum which is the tissue between the anus and vagina.

Cancer of the Vulva
What is It?

Cancer of the vulva is mostly formed in the large outer lips of the vagina. It takes a long time to develop and about 50% of all vulva cancers are caused by HPV which was discussed earlier. Vulva cancer presents mostly in older women and is very rare among the female genital cancers.

Types of Vulva Cancer

- Most are related to the skin and are called Squamous Cell Carcinomas. A smaller number develop in the Bartholin gland which is present at the entrance into the vaginal and usually produces fluids for lubrication
- Melanoma
- Adenocarcinoma
- Basal cell carcinoma

Signs and Symptoms

- Severe itching
- Open sore on vulva
- Burning or pain
- Change in color of skin

Risk Factors for Vulva Cancer

Certain risk factors have been identified and include:

- Smoking
- Infection with HPV and HIV viruses
- History of genital warts (low risk HPV)
- Sex with several sexual partners
- Previous cervical cancer
- Vulval intraepithelial neoplasia (VIN) precancer lesions
- Age greater than 50 years
- *Lichen Sclerosis

*Lichen Sclerosis a condition which causes thinning of the vulva lining and skin, itching, burning, and painful sex, and can sometimes lead to cancer of vulva if it persists and left untreated (See below for detailed discussion).

Treatment of Vulva Cancer

The diagnosis is made after biopsy, various tests, and imaging studies are completed. Treatment includes surgery, chemotherapy, and radiation depending on the extent of the cancer.

Prevention

Vaccination of girls and women up to the age of 45 years with HPV vaccine. It used to be up to age 26 years, but this has been extended to include older women.

Vulva Intraepithelial Neoplasia (VIN)

Vulva Intraepithelial Neoplasia (VIN) is a pre-cancer skin lesion of the vulva. It may turn cancerous after a number of years. It may be the result of infection with the HPV virus especially in younger women (35 to 49 years).

Symptoms

Symptoms include itching, soreness, change in skin color, rough thick skin, a lump, bleeding, ulcer and painful sexual intercourse.

Treatment of VIN

After taking the history and the physical examination, a biopsy of the lesion may be taken and sent to the lab. All VIN are treated with either surgery to remove the cells, or destroy the cells by laser or diathermy (ablation), or topical antiviral cream (Imiquimod). Some women may just be treated with frequent examinations by a doctor if large areas are involved and they do not have any symptoms.

Lichen Sclerosis
What is It?

These are patchy white spots on the skin which occur anywhere on the body like the genitals, arms, breasts, and torso or chest area. The cause is unknown but it is believed that genetics, overactive immune system, or hormones may all play a vital role. When it affects the genitals; it occurs in the vulva, foreskin of the penis in men, and around the anus. Vulva cases are common in post-menopausal women and can change into vulva cancer.

Symptoms and Signs

- Thinning of the skin of the vulva with patchy white spots
- Itching and easy bruising
- Tearing of skin and ulcer formation

Complications

It can lead to vulva cancer, narrowing of the vulva area, painful intercourse, and scarring with the tissues becoming hard and painful.

Treatment

After taking the history and the physical examination, a biopsy of the vulva tissue is taken (a small piece of tissue is removed and sent for Pathology examination). Treatment is with potent steroid creams, immune altering medicines like Tacrolimus or Pimecrolinus, and topical sex hormones like estrogens and testosterone. If there is a lot of scarring in the vulva, surgery may be required. The patient needs to follow-up every 6 months with a doctor for monitoring in case it changes to vulva cancer or complications occur, however, mild cases may resolve spontaneously in some women.

Vaginal Cancer

About 80% of vaginal cancers are from other places of the female reproductive system mainly from the cervix or endometrium (lining of the uterus). Cancer starting in the vagina itself is rare and consists of only about 1–2% of gynecological cancers.

22

Breast Disorders
(References: WebMD, Cleveland clinic.org)

Structure of the Breast
Fibroadenoma
Breast Cysts
Fibrocystic Breast Disease
Mastitis
Yeast Infection under the Breasts (Inframammary Candidiasis)
Breast Cancer
Breast Plastic Surgery

Introduction

....

The breast is unique in females and has a number of disorders, some of which we will discuss in this section. A great deal of time is dedicated to BREAST CANCER, because it is one of the most common cancers affecting women and makes women fearful of developing Breast Cancer.

Female Breast

The exterior structures of female breast are:

Breast tissue
Areolar
Nipple

The interior structures of female breast are:

Lobules (form or produce milk)
Ducts (tubes the milk flows through)
Larger collecting ducts within the nipple
Fatty tissues and supporting tissues (surround the Lobules)
Nerves and Blood Vessels

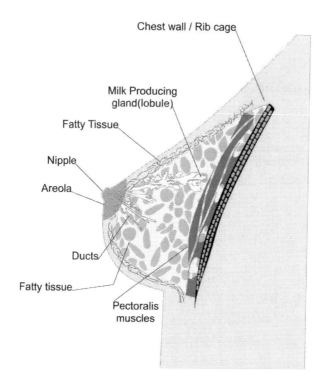

Chest wall / Rib cage
Milk Producing gland(lobule)
Fatty Tissue
Nipple
Areola
Ducts
Fatty tissue
Pectoralis muscles

STRUCTURE OF THE BREAST

Breast Disorders

There are several breast disorders and are classified as:

Benign (not cancerous) or
Cancerous (or Malignant)

Most women get alarmed when they feel a lump or mass in their breasts, however, about 80% of breast lumps are benign. We shall discuss the most common conditions that affect women at different ages of life. These are:

Fibroadenoma
Breast cyst
Fibrocystic Breast Disease

Mastitis
Breast Cancer

Fibroadenoma
What is It?

This is the most common benign breast mass found in women and is known as "Breast Mouse". They are usually round, firm, rubber like, and move freely – not attached to underlying breast tissue. They are formed from the milk – producing glands or lobules – and the stroma or supporting tissues of the breast. They are common in black women and those between the ages of 20–40 years. They may be single or multiple and may be felt in both breasts. They are usually not painful and are not Cancerous. Cause is not known but may be due to Estrogen since it is common around puberty, pregnancy, and in those on oral contraceptive pills. They may disappear in younger women after a while and tend to get smaller during menopause.

Treatment

After an Ultrasound, Mammogram, or Biopsy they can either be left alone or excised (removed) depending on the age of the woman and on the other concerns.

Breast Cysts
What are They?

These are benign fluid filled sacs which may be single or multiple in the Breast. Cause is not known but it's believed that changes in hormonal levels are involved and also perhaps when women have excess Estrogens present. They may or may not be painful and the size or how tender they are may be related to the time of a woman's menstrual cycle.

Treatment

After examination of the breasts, an ultrasound and mammogram of the involved breast can confirm whether the mass is a cyst or a solid mass. An ultrasound is the best imaging to detect a Cyst.

Repeat Ultrasound

A repeat ultrasound may be done after a few menstrual cycles to see how a cyst is behaving.

Aspiration

A small needle is used to drain the fluid out of the cyst and this flattens it. This is used for both diagnosis, confirmation and treatment. If the fluid is clear and the lump disappears then there is no need to worry. But, if it does not disappear or the fluid is bloody, then it has to be removed surgically.

Hormone Use

Use of birth control pills have been found to reduce the incidence of breast cysts.

Surgery

Surgery to remove a cyst is performed if it is tender, changes in size, does not disappear after aspiration, is bloody or of concern.

Fibrocystic Breast Disorder
What is This?

This is due to small cysts forming within the breasts and increased thickening of breast tissue (fibrous) which tend to occur in women of child bearing age. They are considered to be the result of hormonal changes and become symptomatic especially about a week before a woman's menstrual cycle. Excessive caffeine intake also makes it worse, and the condition tends to decrease after women go through the change or become post-menopausal. It is believed about 50% of all women may experience this at sometime of their lives.

Signs and Symptoms

Some women will experience pain, tenderness, enlargement, heaviness of breasts, and feel breasts lumps of different sizes just before and during their menses. These symptoms tend to decrease after menses.

Treatment

Certain lifestyle changes, medicines and supplements may help. These include:

- Lifestyle changes: Avoid drinking too many caffeinated drinks, like coffee, tea, colas etc. Decrease chocolate around that time (these have not been confirmed by studies)
- Avoid wearing firm supportive bras
- Supplements: Vitamin E 400 units daily or Evening Primrose oil capsules
- Needle aspiration of cysts by a doctor

  Medications: Which affect Estrogens e.g. Danazol and oral contraceptive pills
  Make sure your doctor knows whatever supplements or other medicines you
   are taking or wish to take

Mastitis (Breast Inflammation)
What is It?

This is infection or inflammation of the breast. It tends to occur after childbirth when a woman is breast feeding, however, it can happen at any other time to a woman. It is usually caused by bacteria entering the breasts from the nipple area. The fatty tissue is involved and this presses on the milk ducts resulting in the symptoms. You should seek medical attention as soon as possible.

Signs and Symptoms

The breast will become red (inflamed), swollen (engorged), hot, and painful and one may also have fever. There may be enlarged lymph nodes in the arm pit of involved side.

Treatment

The woman who is not feeding breast may need a breast ultrasound or mammogram. In a breastfeeding woman, emptying of the breasts by breast feeding or pumping the milk out will help. It is okay for the baby to breastfeed because any bacteria are destroyed in its stomach.

Warm wet towels applied to the affected breast about 3x a day will help the milk flow especially before nursing or breast feeding. Massaging the breast also helps the milk flow and empties the engorged breasts.

Pain relievers like ibuprofen, paracetamol, acetaminophen, (Tylenol) help with pain.

You will be prescribed oral antibiotics, and nursing mothers should continue to breastfeed.

Yeast Infection Under the Breasts (Intertrigo)
What is This?

Intertrigo also known as Inframammary Candidiasis yeast infection is caused by a fungus and it tends to thrive in moist dark areas like under the breasts, in the groin or vulva areas. It causes itching, redness, weepy, macerated (moist and soft), scaly and peeling skin, accompanied by an odor or smell.

Treatment

This is treated with antifungal topical medications, examples of which are Clotrimazole, Terbinafine, or Miconazole creams. Oral antifungal medications like Fluconazole (Diflucan) or Terbinafine may also be used. Antibiotic creams may also be used if the skin is cracked and looks infected by Bacteria. Sometimes a mild steroid cream is also applied for a few days to relieve itching and redness. If there is no improvement, then other causes must be considered like Bacteria called Pseudomonas and Erythrasma. These bacteria may cause skin infections in those with low immunity. In Erythrasma they appear as red/brown scaly itchy skin patches, and pseudomonas may cause red, ulcerated purple or black skin lesions in the inguinal or genital areas. These are treated with oral antibiotics. A special ultraviolet lamp called Wood's lamp will help identify these depending on how they glow under the light.

Prevention

After the treatment of inframammary candidiasis, to prevent a recurrence one is advised to use medicated body powder or any powder which has menthol or cornstarch in it. Alternatively, an antifungal powder called Nystatin may be applied. After taking a shower or bath, the area under the breasts must be dried very carefully with a towel and then the powder is applied to the dry area. As mentioned above, this should be used only after treatment is completed. That will prevent recurrence of the fungal infection.

Breast Cancer (BC)

References: American Cancer Society, WebMD, National Institute of Health Breast Cancer Home Page, WHO (World Health Organization).

A fair amount of time have been dedicated to research on Breast Cancer because it is a very common female cancer and most women want to know more about it and what is their risk of getting it.

Overview

What is Breast Cancer?
Breast Cancer in resource rich and resource poor countries
Factors hindering early Breast Cancer screening
Who is at risk of Breast Cancer?
Assessing individual risk of Breast Cancer
Modifying risk factors to prevent breast cancer

Types of Breast Cancer and Presentation

Types of Breast Cancer
Signs and Symptoms of Breast Cancer

Diagnosis and Treatment

Diagnosis of Breast Cancer
Treatment of Breast Cancer
Life during treatment of Breast Cancer
Complementary and Alternative Treatment used by Breast Cancer Patients

Life after Breast Cancer

Life after Breast Cancer
Connecting with other Breast Cancer Survivors
Factors affecting Survival in Breast Cancer patients
Prevention of a second Breast Cancer in the other breast
Screening for breast cancer after Breast Cancer surgery

Breast Cancer Screening

Detection of Breast Cancer in women
Self Breast Examination
Clinical Breast Examination
Screening Mammography (Mammogram)
Preparing for a successful Mammogram Examination
Other Breast Imaging Studies

What is Breast Cancer?

"October is breast cancer awareness month, but for a survivor, it's every single day."

—Unknown

"There can be life after breast cancer. The prerequisite is early detection."

—Ann Jillian

"Don't let breast cancer take away the motivation to achieve your dreams."

—Diana Cohen
(sayingspoint.com/breast-cancer-saying)

Breast cancer (BC) in women is the rapid growth of abnormal breast cells in the glands of the breasts or in the milk ducts resulting in a lump, mass, or tumor (these terms are used interchangeably). The cancer can affect either one or both of a woman's breasts, and the cancer cells can eventually travel to nearby glands called Lymph Nodes which are in the chest or under the arm pits (axilla) or locally to the skin or chest wall. The cancer cells can spread through the blood to the liver, lungs, bones, and brain which is known as Metastatic breast cancer.

Incidence of Breast Cancer (BC)

In 2012, BC was the most common cancer worldwide in women contributing more than 25% of the total number of all cancers diagnosed according to International Agency for Research on Cancer. There were about 1.67 million cases in 2012 and out of this 522,000 women died. It is a disease prevalent in both developed and less developed countries. Incidence rates according to WHO vary from 19.3 per 100,000 women in Eastern Africa to 89.7 per 100,000 in Western Europe (GLOBOCAN 2008).

Breast Cancer in Resource Rich and Limited Resource Countries

Resource Rich Countries

Breast cancer is the second leading cause of cancer death among women in the USA. The life time risk of developing BC by a woman is 1 in 8 or 13%. In the USA, it was estimated that 252,710 women were diagnosed with breast cancer in 2017 and 40,610 women died from the disease. According to the research of American Cancer Society, there has been about 39% decrease in deaths in the past 25 years (between 1989 and 2015), with over a third of a million women saved from death due to screening and early detection. BC usually occurs in women above the age of 50 years, with fewer numbers between 40 and 50 years; however, it has been found that more black women compared to white women below the age of 40 years are diagnosed with breast cancer. Even though there have been decline in deaths, the decline among American black women is less than for Caucasians and this is result of many factors including socio-economic factors, access to screening, and the difference in the major type of breast cancers that are found in each group. The type found commonly in black women is called Triple Negative Breast Cancer (TNBC) which tends to be more aggressive with increased death. See details below.

Limited Resource Countries

In limited resource countries (used to be called Developing Countries), Breast Cancer is the leading cancer death among women. Research shows that death rates are higher in these countries because detection and treatment are late. For example, Dr. Florence Dedey, Member of the Breast Cancer Team, Korle-Bu Teaching Hospital, Accra, Ghana, had reported in 2013, that there were about 16,600 cancers cases expected per year in Ghana with some 12,000 deaths from cancer per year. Of these, breast and cervical cancers were the leading causes in Ghana and the deaths have huge socio-economic impacts on both families and the nation. However more recently, according to Professor Joe Nat Clegg Lamptey, Head of the Korle Bu Hospital Breast cancer multidisciplinary team, 2200 women are yearly diagnosed with Breast Cancer in Ghana and only 25% of women diagnosed are cured with the rest dying from it within 5 years; because the vast majority of women who are diagnosed with breast cancer have advanced disease (ghanaweb. com, Oct. 2017). These figures will not be much different for other limited resource countries. In all of these countries, lack of screening and or late detection make early treatment and cure more challenging and therefore, the increased death rate found in these countries.

Factors Preventing Early Screening for Breast Cancer

Early detection and treatment enables a breast cancer patient to be treated and cured, or the disease kept from spreading further (Metastasis). The 5-year survival rate is over 90% if the breast cancer is diagnosed early. Unfortunately, several factors hinder women from going to be screened for breast cancer and some of which are discussed below. They include:

- Fear of the diagnosis:
  Some women say, "I will rather not know I have breast cancer", so will not go for screening. The fact is that with any cancer, it can spread from the breast to surrounding tissues like the chest wall and to distant places like the bone, liver, and brain. This may cause a lot of pain and discomfort for the individual. So, unnecessary suffering down the road can be avoided if it is discovered earlier rather than when it is in the advanced stage

- Lack of knowledge or ignorance:
  This is one of the reasons this book is being written so women can have the right information and know how they can prevent all kinds of diseases like breast cancer, or have them detected early

- Lack of finances:
  It is true that some women may not be able to afford a procedure like a MAMMOGRAM for early detection, but every woman can learn how to do self-breast examinations and get to know how her own breasts feel like. She can also ask a health professional to do a breast examination on her or to teach her how to do this. These latter two ways are not as accurate as Mammograms and has even been discouraged by some experts, but for people in Developing Countries it could be quite helpful in detecting breast lumps. In all countries, there may be non-profit organizations or hospitals which subsidize or give grants to women to get free screening Mammograms especially during the month of October which is Breast Cancer Awareness Month

- Lack of awareness:
  Some women are unaware that breast cancer can affect every woman especially those above 50 years or who are in the post-menopausal era (have stopped having menses). You don't have to have a family history to be at risk for breast cancer. Being a woman and also being over 50 years are two of the most important risk factors for getting Breast Cancer. Family history is responsible for only about 5% of breast cancers

- Fear of Mammogram Examination
  Some women are frightened of pain involved in the squeezing of the breasts between the plates during the Mammogram Examination. One can take a pain pill like Acetaminophen or Ibuprofen (I personally don't think it's that painful)

and also be well hydrated before the examination if one is afraid of pain. The examination is uncomfortable, but far less painful than child birth or even an attack of kidney stones or toothache. The total exam lasts about 15 minutes so it is not a long procedure

Who is at increased risk of Breast Cancer (BC)?

Remember, a risk factor can be anything that increases a person's chance of getting a particular disease. In BC although most women diagnosed have no known risk factors except for their GENDER and AGE, It has been observed that certain risk factors may predispose a woman to breast cancer. These include:

1. Gender
    Being a woman puts one at the increased risk of breast cancer
2. Personal History of Breast Cancer
    Any woman with a history of previous breast cancer has a 3-4-fold increased risk of developing another breast cancer unrelated to the first one
3. Age
    Older women aged 50 years and above, and who are post-menopausal tend to get breast cancer. However, black women have been found to be more likely to get breast cancer before menopause compared to caucasian women
4. Family History of Breast Cancer
    Family history of breast cancer in a first degree relative (Sister, Mother, or Daughter) especially before menopause puts one at increased risk
5. Genetics
    Women carrying certain breast cancer genes which are changed or altered (referred to as "Mutation") are more prone to developing certain types of breast cancer. The most common genes which when mutated can lead to breast cancer are called BRCA (Breast Cancer Genes) genes 1 and 2. Less than 5% of women with breast cancer are found to carry a mutated BRCA gene. A woman with a mutated BRCA gene has up to 7x higher risk of developing breast cancer compared to someone who has a normal BRCA gene
6   Distant Family History of Breast Cancer
    Breast cancer in Grandmother, Aunties, or Cousins puts one at increased risk of developing it, although the risk is less than in a first degree relative

Other less important risk factors for developing breast cancer include:

*   A previous abnormal breast biopsy like one called "Atypical Hyperplasia"
*   Having dense breasts (they have less fat and more connective tissue in them)
*   Age of first childbirth after age 35 years

- Never having given birth (natural birth)
- Early age of beginning menstruation with late age of menopause (long reproductive time frame)
- Starting menopause after the age of 55 years
- Excessive radiation exposure especially to the chest
- History of being on combined hormone replacement therapy for menopause symptoms
- Obesity especially after menopause
- Increased alcohol intake
- Family history of ovarian cancer

Assessing an Individual's Risk for Breast Cancer

Several studies have been done by the scientific community to develop risk assessment tools which can be used by health professionals to assess an individual's risk of developing breast cancer. One has been developed by the American government's National Institute of Health (NIH) and it's called "The Breast Cancer Risk Assessment Tool".

Some of the information that have to be gathered include questions like: age, age at which first child was born, previous breast biopsy, race or ethnicity, age at time of first menses etc. Based on the answers a point system is used to estimate a woman's risk of developing invasive (breast cancer occurring beyond the ducts) breast cancer during the next 5 years of her life and also her life time risk, i.e. risk at the age of 90 years. Although the tool calculates risk, it is unable to indicate for sure who will specifically develop breast cancer. It is usually used by the health professionals.

Prevention of Breast Cancer in Women by Reducing Risk Factors

We have already discussed the risk factors for developing breast cancer. Some of them are modifiable risk factors but others are not. It is important that women take note of the modifiable risk factors and try and reduce them in order to prevent breast cancer. For example, nobody can modify the family history of breast cancer of a patient or the age, but other risk factors can be modified to minimize the risk of developing BC. These include:

- Alcohol Reduction: Reducing intake to not more than one drink a day
- Weight loss if obese: Try eating a healthy diet and exercise regularly to achieve this. Alternatively, use weight loss medications if effort has been made with the other two but without much success. Use of medications should go along with lifestyle changes

- Avoid sedentary lifestyle: Increase activity by engaging in physical activity of any kind
- Hyperlipidemia: Decrease levels of your blood cholesterol by exercise, healthy eating, or taking cholesterol medicines, if needed
- Avoid long duration of Estrogen exposure: Combined Birth Control Pills contain Estrogen and Progesterone which are female hormones. There is increase risk associated with long duration of Estrogen exposure, so if using this, the estrogen should be at a low dose. Alternatively, change to another type of birth control method without estrogen if one already has several risk factors for breast cancer. For example, Progesterone shot, or the progesterone only Mini Pill
- Avoid prolonged use of Hormone Replacement Therapy (HRT): This is medicine used to treat hot flashes and night sweats associated with menopause and contains Estrogen. Avoid prolonged use and limit use to not more than 5 years Post-Menopause. Using topical or patches instead of pills, further reduces one's total exposure to estrogen

Chemoprevention Medicine Used to Reduce Risk of Breast Cancer
What is It?

This is when a drug is used to prevent a medical condition or disease in high risk individuals. For example, daily Penicillin is given to prevent infection in kids with Sickle Cell Disease. Same principle can be applied to women who are at high risk for developing breast cancer. These include those at increased risk due to family history or genetics as well as those whose breast biopsies have shown Atypical Hyperplastic Cells (these cells are abnormal and are regarded as pre-cancer cells). These medicines include TAMOXIFEN (Nolvadex), RALOXIFENE (Evista), ANASTROZOLE (Arimidex), and LETROZOLE (Femara).

Types of Breast Cancer

Breast cancer can occur in different parts of the breast. The most common types of cancer are:

- INTRADUCTAL CANCER – Forms inside the ducts that carry milk to the nipple
- LOBULAR CANCER – Begins in the lobules which are the milk producing glands

Classification Based on Location of Breast Cancer

IN SITU: When breast cancer is localized and has not spread from where it started. For example, we can have Lobular Carcinoma In Situ (LCIS) or Ductal Carcinoma In Situ (DCIS). It is also known as non-Invasive Cancer

INVASIVE: It is invasive when it spreads beyond its original site. For example, from the ducts or lobules and is found in other parts of the breast

METASTATIC: When cancer cells spread beyond the breast tissues and into the chest wall, lymph nodes, liver, lungs, bone, or brain

Hormone and Genetic Influences on Breast Cancer

After cancer is diagnosed and the individual has surgery (will be discussed in detail later), Doctors test samples of tumor tissue to find out if the cancer cells are sensitive to different female sex hormones or not. These will have an impact on treatment regimens used.

Estrogen and Progesterone Receptors

On the surface of cancer cells there may be proteins called Estrogen (ER+) or Progesterone Positive (PR+) receptors. They attract these female hormones which make them grow and negatively influence the course of the disease. In those with the hormone positive receptors, anti-hormone therapy can be used for treatment and they act by blocking the influence of these female hormones and slow the growth of the cancer.

Human Epidermal Growth Factor Receptor 2 (HERS 2 Gene)

Another test that is done is to look for presence of the HERS positive gene called HER2 or HER2/neu. This is a gene which sends messages to the breast cells via the HER-2 protein to make them multiple, grow, and make repairs. Each normal breast cell has 2 copies of these genes, however, with age, and probably as a result of effects of environmental factors, some breast cells develop several copies of the genes and so there is excessive production of the HER-2 protein and this causes the breast cancer cells to multiple excessively. There are specific medicines which work to block the growth pathways on or inside the cancer cells.

Triple Negative Breast Cancer (TNBC)
What is It?

Some BCs do not have any hormone receptors at all and are called Triple Negative Breast Cancers (TNBCs). In the USA, it is seen in about 15% of all breast cancers cases. It is interesting that in research and studies to find out what types affect the different races, it has been found that black women in sub-Saharan Africa and African Americans in America (they have common ancestry) have increased risk of being diagnosed with TNBC and as well as those with BRCA1 mutations. TNBC tends to be more aggressive and occur in younger women (premenopausal). It however can occur in all

"It has been clearly demonstrated that African American women have about a two fold higher incident of triple negative breast cancers compared with caucasian American breast cancer patients"

—Dr. Lisa Newman (State of the Art treatment for Triple Negative Breast Cancer. Medscape Oncology/Triple negative Breast Cancer foundation)

races. One such researcher is Dr. Lisa Newman, a surgical oncologist from Michigan, USA who specializes in breast cancer and is working with doctors at a Teaching Hospital in Kumasi Ghana, and in Ethiopia to find out why this is so. During an interview with CNN media network, she said, "It's heartbreaking that we see many advanced stage of cancers in the women of Ghana, but it's a tremendous opportunity to make a difference and to be able to share what we have in the United States with the women here, with our family, our extended family". Extensive information on TNBC is found at the website: www.tnbcfoundation.org

Among the three types of cancers described above, Hormone-Receptor-Positive Breast Cancer is more common and has a better prognosis than HER2-positive and Triple-Negative Breast Cancers. This is because the Hormone Receptor-Positive Treatment blocks the receptors leading to slowing or stopping the growth of the cancers.

Signs and Symptoms of Breast Cancer

Breast cancer can present as:

- A hard lump under the skin of the breast
- Change in size, shape or surface of the breast
- A new dimple in the skin of the breast
- Pain or tenderness, (not seen very often)
- A lump under the arm pit
- Redness or swelling of the breast
- Bloody, pink, or clear discharge from the nipple
- Change in the skin presenting as a scaly, red, swollen, or indented area

Not all breast lumps are cancerous but if a lump is present, it needs to be checked by a health provider and individual sent for Mammogram and an Ultrasound, and possibly a Biopsy if needed to confirm this.

Diagnosis of Breast Cancer

Once a lump is discovered in the breast either by yourself, doctor, husband, a screening mammogram or presence of some of the other symptoms and signs mentioned above, you need to consult your health care provider immediately. The health provider will order a Mammogram, which is a special type of x-ray which takes pictures of the breasts. Screening mammograms (will be discussed later in detail) are used as a preventive tool to detect breast cancers. However, when a lump or some of the other symptoms and signs mentioned above are discovered, then the patient has to have a DIAGNOSTIC MAMMOGRAM. This type of mammogram is used when a particular breast needs more detailed study due to a density or mass in the breast and additional views of the breast are taken compared to a screening mammogram. The Diagnostic Mammogram is ordered together with an ULTRASOUND of that breast to help radiologists have a better look at the mass or lump and it may help distinguish between a Cyst (fluid filled sacs) and a Solid Breast Mass. After the Diagnostic Mammogram and Ultrasound, if the mass is found not to be a simple cyst, or it is suspicious, then the doctor will refer patient to a surgeon to have a Biopsy. A simple cyst may be aspirated with a needle and the contents sent for analysis in the lab. A biopsy may also be done by a procedure called Ultrasound Guided Biopsy.

Ultrasound Guided Biopsy

Some biopsies may be done with the aid of an Ultrasound in the Radiology department. If the mass is deep in the breast and is not palpable but was discovered by a screening mammogram or by palpation, then a mammography is used to aid the doctor to do what is called a Stereotactic Breast Biopsy.

Stereotactic Breast Biopsy

The mammogram identifies the position of a mass in three dimension and the biopsy needle is guided to the exact location of the mass. One has to lie face down and the breast is compressed between two plates to flatten it and get the needle to go into the right location where the lump is present, and then a biopsy is taken. It is then sent to the lab and if the pathology examination of the breast tissue shows that it is breast cancer, then many more studies can be done on the tissue e.g. test for Estrogen or Progesterone positive receptors; which eventually determines what therapy patient has to be given.

Other Studies

Other studies include MRI of the breasts which may identify masses of the breast that may have been missed by Mammogram. An imaging study called PET/CT may be done on the whole body to check for signs of Metastasis to other parts of the body.

Treatment

We will discuss some of the therapies used to treat breast cancer. Treatment depends on the stage of disease (localized, invasive, or metastatic), type of breast cancer, and presence of hormonal receptors or immune factors. Treatments include:

- CHEMOTHERAPY (KI MO THI-RAPY) or CHEMO for short
- RADIOTHERAPY (RADIATION)
- SURGERY

- HORMONAL THERAPY
- IMMUNOTHERAPY

Chemotherapy

These are various anticancer medications given intravenously (into the veins) or orally (by mouth) to destroy cancer cells or to stop the chance of the cancer recurring. The chemotherapy can be used in a number of ways:

1. May be added to surgery and or radiation to kill cancer cells
2. To shrink the size of a big tumor before surgery is performed
3. To treat breast cancer which has spread beyond the breast and the lymph nodes in the axilla (armpit)
4. To prevent recurrence of the disease

In the process of destroying the cancer cells, chemotherapies tend to destroy fast growing regular body cells like hair, the lining of the mouth, stomach, or intestines. In essence there is "collateral damage" to these cells and the result is that these body areas are adversely affected, contributing to the side effects that occur with treatment.

Side Effects of Chemotherapy

1. Hair Loss (Chemotherapy Induced Alopecia – (Alo pee cia))

A woman's hair is the source of attraction and beauty and some women get very devastated when they see their hair falling off during treatment. One may lose eyebrows, eyelashes, and body hair as well. The good thing is that the hair grows back after the treatment is over.

For scalp hair the following choices are available:

Some women just cut their hair short even before they start treatment
There are wigs which patient can buy and wear if she prefers that
Some women prefer going bald without covering the scalp and that is also fine
There are new therapies called Cooling Cap System being used to prevent hair loss

Cooling Cap System

In 2015, the United States FDA approved a cooling cap system which helps reduce hair loss. In a recent clinical trial using the cap, after four cycles of chemotherapy some women still had hair preservation. The cap reduces the temperature to below 66 degrees F and decreases blood flow. Therefore, there is minimal chemotherapy to the scalp, resulting in less hair loss. It is believed the cooling cap does not interfere with the chemo effect of killing the cancer cells. It is worn before, during, and after treatment for each cycle. (Dr. J. Nangia, San Antonio Breast Cancer Symposium Dec 2016)

The important thing is that a patient can do whatever she is comfortable with. There is no need to be ashamed about hair loss or let it affect one's self esteem. It will GROW BACK.

2. Nausea and Vomiting

It can be very difficult to prevent this side effect. Patients are usually given anti-nausea and vomiting medicines e.g. Promethazine or Ondansetron prior to treatment. It may still occur in spite of this. A herbal medicine like GINGER ROOT may be useful taken as a capsule or tea. To minimize or prevent these effects patient can eat dry foods like crackers or cabin biscuits which are not too sweet, sip small amount of water or clear fluids, avoid fatty or greasy foods, and eat small frequent meals.

3. Digestive Problems

Many digestive problems may take place and these include loss of appetite, changes in sense of taste or smell, constipation or diarrhea, dry mouth, soreness in the mouth, sore throat and trouble swallowing food.

Solutions

- Soft foods and liquids:
  To help with most of these digestive problems, a patient has to eat foods that are gentle on your mouth and stomach. Examples of these are fruits which are juicy and have plenty of water – like water melon, papaya/pawpaw, pineapple, or grapes. Avoid citrus fruits if they sting your mouth. Other foods to eat include soft cooked cereals like oats, cornmeal, sorgum porridge, grits, soups, yogurt, boiled eggs, cheese, peanut butter, brown or whole wheat bread. Chicken or fish can be baked or grilled instead of fried, and these can be used in vegetable soups. It is important that one should drink plenty of fluids in the form of water, coconut water, broth, and juices to provide needed sugar and nutrients
- L-glutamine supplement for sore mouth:
  This is an amino acid (protein building block) naturally produced in the body and is also available as an OTC supplement. This is used by some to treat inflammation of mouth and intestines caused by Chemotherapy. Always talk to your doctor before using OTC medicines
- Stool softeners and laxatives for Constipation
  Effects of pain medications can be bothersome and so stool softeners or laxatives may help one have regular bowel movements

4. Dry Mouth

This is the result of chemotherapy and radiation to the head and neck areas. There is decreased saliva production and it can lead to sore mouth, teeth, and dental problems. To avoid this, a dentist can give you a prescription to get a rinse for dry mouth. Rinsing the mouth using a little water with added lime or lemon can help keep the saliva flowing. Other tips include: chewing sugar-free gum, sucking a sugar-free hard candy, dry mouth lozenges, and use of a mouth rinse with fluoride. Products that help with flow of saliva include but are not limited to XyliMelts, Salese, Oramoist, and Biotene rinse. All of these products contain XYLITOL which promotes saliva flow. The use of a humidifier in the room, limiting intake of alcohol, caffeine, and sugar also help decrease symptoms of dry mouth. Good oral hygiene by regular brushing the teeth with a fluoride containing toothpaste at least twice a day will also help.

5. Fatigue

This fatigue is also called "Cancer Related Fatigue". The treatments cause extreme fatigue during and after treatment for breast cancer and other cancers. It is believed to be a result of side effects like anemia, pain, the cancer itself, medications, lack of exercise and emotional stress of the illness. It can unfortunately persist for years; however, getting plenty of rest may help with this. Other interventions include exercise both aerobic and resistance training, psychological therapy, and prescription medications. These medicines include Steroids, Ritalin, Dexamphetamine, Modafinil, Armodafinil and the antidepressant Paroxetine.

6. Chemobrain (foggy brain)

This is when after chemotherapy; patients have problems with memory, concentration, thinking clearly, attention, finding words, remembering things, and difficulty with multi-tasking and performing daily activities. This may affect up to 75% of breast cancer patients. It is believed that several factors contribute to the problem and not just the chemotherapy. The latest research shows that the Cancer itself is a contributing factor. Knowing that this can happen prior to start of treatment may help some individuals prepare for it.

Things that contribute to Brain Fog include:

Cancer itself
Stress, fatigue and anemia
Post-menopausal state
Anxiety, depression, and sleep problems
Therapies like radiation, surgery, immunotherapy and hormonal therapy
Proteins called cytokines which cause Inflammation

Treatment of Brain Fog

There is no specific treatment for the Brain Fog, however, the following have been used. It may resolve within a year after treatment, but can persist in others:

- Treatment of symptoms like sleep problems, depression and anxiety may help minimize its effects
- Use of occupational therapy has given some favorable results
- Some medications that have been used include medicines used to treat Alzheimer's dementia like Donepezil (Aricept) and Memantine (Namenda)
- Drugs for excessive drowsiness: Use of Modafinil and Methylphenidate which is usually used to treat Attention Deficit Hyperactivity Disorder (ADHD)
- Playing brain games or doing cross word puzzles to stimulate the mind may also help
- Complementary and Alternative (CAM) supplements like Ginkgo and Vitamin E have been studied but no benefits have been found. Patients should always let the doctor know if planning on trying some CAM supplements like those

Other simple but effective ways which may help include:

- Avoid multi-tasking, try and do one activity at a time
- Write things down like a "To do List" so you don't forget
- Try to keep every day things after use at the same place
- Don't forget to exercise, and simple walking is good enough and it is free
- Get enough rest and pace yourself, but don't social isolate
- Do difficult tasks when you are most alert
- Eat healthy foods especially brain foods rich in Omega 3 (see list under Brain diseases/Dementia)
- Mindfulness meditation

7. Weight Gain or Weight Loss

For unknown reasons some women gain weight while others lose weight. To help build muscles some people use L-Glutamine powder one-teaspoon daily. This is an over the counter supplement and one should consult the Cancer Doctor before starting it.

8. Numbness/Tingling or Pain in Extremities (Neuropathy)

Some chemotherapy medicines may cause numbness and tingling or even pain especially in the lower extremities – legs and feet. This condition is known as NEUROPATHY. Let the doctor know if this happens since there are medicines which can make it better or it may improve with time.

Prescription medicines recommended by the American Society of Clinical Oncology (ASCO) include Duloxetine, and they consider it reasonable to use Tricyclic Antidepressants, Gabapentin, and a topical gel compounded containing Baclofen, Amitriptyline, and Ketamine (ASCO guidelines, 2014).

ASCO does not advocate for Vitamin E, Omega 3 fatty acids, or Venlafaxine due to limited studies, but they have helped some people.

L-Glutamine is used by some for neuropathy. Some patients indicate that over the counter Vitamin B6 100 mg one daily is helpful, as well as Vitamin B complex

9. Taste Changes in Mouth

Chemotherapy can make food taste different leaving a metallic taste in the mouth. Since chemotherapy attacks cells that grow or multiple fast, it attacks the cells lining inside the mouth as well; resulting in soreness in the mouth. Some people on chemotherapy have used the local Ghanaian berry known as "Asaba" (Fanti) or "Thami" (Ga) or Miracle Berry to help them overcome the metallic taste, and enjoy their food. Miracle Berry fools the taste buds so that any bitter or sour food or drink will taste sweet.

10. Increase Risk of Infection

Due to the destruction of cells that protect the body from infection, people undergoing chemotherapy may be at increased risk of infection. Patient has to be careful being around people with infections so that one does not get their illnesses. Sometimes, you may have to wear a mask in crowded areas. Any fever or chills has to be reported to your doctor or go to emergency room right away.

11. Decrease In White Cell Count
(Infection-fighting cells/Neutropenia)

Chemotherapy can result in a decreased number of infection-fighting white blood cells (neutrophils). This makes one prone to infections. This may start as a low white cell count seen in a blood test and associated with fever. This is known as FEBRILE NEUTROPENIA (fever and low white cell count). To prevent this, patient may be given a medicine called Pegfilgrastim (Neulasta), which stimulates or boosts the growth of white cells in the bone marrow and it may be given in-between Chemotherapy treatments. One common side effect is that it can cause some bone discomfort. Taking Acetaminophen may help with the discomfort.

12. Decrease in Bone Mass (Thinning of the bones)

Some chemotherapy medications may cause the density of a woman's bone to decrease. There is a special test called DEXA SCAN or BONE DENSITY SCAN that can be done to check if the bones have been weakened by the chemotherapy.

Weak brittle bones can lead to fracture of bones and a long stay in bed which also further weakens the bones due to lack of movement. Checking blood Calcium and Vitamin D levels is also a good idea since they affect bone density. If the bone density is found to be low, there are treatments available to help with that.

13. Damage to Heart

This is ongoing research by Cardiologists, since it has been found that certain chemotherapy drugs called Anthracyclines have caused decrease heart function. But, this also depends on the dose used to treat a breast cancer patient. In some centers, a heart test to determine the heart function is done before and after therapy with this type of drug and if found to have affected the heart, appropriate medicine is given to treat this.

14. Anemia

Anemia is low hemoglobin. Hemoglobin is found in the red blood cells and it is what carries Oxygen to the different organs in the body. Cancer itself may cause anemia, and other causes of anemia are Chemotherapy and Radiation treatments, previous kidney problems, and low iron and other minerals needed to produce the hemoglobin. Low hemoglobin as found in a blood test may produce symptoms like fatigue, palpitations, shortness of breath, swelling of the feet, dizziness, and chest pain. Doctors may treat this if the levels are very low with blood or iron infusions.

Breast Surgery for Breast Cancer

Most people who have breast cancer will have some type of surgery depending on the type of cancer, the location of the tumor, and the size of the cancer.

Types of surgery

1. LUMPECTOMY
    This is when the tumor or lump is removed together with the surrounding healthy breast tissue. This is used when tumor is a small size and limited to the breast. Advantage is the preservation of the breast
2. MASTECTOMY
    This is the removal of the breast or sometimes both breasts together with lymph nodes in the arm pits (axillae). Lymph nodes are part of the lymphatic system which is the part of the body's defense system against bacteria, other microbes, and cancer cells. Like a sieve the lymph nodes will filter these foreign invaders and prevent them from entering the blood system and spreading. Cancer cells also accumulate in the lymph node and at surgery some of these lymph nodes present in the arm pits are removed and examined for cancer

cells. If present in these cells, then surgery will involve the extensive removal of most of the lymph nodes in the arm pit or axilla

3. DOUBLE MASTECTOMY

    This can be done when there is breast cancer in both breasts, however, it is also done when one has breast cancer in one breast but decides with her surgeon to have a double mastectomy to prevent another cancer developing in the other normal breast. It is then known as Contralateral Prophylactic Mastectomy. Many women are getting this done, however unless patient has certain risk factors, research has shown that it does not improve survival or prevent metastasis or spread from occurring

Contralateral Prophylactic Mastectomy

It may be recommended to those with:

A strong history of Breast Cancer in the family
Those who have genetic mutation of the breast cancer genes BRAC 1 and BRAC 2
Those who have had radiation treatment of their chest for other medical conditions

Risks of prophylactic mastectomy: Double mastectomy may cause increased side effects and more surgical complications. A woman should make sure she has the necessary risk factors before having prophylactic mastectomy done on the normal breast

Side Effects of Breast Cancer Surgery

A. PAIN: Severing/cutting of nerves may lead to pain which may resolve or persist
B. INFECTION: If the surgical wound is extensive there may be infection and slower recovery from surgery
C. LYMPHEDEMA (Leaf-e-dema): When surgery for breast cancer involves removing part or the entire breast, plus the removal of lymph nodes from the axilla; this results in swelling of the shoulder region and arm on the involved side of the body. This is called LYMPHEDEMA. It may result in heaviness of the involved arm, numbness or tingling of arm and fingers, and sometimes there may be ulcer forming on the swollen arm

How to Avoid Lymphedema

Risk factors have been identified as contributing to development of lymphedema. These include:

Hypertension history and obesity
Extensive removal of axillary lymph nodes

Older women
Lack of movement and previous injury to the involved arm

Before surgery:

One should know about lymphedema and ways to minimize its development after surgery

Soon after surgery:

- Keep the arm elevated or above your heart level by supporting it on a pillow when sitting or lying down, this prevents fluid from accumulating in the lower arm or hand
- Regular exercise of the involved arm with movement of the arm and shoulder joint are important. Good blood pressure control and weight loss in general are useful in avoiding lymphedema

Long term care after surgery:

- One should keep that arm from extremes of temperature
- Avoid tight sleeves
- Prevent having a BP cuff put around it to check blood pressure
- Prevent having drawing of blood from that arm
- Identify early signs of lymphedema development like tight clothing, and heaviness of arm, swelling, tiredness, or pain in the involved arm
- Avoid lifting heavy objects with that arm
- Avoid dry skin which can easily chaff and split open
- Avoid injury to the skin and muscles of the arm by maintaining good skin care and adequate moisturizing of skin
- Get treatment as outlined below

Treatment of Lymphedema

Patient should use special compression sleeves known as lymphedema sleeve on the arm and there are separate ones for the hand and fingers. They come in different sizes and can be measured for the appropriate size. It compresses the arm and prevents or keeps the swelling down. The earlier the sleeve is used after surgery, the less likely swelling of the arm will occur.

Keeping the arm from hanging down also helps to reduce the swelling. If the arm keeps swelling a physical therapist is needed to treat it and reduce the swelling with special treatments with a compression pump and arm sleeve. Some patients may have the pump system which they use at home periodically.

Hormonal Treatment
What is It?

Certain breast cancers are sensitive to female hormones called Estrogens and Progesterone. These hormones cause these particular breast cancer cells to grow. Once it is determined that the cancer is the type that can thrive on these hormones, then efforts are made to deprive the cells of the hormones by using drugs that compete or block these hormones. Hormonal therapy is usually an added treatment to prevent cancer from re-occurring.

These drugs are usually given after the initial treatment of the breast cancer by surgery, chemotherapy, or radiotherapy. Not everyone with breast cancer receives hormonal therapy; it is for those whose cancer cells test positive for the female hormones receptors. Examples of these medicines are TAMOXIFEN, TOREMIFENE, and FULVESTRANT.

Tamoxifen (Nolvadex)

It can be used in both pre-menopausal and post-menopausal women. This attacks to cancer cells and prevents or blocks estrogen from getting to the cells, thereby hindering multiplication and growth of cancer cells. It is a pill which is taken daily for between 5 and 10 years. It works by:

- Preventing breast cancer from recurring in women who have been diagnosed and treated for breast cancer
- Preventing breast cancer from developing in the other breast
- Preventing breast cancer in women who are at high risk for developing breast cancer
- Decreasing the size of breast tumors in women who have Metastatic breast cancer
- While suppressing Estrogen in the breast, it actually also increases estrogen in some other tissues like the Endometrium (lining of the uterus)

Side Effects of Tamoxifen

Tamoxifen has side effects like any other medicine and the common ones include:

- Tiredness, vaginal discharge, hot flashes, night sweats, amenorrhea, menstrual irregularities, cataracts, bone pains, and mood swings. These symptoms are similar to those peri-menopausal women experience when going through the change

- Other side effects include blood clot in the legs (deep vein thrombosis – DVT) or in the lungs (Pulmonary Embolism – PE)
- DVT will present with redness, pain, and swelling in the calf area of the legs, and PE presents with shortness of breath, difficulty in breathing, and chest pain. Any one on Tamoxifen who experiences any of the above has to go to the emergency room or see their doctor as soon as possible
- Rare but serious side effects include, thickening of the lining of the endometrium and possible Endometrium Hyperplasia or Endometrial Cancer in mainly post-menopausal women (incidence is less than 1%). Any bleeding from the vagina in a post-menopausal woman has to be reported to a health care provider. However, it has been found that the risk of Endometrium Cancer in pre-menopausal women is not any greater than in other women who are not taking the medicine

Aromatase Inhibitors (AI)

Examples are Anastrozole (Arimidex) and Letrozole (Femara). These are used in post-menopausal women who have had breast cancer or in women who have already taken Tamoxifen for over 5 years. They work by blocking an enzyme called Aromatase which converts other hormones or substances to Estrogen; thereby decreasing the amount of estrogen in the body; and preventing the cancer cells from growing. These may be used for five or more years. They have been found to prevent recurrence and prolong survival in post-menopausal women.

Side Effects of Aromatase Inhibitors (AIs)

AIs can thin the bones resulting in decreased bone density and so it has been suggested that any woman before starting an AI should be evaluated for fracture risk, by having a bone density test. If found to have abnormal bone density, then treatment with injectable Osteoporosis medication is preferred as well as exercise which increases bone density. Other side effects include fatigue, nausea and vomiting, bone pain, stiffness of the joints, hot flashes, vaginal dryness, and mood problems. Let your doctor know if you are on this and it is causing side effects.

Hot Flashes and Night Sweats in Breast Cancer Survivors

Breast cancer survivors may develop bothersome hot flashes, night sweats, cold sweats etc. as a result of ovaries removal, chemotherapy induced artificial menopause, or when they are put on Tamoxifen or Aromatase Inhibitors. These are very bothersome for survivors, but unfortunately they cannot take Estrogen and so need to use non hormonal medicines or changes in lifestyle to control these symptoms.

Treatment of Menopausal Symptoms Associated With Breast Cancer

- Lifestyle changes:
  exercising, dressing in layers, avoiding hot showers or beverages, drinking ice water, taking a thermoflask or stainless steel insulated water bottle filled with water and ice with you to bed
- Weight loss may help: achieved by small food portion sizes, exercise and healthy foods
- Medicines Antidepressants (which are not necessarily being used to treat depression in this case) like Venlafaxine and Paroxetine. However, if one is still on Tamoxifen, one should not use Paroxetine because it reduces the effect of Tamoxifen. Other medicines used are Gabapentin (used to treat many other conditions), Clonidine and Methyldopa (blood pressure medications)
- The use of CAM supplements like, Black Cohosh, soy, or isoflavones (Phytoestrogen) have been found not to be anymore effectiveness than placebo. Soy and isoflavones may have Estrogen like effects and so should be avoided.

Immunotherapy

What is It?

This is when chemicals are used to boost the ability of the body's immune system fight the cancer cells. Immunotherapy is also known as biological therapy. It works by using the body's immune system to fight the cancer cells and has been used for lung, kidney, and bladder cancers and now its being used for breast cancer, especially the HERS positive and Triple negative breast cancer. Another subsets are called Immune Checkpoint Inhibitors.

It is believed immune therapy works by:

- Stimulating the immune system to produce cells to fight the cancer cells
- Antibodies are introduced to attack the cancer cells and destroy them
- Antibodies may be attached to a toxic substance
- Others are proteins which help the immune system to recognize non cancer cells and do not attack them, but attack only cancer cells
- Examples of antibodies with antitumor activities include: Ado-trastuzumab (Kadcyla) which is used to treat metastatic breast cancer in women who are HERS2 positive. Another is Pembrolizumab (Keytruda) which is an immune checkpoint inhibitor and has been used for treating Metastatic Triple Negative Breast Cancer

Targeted Cancer Therapy
What is It?

According to the National Cancer Institute (a US government organization), Targeted Cancer therapies are drugs that block and decrease spread of cancer cells by working at the molecular level on just the cancer cells and not on other cells of the body, for example, hair cells which standard chemotherapy affects. The medicines against HERS 2 positive breast cancer target the high amounts of the protein receptor produced by the cancer cells and block them from receiving signals to grow and multiple.

Examples: Trastuzumab (Herceptin), Pertuzumab (Perjeta), and Palbociclib (Ibrance). Targeted therapies are started after regular treatments and these have fewer side effects and can be used for longer periods of time.

Life During Treatment of Breast Cancer

During the fight with cancer, not only should the disease be fought with the methods described above, but there is often a mental and spiritual struggle as well which needs to be tackled. It is important to get support from family, friends, and other breast cancer survivors. Due to early detection and aggressive treatment of breast cancer, most women are surviving after defeating breast cancer. In developed countries, the 5 year survival rate for breast cancer is greater than 90%. This means on the average, if 100 women are diagnosed with breast cancer and they are treated, after 5 years it is expected about 90 of them will be still alive.

A woman who survives from breast cancer has much to teach other women, however; she has to have gone through or be going through her own recovery physically, mentally, and spiritually to be able to teach or help another woman.

We have previously discussed some of the physical distress which may occur and how they can be handled during Chemotherapy, Radiation and Surgical treatments. Have a positive attitude and stay informed about your treatment protocol. Getting information about your disease and treatment is a great way of getting informed.

Remember to pose questions to your breast cancer treatment team. Keep a notebook and write down questions and answers which come up.

Many women also do "journaling" by documenting their journey through breast cancer diagnosis and treatment. This helps remind them about how far they have come.

Life After Breast Cancer

After breast cancer or gynecological cancers in women who have been cured or they have been rendered disease free, there are certain medical problems which are unique to them. These include:

- Infertility (not able to have children)
- Sexual dysfunction
- Early menopause

Women may find themselves in a dilemma because their oncologist or cancer doctor during follow up may not bring up these issues or counsel them about these problems. This is even a problem in developed countries where only about 50% of cancer survivors receive any counseling on reproductive health, fertility, and sexual health according to the North American Menopause Society.

The issues which Doctors, Oncology nurses, or Nurse navigators have to address with survivors include:

- Issues relating to long term effects of cancer treatment
- Ongoing side effects of cancer treatment (those mentioned above)
- Psychological issues e.g., depression, anxiety, or fear of recurrence
- Fear or shame of letting people know about their disease
- Chronic diseases they may have e.g., hypertension, high cholesterol, diabetes, or heart disease etc.
- Lifestyle changes which will prevent development of chronic diseases
- Screening for other cancers e.g., Pap smear for Cervical cancer and Colonoscopy/Sigmoidoscopy for Colorectal cancer

Preventive Health for Cancer Survivors
Cancer Screening

If one has cancer of one part of her body, there is a greater chance of developing cancer in another organ of the body and so approved cancer screening tests if available should be performed. For example, if a woman has cancer of the breast she should be regularly screened for other cancers like, Colon or Cervical cancer.

Attention to Chronic Diseases

Apart from screening for cancers, a survivor also needs care for chronic diseases which may develop or which she already has. Just like the general population, preventive health is important for cancer survivors. Recently, the Siteman Cancer Center at Barnes-Jewish Hospital and Washington University School of Medicine in the USA have developed a brochure for cancer survivors:

"Cancer Survivors' 8ight Ways to Stay Healthy after Cancer"

It encourages cancer survivors to do the following;

1. Don't smoke
2. Avoid secondhand smoke
3. Exercise regularly
4. Avoid weight gain
5. Eat a healthy diet
6. Drink alcohol in moderation, if at all
7. Stay connected with friends, family, and other survivors
8. Get screening tests and go for your regular check-ups

At regular checkups you must have blood pressure, cholesterol and blood sugar checked periodically so that if any of them is abnormal it can be treated quickly.

(Siteman Cancer Center at Barnes-Jewish Hospital and Washington University School of Medicine, 2013).

Complementary and Integrative Medicine (CIM) Use In Cancer Patients

What is It?

This is the use of products and practices of non main stream origin (complementary), or when complementary approaches are incorporated into mainstream health care (Integrative) in a coordinated way.

Studies on CIM Use and Survival Rates in Cancer Patients

It is well known that a number of cancer patients may use CIM therapies during treatment to help with side effects of therapy, for example, nausea and vomiting, or to help with pain control. Recent reviews of several studies by Dr. Moshe Frenkel and others, on the effect of complementary and integrative medicine (CIM) use during and after cancer treatment indicate that, some of them prolong survival if used alongside conventional medicine. Examples of these therapies are physical exercise, body mind practices (like guided imagery, meditation, and yoga), nutrition, supplements, and stress reduction. Increased vegetable intake has also been found to prevent recurrence in breast cancer patients. In other studies, body and mind practices which tend to reduce stress led to increased survival rates. Therefore, it's important that exercise, diet, and stress reduction must be a part of strategies to prevent recurrence in cancer patients. (Frenkel, M., Sierpina, V. & Sapire, K. Curr. Oncol. Rep (2015)17: 21).

Certain Oncologists (Doctors who treat cancer patients), include these therapies in their treatment of cancer patients right from the beginning. For example, some studies have shown that in breast cancer patients, Tamoxifen (a hormone therapy) can prevent risk of recurrence by 40%; however, physical exercise if performed regularly prevents risk of recurrence by 50%. However, this is not stressed or made known to breast cancer patients so they can make physical exercise a serious part of their prevention action.

Self Help Things You Can Do to Help Your Survival

- Self-help through self-education, self care, and socialization
- Self education by reading about the disease on line, in books, or magazines
- Self care physical attributes especially exercise and diet
- Mental and Spiritual well being are important because it is important to nurture and feed your soul and spirit
- Your soul has to do with your intellect, feelings, emotions, and will. Find ways of enriching these areas through stimulation of your mind and having healthy relationships with family and friends
- Minimize stress in your life
- Having a social support system is a great way to help you continue on your journey of being a survivor
- Spiritually, get connected with God your creator and others of like faith

Connecting With Other Breast Cancer Survivors

- A breast cancer support group can be a great support system for you and connecting with other breast cancer survivors cannot be over emphasized
- You are able to help others who have just started the journey of living after breast cancer or who are going through treatment. There is no need to be ashamed of having had the disease
- Groups like these help to create awareness of the disease and also help other women to recognize the importance of early detection through screening

Anti Inflammatory Drugs (NSAIDS) and Breast Cancer

In a recent study in 2014 published in a breast cancer research journal, researchers found that in post-menopausal women with Estrogen-Receptor-Positive breast cancer who are overweight or obese, the risk of the breast cancer recurring or returning is reduced when they were taking daily Non-Steroidal Anti-Inflammatory Drugs (NSAIDs) such as, Aspirin or Ibuprofen. They also were found to be disease free for a longer time. Therefore, it may be a good idea for women in this subset of cancer survivors to take NSAIDS. Whether other women with other types of cases may have similar benefits is yet to be determined (AACR Cancer Research, Bowers, L. et al. Aug. 2014. vol. 74, issue 16). However; discuss all medicines with your doctor first.

Weight and Breast Cancer

Studies have shown that being obese at the time of breast cancer diagnosis is associated with a higher risk for cancer-related death. This may be because of elevated levels of inflammation cells found in obese patients. Recent study results have shown that low fat diet associated with weight loss after breast cancer diagnosis led to increased survival in a subset of breast cancer patients with Estrogen and Progesterone Receptor Negative disease. This is quite a common type of cancer in black women and this type of breast cancer tends to be aggressive. Therefore, survivors in general should eat low fat diet and exercise to lose weight.

Prevention of Second Breast Cancer in Other Breast

Research has shown that breast cancer survivors have a two to six fold higher risk of developing breast cancer in the other breast. To prevent the disease, following points are helpful:

- Work on changing these lifestyle risks: Obesity, excessive alcohol intake, and smoking
- Chemotherapy and Hormone therapy use: Tamoxifen and Aromatase inhibitors (for example Anastrozole (Arimidex) and Letrozole)
- Prophylactic double mastectomy in preventing Ductal Carcinoma Insitu (DCIS) breast cancer in the opposite breast has been questioned ('Unique' DCIS Study: Double Mastectomy Not Needed – Medscape – May 02, 2017)
- Bilateral prophylactic mastectomy: For women who have inherited defective BRCA1 and BRCA 2 genes, or other genes which put one at increased risk for breast cancer, or have a strong family history of breast cancer, their risk can be decreased by having this surgery (https://www.cancer.gov/types/breast/risk-reducing-surgery-fact-sheet)

The surgeons will examine the total risk factors of a woman and accordingly after discussion with the patient will take the best decision.

Screening for Breast Cancer After Surgery

There are different scenarios depending on type of breast surgery and or reconstruction of the breast.

- For those who have had a mastectomy and breast reconstruction using fat, there is no need for screening mammograms on a continuous basis. It is important to have yearly clinical breast examinations and the survivor can also do monthly self-breast examinations

- For those with mastectomy without reconstruction, there is no need for mammograms of that breast because there is not enough breast tissue available
- If one had a lumpectomy one still needs annual screening mammogram
- If there is reconstruction after a simple, modified radical, or radical mastectomy, there is **no need** for routine mammograms, according to the American Cancer Society unless there is an area of concern, and in that case diagnostic mammogram, ultrasound and MRI can be done
- Those who have skin sparing mastectomy when the nipple and tissue underneath it are preserved, there is **still need for** annual mammograms (American Cancer Society) https://www.cancer.org/cancer/breast-cancer/ screening-tests-and-early-detection/ mammograms/having-a-mammogram-after-youve-had-breast-cancer-surgery.html)

Detection of Breast Cancer

In effect, this is screening for breast cancer in someone without symptoms. Early detection is the key to successful treatment or cure. To have a successful outcome, there should be screening for breast cancer so it can be detected early. The death rates from breast cancer in developed countries have been decreasing over the last few years due to increased awareness, screening, and improved treatment methods. The recognized ways to screen for breast cancer include a three part action plan, according to the American Cancer Society.

Self-Breast Examinations (Breast Awareness)

Although it has been debated whether this saves lives, it has been found to lead to early treatment. Some experts do not recommend it, however it is good for a woman to know what her breasts feel like so that if there is a new lump, mass, or thickness she quickly recognizes it. Those in countries without regular Mammogram availability need to do this. The best time to do this examination, if you still menstruate is about 7–10 days from the start of the period. If you are post-menopausal just fix a particular day of the month and do it at that time; for example, you may choose the first day of each month or the last day of each month.

Learn How To Do Breast Self Examinations

It is important that prior to starting breast self-examinations one goes to a health professional for an examination and be taught how to do the examination properly. The health professional after examining and declaring that there is nothing of concern in the breasts, will then make you confident to do your own self breast examinations. You can also look at videos on the internet which teach how to do self-breast examinations.

Breast Examination Using A Breast Light

Several devices have been developed to enhance a woman's self breast examination and a prototype consists of a hand held infrared light which one shines in a systematic way on different parts of the breast in a darkened room. Veins and blood vessels appear as dark lines and any tumors/masses may show up as shadows. However, experts believe it gives women a false sense of assurance and the mammogram should be the screening choice. On the other hand, in low resource countries where mammograms may not be readily available, this may be useful in the hands of a health professional. Examples are:

The Breastlight device

Sold in the UK and other countries for women to use alongside with self breast examinations. It has been criticized as making false claims about what the device can do. (http://www.dailymail.co.uk/health/article-2215339/Breastlight-Thousands-misled-torch-claims-detect-breast-cancer).

Breast-i

This is an improved version of the Breastlight device. It is a handheld optical device which uses red light to illuminate the breast in a dark room. It has been described as effective and reliable Adjunct Screening Tool to clinical breast examination for detecting breast cancer. A study in Ghana in 2018 found that screening using Breast-i discovered an additional 22 suspicious lesions which could not be detected with an examination by a health professional (CBE). After biopsy it was found that Breast-i detected 24 cancers giving it the sensitivity of 92.3% at detecting breast cancer. The health professional examination picked up 19 cases and thus had a sensitivity of 73%. (https://www.hindawi.com/journals/ijbc/2018/2539056)

Health Professional Examination (Clinical Breast Exam – CBE)

If you don't have access to regular mammograms, you will have to consult a trained health professional to do your breast examination. This is known as a Clinical Breast Examination (CBE). Some doctors, especially in developing countries, are not proactive in conducting preventive examinations like, breast exams. So, you need to go and ask your doctor to do your breast examination and to refer you to go and have the BILATERAL SCREENING MAMMOGRAM test done. Explain to them that you want to do self-breast examinations by yourself, so, you would like him/her to check your breasts for the first time, and secondly teach you how to do it properly. Once you get to know how to do this self examination, then you can do it on your own with confidence. A CBE can be done once a year after the age of 40 years and at interval of every 3 years between the age of 20–40 years.

Screening Mammography
What is It?

This is the main or gold standard screening test for breast cancer. A Mammogram is a special x-ray imaging to detect abnormal growths in breast tissues. These include infection, benign tumors, cancers, or fluid filled sacs (cysts). Before your examination, you may have to fill a questionnaire asking you about your breast history, for example, previous breast issues like biopsies, surgery, etc. and family history of breast cancer.

What does the examination entail?

During such an examination, the technician compresses each breast between 2 plates and takes two pictures of each breast. It may be a little uncomfortable but lasts less than 15 to 20 minutes and most women don't have any problems with it. It is important that the breasts are flattened so that any lump present can be detected. If the radiologist who reads it is unsure of a particular dense spot or image, he will request more images to be taken or he/she may recommend an additional ultrasound or MRI of the breast.

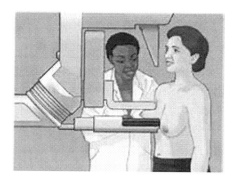

(www.onlinehealthcareservices.wordpress.com/tag/mammography-test)

Please, get a mammogram done if available in your community because it may save your life. Your children, husband, and loved ones will want you around for many years. The United States Preventative Services Task Force (USPSTF) recommends women at average risk aged between 50 to 74 years to have a screening mammogram every two years and for careful consideration before starting between 40 and 49 years for those with average risk. Some other organizations advocate starting at age 40 years. Most medical organizations recommend stopping screening mammograms at age 75 years, however; many issues like life expectancy, frailty, and medical or ill health have to be taken into consideration. Someone who is bed bound with severe chronic diseases may not need them, but someone who is 80 year old, healthy and active may continue with screening.

A study in 2008, showed that those who were 80 years old and above and had regular mammograms tend to have early treatable breast cancer compared to those who did not have regular mammograms (zero or one exam in 5 years). They were also likely to be living 5 years after diagnosis compared with the latter group. In effect, there is no upper age limit (http://www.breastcancer.org/research-news). A recent study on those who are above 75 years also showed that cancer was discovered at an earlier stage and gave them better prognosis (Malmgren, J., Parikh, J, Atwood, M. et al. Improved Prognosis of Women Aged 75 and Older with Mammography-detected Breast Cancer. Radiology Aug. 2014, Vol. 273, No. 3).

How to Prepare for A Successful Mammogram Examination

Some women refuse to have a mammogram because they have heard horror stories of how painful the exam is. Most women who have had a baby naturally have experienced labor and delivery pain which is far more painful than a Mammogram exam. There are a few things a woman can do to make the exam a more comfortable or tolerable experience.

1. Arrive early to have time to fill the necessary paperwork
2. Have information about your breast health and previous mammograms. If possible bring copies of previous mammograms with you because if you are using a new facility, they would want the previous ones to compare with the new one
3. Drink lots of fluids, so you are well hydrated
4. For a woman who is still having menses, the best time to have a mammogram is about a week after your period when the breasts are not swollen or tender. This will reduce the discomfort when the breast is squeezed between the 2 plates of the machine
5. On the day of the exam if possible don't wear any powder or deodorant under your breasts or under your armpits. If you have to, remember to go and wash them off before the exam. These can interfere with the reading of the mammogram
6. Instead of a dress, wear something that is 2 piece so that you take off the top and keep your lower part on – whether it is skirt, trousers/pants or long skirt
7. Each breast will be placed between two plates and then pressed briefly. The different views of each breast will be taken, and the whole process will take 20–25 minutes
8. After the mammograms are read or reviewed by the radiologist, they may sometimes ask you to have additional studies done because of some shadow or very dense breast tissue present. He or she may ask for additional views of mammogram and or ultrasound of the breasts

9. Mammograms do not detect all breast cancers. About 10% of breast cancers are missed by Mammograms

Other Breast Imaging Studies

DIAGNOSTIC MAMMOGRAM: When a screening mammogram shows some abnormality and the particular breast needs more detailed study, then a diagnostic mammogram is ordered together with an ULTRASOUND of that breast. The diagnostic mammogram involves taking additional views of the breast to get better views of a density or mass seen in the breast.

ULTRASOUND is often used along with a diagnostic mammogram to help radiologists have a better look at a mass or lump identified in the breast. For example, it may help distinguish between a Cyst (fluid filled sac) and a solid breast mass. It is also used to aid or guide doctors to do a biopsy of a breast lump right in the Radiology department.

MAGNETIC RESONANCE IMAGING (MRI) is used for women with dense breasts and has recently been recommended for normal screening. It has been found to be more sensitive in detecting small breast abnormalities, than traditional mammograms. The advantage is that it does not expose women to radiation; however, it may lead to more unnecessary breast biopsies since most lumps seen tend not to be cancerous but benign.

3-D Mammography (Breast Tomosynthesis).

This is known as 3-D Mammography, or Digital Breast Tomosynthesis (DBT), and it overlays 3-D optical mammogram images with x-ray to acquire three-dimensional images of the breast with more layers of breast tissue, while a conventional mammogram produces a 2-dimension image of the breast. 3-D mammogram is used as screening to evaluate women with dense breast tissue as well as women at high risk of breast cancer due to family history or if they have certain breast cancer-causing genes present. It helps differentiate benign lesions from malignant ones to a greater extent, and studies show it discovers more cancers and have less false positives compared to conventional 2-D mammograms and so less recalled patients for additional studies. It also shows a decrease in interval cancers (JAMA Oncology, Feb. 2016). It is being used for routine screening in some places and women are offered that option. It costs more than a regular mammogram.

23

Changes Women Go Through The Years (Transitions)

Women go through physical and physiological changes throughout their lives and this is mostly dependent on their female hormonal status. The levels of these hormones change with age. They are low in the pre teen and teenage years, maximum during the reproductive years when childbirth is possible, and then they decrease in the peri, menopausal, and post-menopausal transitional years. Each of these will be discussed in detail and it is advisable that you discuss the information from the premenarche to adolescent health portions with your daughters, grand daughters, or any young girl in your life.

The major different stages are listed below:

Premenarche
Beginning of menstruation (MENARCHE)
Adolescent Health
Reproductive years
Infertility
Adoption
Ovulation and Conception
Preconception
Pregnancy
Family planning/contraceptives
Perimenopause
Menopause
Post-menopause

Sources of Information for This Entire Section

(Medscape.com, WebMD.com; Family Planning Program CHC Inc. Channing Bete Company, 2010; Familydoc.org, North American Menopause Society). Others are mentioned within the topics.

Premenarche (Before Menarche) – Maturation Period
What is It?

This is the time in the life of a female before menstruation starts. It is a time of maturation and growth of the body and mind and its known as puberty. About a year prior to menarche, there is a rapid increase in reproductive hormones in the brain which affects a female child's body and mind. The changes in the body, reproductive organs and emotions were discussed in the first part of the book, however we will mention some of the challenges that occur during puberty.

Challenges

Physical and Emotional: The physical changes can cause them to be embarrassed or confused. The changes in the mind during this time cause the pre teen and teenage girl to have fluctuating emotions. Mothers or a female guardian may play a significant role by helping a young girl cope with and get a better understanding of the avalanche of changes.

The areas they can be helped with include emotions, relationships, body changes and body image, sex, along with illegal drugs, alcohol and tobacco use (substance abuse). Resources like: familydoctor.org; girlshealth.gov, and www. cdc.gov/ncbddd/childdevelopment, are helpful resources adults in their lives can access to gain information on how to help them cope during this time.

Precocious puberty: This is starting puberty before 8 years in girls and may be a sign of some abnormality in the brain (e.g. tumor, infection or injury), tumors of ovaries in girls or abnormalities of the adrenal glands. (The adrenals are part of a system called "endocrine" system which was discussed earlier on). The parents should let a pediatrician or endocrinologist be consulted if this happens. Various tests and measurements have to be done and if the diagnosis is made the girl will have to be treated.

Beginning Of Menstruation (Menarche)

The time of a girl's first period is known medically as MENARCHE. This typically starts at the age of 12-years when a preteen female will start having her menses. This is about 2 to 3 years after breast development starts.

Menstruation Challenges
Irregularity

The first initial years the menses may be irregular. It will not necessarily be a monthly occurrence and a guardian and the girl herself may get concerned. The reason is because the female hormones which regulate the monthly cycle are not fully operational. There is no need to worry, and reassurance of a girl explaining that with time the periods will be more regular is what is needed. Simple tips like keeping record of when the period starts and ends on a calendar or cell phone can be practiced.

Sanitary and Hygiene Care

Girls have to be taught how to take care of themselves when the period is on. For example, they have to change pads regularly, have to be aware that the second and third days may be the heavy flow days, and that during the period one needs to probably avoid wearing white or light colored clothing during the days of heavy flow.

Menstrual Cramps or Pain (Dysmenorrhea dis-meno-reah)

Menstrual cramps of lower abdomen and or back pain is also known as dysmenorrhea (dis-men-o-ria), and may be accompanied by nausea,vomiting or diarrhea. It may be so severe, that it may affect school and work attendance, and this needs to be addressed by a health care provider. Use of an NSAID like ibuprofen, naproxen, etc. will help decrease both the cramps and the amount of blood flow. (Acetaminophen helps pain but not the flow and is not as helpful as the NSAIDS). There are other OTC medicines like Midol etc. which people use for pain and bloating. Midol, depending on the type may contain acetaminophen, naproxen, ibuprofen, pamabrom, caffeine, and pyrilamine maleate. If these do not work, an older adolescent may be put on birth control pills, which will decrease the pain and amount of flow at the same time. The adolescent should be cautioned that it is not a "license" for sexual activity, and if they choose to be, birth control pills do not protect one against STDs.

Adolescent Health

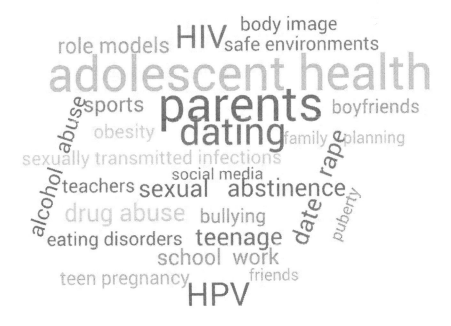

Adolescence: Challenges and Solutions
Introduction

Early Sexual Activity
Eating Disorders
Sexual Transmitted Infections (STIs) and HIV
Pregnancy
Illegal Abortions
Birth Control and Contraceptives
Immunizations
Sexual Education
Body Image Issues
Mental Health Challenges
Suicide Attempts
Drug and Alcohol Abuse
Tobacco Abuse
Social Challenges
Bullying
Peer Pressure
Sexting
Violence
Sexual Abuse and Rape
Dating Violence
Challenging Educational Issues for Girls

Introduction

An adolescent (from word adolescence meaning "grow up" in Latin) is a young person who is developing into an adult. Other synonyms are youth, teenager or juvenile, and it's a transitional stage when there are changes in body, thinking, emotions, and one may add spiritual life as well. It generally starts around puberty which is around 10-years, and goes up to 19-years according to the World Health Organization. However, ages may vary according to culture and country. This period may also be divided into:

Early Adolescence (10–13): They grow quickly, with body changes described under puberty. They become self conscious and may have anxiety about these. They think in concrete terms and get "selfish" or egocentric. There may be conflict with parents as they seek to be independent and test their boundaries.

Middle Adolescence (14–17): They continue with physical changes and may develop acne, with periods becoming regular now. They become sexually attracted to boys, with image issues and Peer Pressure becoming prominent. Struggles and defiance of adults in their lives continue. Mentally although aware of consequences of risks, they let emotions and impulsivity control most decision making, resulting in risky behavior like early sexual activity and substance abuse.

Late Adolescence (18–21) years: Physically have attained their maximum height and completed physical development. Mentally, they are less impulsive and think more maturely about the consequences of their actions. They have a better relationship with adults in their lives, and relationships with opposite sex are more stable. They develop goals and plans for their future, becoming more independent. (https://www.healthychildren.org/English/ages-stages/teen/Pages/Stages-of-Adolescence.aspx).

In every stage, they face a lot of pressures from changes in physical, sexual, emotional, mental state, as well as from social media issues which is of great importance these days. What girls face today is a far cry or enormous compared to what their parents or even ladies born in the 1980s faced growing up. We will address some of these in this section.

Help for Adolescent Girls

There are things girls can do to avoid some of the upheavals or disruptions during this time, and there are things girls and adult figures in their lives can do to minimize risks, protect them, and promote their health. To help them, a collective effort should be done on the part of:

Parents and Guardians
Schools
Government at Local and National levels
Community in which they live

Health risk behaviors and issues facing adolescents and strategies and solutions are briefly discussed in this section. There is no doubt the home environment plays a very important role in nurturing, encouraging, and affirming the adolescent. If no responsible or caring adult is in the home, then caring adults in the community can help a young person as they go through these challenging times. This is when teachers, school counselors, adults who are leaders of church, social, or athletic groups which young people are involved in, can step in, and complement what the youth is getting from home; or even take up this task if there is no support from home.

Early Sexual Behavior

This can lead to transmission of STIs/HIV, Pelvic Inflammatory Disease (PID) and also result in pregnancy. Pregnancy is a high risk physical and psychological state for girls who are now developing; and physically may not have a wide enough pelvis to deliver a baby naturally. Psychologically, they may not be mature enough to take care of a baby, and it can also cut short schooling opportunities leading to lack of economic mobility and poverty. Sex and health education are important to keep them informed and prevent this. Teaching appropriate sexual health education to girls does not mean you are giving them a "license" to start engaging in sex (referred to as being sexually active), rather this empowers them to know about the consequences of early sexual activity, and advantages of delaying sex.

Eating Disorders: Anorexia Nervosa and Bulimia

Anorexia Nervosa (A-no-rez-sia)
What is It?

Societal pressures which equate beauty with thinness has put pressure on young women to try and be thin. However, there are other factors like psychological ones that predispose a girl or woman to become anorexic

Anorexia is an eating disorder which is believed to be more an emotional problem rather than a food problem. This is common and in the USA about 3 million cases are diagnosed each year. Most are young girls and women, and these include models, ballet dancers and female athletes. It may usually start between age 16 to 17 years, but girls as young as 12 years have been diagnosed with it. It occurs in males as well.

Risk Factors

There are many factors that can cause a girl or women to become anorexic, and some identified are genetics, dieting, perfectionism, low self-esteem, obsessive compulsive trait, and social perception of equating beauty with "thinness".

Presentation

In anorexia, there is very low body weight, fear of gaining weight, restricted amount of food eaten, and an altered view of Body Image, as sufferers see themselves as fat. They try every means to lose or maintain their low weight by vomiting after eating, taking laxatives, purging and use of diuretics and enemas.

Complications of Anorexia

This can lead to serious complications like abnormal chemical concentrations in the body, irregular heartbeats, damage to brain, heart and kidney, irregular or no menstruation, osteoporosis (thinning of the bones) fractured bones, and even death. Mental or psychological issues associated with this are depression, anxiety, and low self-esteem.

Bulimia

In bulimia which is another eating disorder, there is binge eating (when a person seems to be out of control and eats a whole lot of food at a time on a regular basis) followed by purging using forced vomiting or extreme exercise to lose weight in order to get rid of excess calories.

Treatment

There is treatment for both conditions including psychological, and medications, either on outpatient or inpatient's basis. It includes counseling, structured eating schedule, healthy eating habits and medications to help correct the emotional aspect.

If you are a young girl and feel you are experiencing either of the above, you don't have to be scared or ashamed but seek help; by letting your parent, guardian or another adult you trust know, and you can be offered treatment. There are support groups available that sufferers can be connected to.

Sexually Transmitted Infections (STIs)/Human Immunodeficiency Virus (HIV)

The STIs Chlamydia and Gonorrhea tend to affect women aged between 15 to 24 years and all of them are discussed in the chapter on Pelvic Conditions and Diseases. Human Papilloma Virus (HPV) is the commonest STI, and about 50% of new HPV infections occur in the age group from 15 to 24 years. Most infected young persons below 21 years will clear the HPV virus from their body through the help of their immune system, however; for some, it can persist leading to genital warts, vulva, vaginal and anal cancers, precancer lesions on the cervix, and even cervical cancer. Cervical cancer is the most common genital cancer in women in Limited Resource Countries with 270,000 women dying every year worldwide. In rich countries, thanks to preventative measures and early treatment the incidence of cervical cancer has decreased. Measures used are education, screening and early detection through VIA (Visual Inspection with Acetic acid), pap smears, HPV testing, and Immunization against the high risk HPV viruses. Immunization in preteens and teens is very important.

How do adolescents prevent STIs and HIV?

By practicing ABCI of sexual disease prevention. These stand for:

1. Abstinence from sexual intercourse
2. Being faithful to one partner
3. Condom use

4. Immunization against the common STIs for which vaccines are available. These include vaccines for HPV, and Hepatitis A and B

Some STIs like HPV and Herpes Simplex can be spread by body to body contact of infected genitals and areas on the penis where condoms do not cover. Improper use of condoms can cause them to slip off, or old ones can also break, however; condom use is important even IF YOU ARE ON BIRTH CONTROL TO PREVENT PREGNANCY, because Birth Control Pills, implanon, or IUD do not protect against STIs and HIV infection. Early treatment if infected also prevents one from developing complications associated with the infections, so if a sexually active young person has vaginal or penile discharge, or wart like growth around the genitals, they should go and get checked at a clinic. Tests can be done to check if you are infected with any STIs and then you can be treated.

Adolescence Pregnancy

"The leading cause of death for girls 15 to 19 worldwide is not accident or violence or disease; it is complications from pregnancy. Girls under 15 are up to five times as likely to die while having children than are women in their 20s, and their babies are more likely to die as well".

—Nancy Gibbs, former managing editor for Time magazine. (quotesgram.com)

Teen pregnancy is common due to reasons which include consented sex without use of a condom or other forms of birth control methods, sexual abuse, assault, and rape. The practice of child/teen marriage occurs in in many countries, and according to UNICEF, the percentage of girls married by the age of 15 years between 2012–2018 varied between 0 to 30%, with highest numbers recorded in Subsaharan Africa. Countries with high percentages – greater than 10% include: Central African Republic, Nigeria, Chad, Bangladesh, Dominican Republic, Eritrea, Ethiopia, Guinea, Mali, Mauritania, Madagascar, and Niger. (https://data.unicef.org/topic/child-protection/child-marriage/).

According to WHO Fact Sheet on Adolescent Pregnancy (World Health Organization. Adolescent pregnancy Fact sheet January 2018) the following occur:

Key facts

- Every year, about 21 million girls aged between 15 to 19 years and 2 million girls less than 15 years become pregnant in low resource countries. About 16 million of the older girls and 2.5 million girls in younger age group give birth each year in these countries

- Worldwide, complications during pregnancy and childbirth are the leading cause of death for 15 to 19 year-old girls. About 3.9 million girls in this same age group undergo unsafe abortions to get rid of unwanted pregnancies
- Adolescent mothers (ages 10 to 19 years) face higher risks of all or most complications associated with pregnancy and delivery. Unfortunately babies born to adolescent mothers face higher risks of low birthweight, preterm delivery, and severe new born conditions than those born to older women (WHO January 2018)

Pregnancy in Teenagers is Dangerous !!!!!

Therefore my advice to adolescents is that they should know the consequences of early sexual activity and make the right choice, knowing that their choices have consequences. If they chose to be sexually active, they should try to minimize the chances of pregnancy by consistent and correct use of condoms and use of a birth control method to prevent pregnancy. Young girls who are forced into marriage unfortunately may not have the means to prevent this, however; at government levels one hopes laws and regulations will be put in place, and women's advocacy groups will help make this practice a thing of the past or at least minimize its occurrence.

Illegal Abortions

Abortion is illegal in many countries due to many reasons including religious, cultural and social. For this reason many young girls who get pregnant and do not want to carry the baby to term can be persuaded by parents or boyfriends to have illegal or unsafe abortions performed. This leads to serious complications like: perforation of the uterus, bleeding, infections and or death of the teenage mother. According to WHO, every year, about 3 million girls aged between 15 to 19 undergo unsafe abortions.

Community Resources for Pregnant Teens

There are many ways governments and communities can help pregnant teenagers. My advice to teenagers who are pregnant and do not want to keep the baby is to consider the following first before making a decision to abort the baby:

- Seek out centers or organizations which take care of pregnant teens: Organizations like Catholic charities, pregnancy crisis centers and other social or religious non-profit organizations are available to help teenagers during the antenatal time (pre delivery), delivery, and arrange adoption or foster care. Some also help the teen mother to either go back to school or enter vocational training, as well as provide daycare for the child

- Consider having the child adopted because there are many childless couples who would love to raise your child
- Talk to a trusted adult about your situation, they may have solutions for you

Psychological Consequences of Abortion

Some women after an abortion have regrets, feel guilt or depressed and may even have Post-Traumatic Stress Disorder. If you have an abortion, whether legally or illegally and you are feeling depressed or guilty, please get help from a counselor, pregnancy crisis center, female pastor or minister, or from a trusted adult.

Birth Control/Contraceptives

Many countries have organizations like Planned Parenthood, other Family Planning/birth control organizations, or Government Clinics which make different birth control methods available for young people who choose to be sexually active. It is advisable for young people to be sexually abstinent until they are in committed relationships like marriage, however; if they choose to be sexually active they need to protect themselves from STIs by using barrier methods like a correctly worn male or female condoms, and from pregnancy by using a suitable birth control method. The various methods are discussed in the section "Changes though the Years" under Birth Control/Contraceptives.

Immunizations/Vaccinations (shots)

There are regular immunizations which are given during the adolescent years and some are routine in economically developed countries and may not be available in Limited Resource Countries. If they are offered, parents are usually encouraged to take their teens for the shots. In some developed countries kids are expected to have their shots before they can be enrolled in middle school. For example in the United States, Preteens and Teens are expected to have:

Tdap (Tetanus, Diphtheria and Pertussis) at age of 11 to 12 years
2 shot HPV series at least 6 months apart at age of 11 to 12 years, or
3 shots with second one 2 months after the first and third one 6 months after the first one
A Meningococcal conjugate vaccine at age of 11 to 12 years (this prevents meningitis)
Group B Meningococcal vaccine booster shot may be given to 16–18 years old
The flu shot is encouraged every year starting around September/October to prevent the influenza virus infection or influenza

Different countries may have other vaccination schedules and so the important thing is to make sure parents take their teenagers and preteens for the shots. I also encourage adolescent girls who read this section to ask their parents about whether they are up to date with their shots, depending on which country they live in.

Lack of Sexual Education

Many countries have some sexual education component included in their education curriculum for students, however, some may not; and some teenagers may get information from the internet, books or from programs organized by nonprofit organizations (NGOs) (for example, my non-profit organization is called Gateway of Hope Inc., and we do health and sexual health education in high schools and for women's groups on our medical mission trips). It is important that young people get reproductive health education from the right sources. Input from religious and civic society need to be included in national reproductive health education for young people.

Parents and Sexual Health Chats with their Kids

Parents and guardians are encouraged to have age appropriate sexual health conversations with their children or wards. I have written a book to help adults feel comfortable and talk to their kids about this so as to prevent sexual abuse. The book is called "A parental Guide on teaching children how to avoid sexual abuse". There are many other books and resources on line which can help parents bring up or initiate the conversation. If parents do not do so, the preteens and teenagers may get the wrong information from friends and other unreliable sources. Formal sex education helps kids delay sexual activity according to a study involving 2,019 teens, aged between 15 to 19 years, who responded to the 2002 National Survey of Family Growth in a 2007 study by the CDC (Trisha E. Mueller, MPH, epidemiologist, Division of Reproductive Health, CDC, Atlanta. Mueller, T. Journal of Adolescent Health January 2008; vol. 42: pp 89–96).

Examples of credible sources are:

CDC – www.cdc.gov/healthyyouth/sexualbehaviors; www.cdc.gov/HealthyYouth
WHO – www.who.int/reproductivehealth/topics/adolescence
UNICEF – www.unicef.org/adolescence/index_73651.html
Familydoctor.org/family-health/kids-and-teen
Your own country's ministry of Health

Remember if you the adult, have religious beliefs which you adhere to, do not expect the authorities, schools, or agencies to necessarily adhere to your views, that is why your talks with your teen are important. One cannot legislate morality and force that on people in general, but you can at least start at home and let your kids know what you believe in and why.

Body Image Issues

Body Image or the way one's body looks is a big issue among teenagers especially in developed countries. As a result of images portrayed on social media, magazines, and TV, societies tend to equate fashion models thinness with beauty. Dieting and losing weight is a big issue and also a big business and teenagers must realize that because they are still growing and need important nutrients for their body, dieting may not be a good idea. Healthy eating is important and that may mean cutting out some sugary drinks or foods that have too much "empty calories". Empty calories foods and drinks supply calories but not beneficial nutrients like vitamins, and proteins.

Overweight and Obese Teens

For teens who are obese or overweight, negative messages and teasing by friends and peers on social media etc. add to their distress. Talk to your doctor or parents if you are facing such issues and get help from trusted people. You can also start cutting back on sugary drinks, empty calories, sugary desserts and eat more fruits, and vegetables. Start walking 3x a week and do a sport you enjoy. That may help you lose some weight gradually, as opposed to that seen on yo yo diets which one cannot maintain.

Downside of "Dieting"

Issues like eating disorders described above may result as teenagers try to look like models seen on the TV and other media. This may lead to conditions like anxiety, depression, low self-esteem and even self-harm or injury practices like "cutting" when people use razor blades or pocket knives to cut their wrists and burning. Remember the models one may see on magazine covers may sometimes have their pictures altered by Photoshop, and some of those thin looking models are suffering from anorexia or bulimia in secret.

Mental Health Issues

"Mental illness is an illness. When you start to understand that, you can start to fix the stigma. When someone is courageous enough to start talking about it, then it opens the doors for treatment and healing."

—Kay Warren, pastor Saddleback Church

All the mental illnesses discussed in the second section of the book under section MENTAL HEALTH can affect teenagers and young adults. These include depression, anxiety, obsessive compulsive disorder, post traumatic stress disorder (PTSD), bipolar disorder, schizophrenia, and chronic stress. Others often found in young people are ADHD (Attention Deficient Hyperactivity Disorder), self-injury, and addiction to illegal drugs and tobacco. There are telephone hot lines available in many countries, however; if this is not available for you, talking to a trusted adult, or your health care provider or your parents may lead you to get help. There is no need to be ashamed if you have a problem with your mind or emotions, there are often many reasons this may happen and your health care provider can explain things to you. A good website to help people who are affected with mental illness is that of Saddleback church in California, where the pastors young son committed suicide after suffering from depression for many years. Now, since then, both pastors have embraced mental health and are encouraging churches to help those affected (http://kaywarren.com/mentalhealth. https://saddleback.com/connect/ministry/mental-health-ministry).

Suicide Attempts

Suicide is the third leading cause of death for adolescents 15 to 19 years old in the USA and it is often a result of depression, and other mental illnesses like bipolar or borderline personality disorder, drug abuse or social isolation. Of late the importance of bullying related suicides or suicide attempts or thoughts have been documented in studies in the US and Great Britain. The types of bullying include emotional, physical, cyberbullying and sexting. Adolescent boys 15 to 19 years old had a completed suicide rate that is 3 times greater than that of females. However, girls' suicidal attempts are twice the rate of that of boys. Each year according to the CDC, about 4,600 young people commit suicide in the US, and for every completed suicide there are at least 100 suicide attempts. Data compiled by CDC in 2017, showed that in 1975, in the United States, there were 1,289 suicides among males and 305 suicides among females aged 15–19 years. In 2015, there were 1,537 suicides among males and 524 among females aged 15–19 year with the female rate doubling in 2015 (CDC. National Vital Statistics System, mortality data. https://www.cdc.gov/nchs/nvss/deaths.htm).

The leading methods of suicide for the 15 to 19 years age group in 2013 were suffocation (43%), discharge of firearms (42%), poisoning (6%), and falling (3%) according to the CDC.

Prevention of Suicide

Involvement of the whole Community

Suicide is preventable if friends, school teachers, and family detect behavior and statements that signify trouble.

They have to look out for an adolescent(s) who is(are):

- Showing signs or communicating on social media that they plan to harm themselves

- Those who are being bullied, taunted, teased or made fun of
- Making statements like "they are fed up with life" and "not happy"
- Show no interest in things they used to do or isolate themselves
- Such youth need to be reported to guidance counselors or responsible adults and then be referred to appropriate places for help
- Depressed or showing signs of changes in their moods and social interaction

Teaching kids in Schools Suicide Prevention Strategies

Additionally, there are suicide prevention strategies which should be taught in schools to students and in communities to parents, coaches, teachers and guardians. These include:

- Taking shame out of mental illness
- Diagnosis and treatment of mental illnesses
- General suicide education for students in schools like, giving students information, what the warning signs are, and how and where to seek help if needed
- Information about Peer support groups, suicide hotlines and crisis support centers
  (CDC, youth suicide prevention programs A resource guide 9/1992). This resource may be applicable to adolescents in all countries and not just the USA.

Risk factors for Suicide

These include the following:

Mental illness especially depression
Situational stress at school e.g. bullying
Conflict at home
Presence of a firearm in the house
Physical and previous or current sexual abuse
Family history of suicide
Excessive despair and depression after break up with a girl or boy friend, with verbalization of harming themselves or dying
If a teenager has a plan in place to kill themselves, and discusses desire to die with others

It is important that if any of the risk factors and warning signs mentioned above are present, adults, and peers should be vigilant and get help for them. The help may include medication and ongoing counseling with a trained therapist or psychologist.

Drug and Alcohol Abuse

According to the National Institute of Drug Abuse in the US, by the time adolescents are in last year of high school, almost 70 percent of students will have tried alcohol, and 50% would have used an illegal drug. About 40 percent would have smoked a cigarette, and more than 20 percent would have used a prescription drug for a nonmedical purpose. In other countries the same trend is seen and youth are being exposed to illegal drug use leading to addictions (e.g. high dose Tramadol and codeine containing cough syrups in some African countries), wrecked lives and death from overdose.

Spike in Opioid Drug Abuse

There has been a rise in opioid abuse use especially in the USA, namely oxycodone, hydrocodone, fentanyl which are legal, but the worse is heroin with 15,466 deaths in 2016. Fentanyl is a synthetic opioid drug which is either used alone or it is mixed with other drugs like marijuana and cocaine and that leads to overdose deaths. It is mainly imported illegally from China. According to the CDC 64,070 people died of drug overdose in 2016, and on average 115 Americans die every day from an opioid overdose (www.cdc.gov/drugoverdose/epidemic/index). Data is even worse for 2017. CDC found that in 2017 over 70,000 Americans died from drug overdose and this is more than deaths from HIV, automobile accidents and gun violence. Fentanyl deaths increased by 45%, and drug overdoses are the leading cause of deaths for adults under 55 years (www.cdc.gov/nchs/data. NCHS Data Brief. No. 329. Nov. 2018). Between 1999 and 2015, teens aged 15 to 19 years had double the drug overdoses seen previously. Deaths from overdose continue to rise and it has been termed an "opioid epidemic".

Reasons for Drug and Alcohol Abuse

Most adolescents may engage in risky behavior of abusing drug and alcohol because of several reasons including; tendency to feel invincible, peer pressure, family environment (others are using them, or dysfunctional family associated with abuse, violence etc.), genetics, and school and neighborhood environments to name a few. The adolescence brain up to age of early 20s is still developing and the area of the brain – front part or frontal lobe – which controls judgement and self-control is still not mature, so irrational actions and ideas may prevail.

Prevention

This can be tackled on several fronts and these include:

Reversal of Criminalization of Drug Abuse

The "war on drugs" approach of criminalizing drug abuse where resources and funding are channeled to punitive measures against those addicted to drugs does not work, rather prevention, treatment, recovery support, overdose reversal and preventing pharmaceutical companies from flooding the market with opioids should supersede the "war on drugs".

Halting Supply Chain

The over prescription by doctors and the "pill mills" which are medical offices who "treat" chronic pain with prescription painkillers or narcotics without adequately assessing the individual have also fueled the excessive use of legal narcotics and overdose of these drugs. Pharmaceutical companies have played down the addictive potential of narcotics and have provided incentives for some doctors to prescribe them. The arrest and prosecution of doctors involved and shut down of pain clinics have occurred in many states. In the US many States have guidelines and policies in place to discourage long term narcotics prescription for noncancer pain, for example, verification of patients supply from other doctors and limits on quantity prescribed.

Use of medication for reversal of overdose

In many developed countries including the US there is availability of Naloxone (Narcan) which is the antidote for opioid overdose and blocks their effects. It is available without a prescription for drug abusers, family, and friends to buy and use to reverse the effects of opioid overdose which includes respiratory depression or slow breathing leading to respiratory arrest; which often is the cause of overdose deaths. It is available as a nasal spray or injectable form.

Programs to help teens stay away from gangs

Teens may join gangs looking for acceptance, "family", approval, and affection and may be introduced to crime, drugs and alcohol. Countries and local governments should invest in programs which will help young people with drug problems. Young people with addiction problems should seek help or be encouraged to do so through treatment and counseling to overcome this problem; and provision of job training programs, and social support systems to help them.

Decriminalization of Marijuana

Decriminalization of drugs like marijuana in small amounts or for personal use, use of medical marijuana and other measures have helped some countries decrease drug related crimes. The resources are then channeled to programs and other things that can help drug addicts; however, there is still debate about decriminalization of marijuana in many countries.

Tobacco Use

Worldwide about 80,000 to 100,000 young people start smoking every day. Tobacco use through the many modalities and electronic cigarettes (e-cigarettes and use is called Vaping) are all abused by teens. The e-cigarette is supposed to help smokers quit smoking, but most times, they continue to smoke and do Vaping as well.

- Tobacco Products
  The main substance in tobacco is nicotine which is extremely addictive, and tobacco smoke has over 60 cancer causing chemicals (carcinogens) in it. The tobacco and nicotine products come in many forms, and people can smoke, chew, sniff, or inhale their vapors. The smokeless tobacco are chewed or sniffed but it tends to be mainly used by men and boys
- Vaping
  Electronic cigarettes or e cigarettes are devices that contain nicotine and flavorings and are battery operated. Puffing activates the heating device without burning tobacco, but vaporizes the liquid in the cartridge. The resulting vapor is then inhaled (called "vaping"). According to the CDC, in 2016, more than two million US middle and high school students used e-cigarettes each month, and they seem to be using it more than regular cigarettes. Research about e-cigarettes show they are not harmless, and the tobacco industry is using fruit and sweet flavors to attract young people to use them. Recently, in 2019, there have been a rush of deaths and serious lung problems with admission into hospital ICU of young people who had been Vaping. It is believed that the Vaping liquid may have been spiked with THC oils (psychoactive substance in marijuana) or other substances. The CDC has asked young people to stop Vaping. Although the regular e cigarettes contain less nicotine than regular cigarettes, the actual nicotine intake by e-cigarette smokers is about the same as regular cigarette users (Johns Hopkins Bloomberg School of Public Health, 2015)

Side effects of Nicotine

- Nicotine can affect the developing brain in fetuses as well as in the maturing brains of kids up to the age of 20 years
- Nicotine can affect the lungs, making people more susceptible to developing pneumonia by causing inflammation of the lung tissues
- Nicotine affects the immune system in a negative way
- Vaping may release some heavy metals from the heated coils in the device into the body

- Second hand smoke may release particles into the environment which may affect the lungs and heart of others (teens.drugabuse.gov/drug-facts/tobacco-nicotine-e-cigarettes)
- People have had burn injuries from defective vaping devices catching fire
- Young people who Vap may graduate to smoking regular cigarettes later on in life

All the above show that nicotine in whatever form it's consumed is harmful and young people have to be discouraged from starting the habit in the first place, since nicotine is very addictive. Important message to the youth is that using nicotine in whatever form is not "cool" and there are many health issues associated with it.

Helpful Tips for Quitting Nicotine abuse

Those already smoking can get help with smoking cessation by:

- The use of nicotine replacement therapy like nicotine patches, gum or lozenges Counseling on phone or in person
- Approved medications like Bupropion (Zyban and Wellbutrin) and Varenicline (Chantix) which can help with the cravings associated with nicotine withdrawal
- Others like Acupuncture, laser and Hypnosis have been advocated for smoking cessation, but there is not any good research about their effectiveness

These methods are sometimes helpful but most times are not effective in the long term according to a study which reviewed several tobacco control programs for adolescents (Fanshawe et al., Cochrane database of systemic reviews, 2017, issue 11). It is therefore important that adolescents do not start smoking or use nicotine in the first place because quitting nicotine is very hard since it is so addictive.

Social Challenges Teenagers Face
Bullying

Social Media interactions with other young people and even predatory adults is on the rise and parents have to set limits on use of cell phones, tablets and other devices according to age of the youth. Adolescents face a lot of pressure to conform to lifestyle of others or they may also be bullied and shamed by school mates and other young people. Many incidents of youth suicide have occurred all over the world due to social media bullying and shaming. Bullying can also occur in person at schools and other social gathering and young people who are being bullied must not be scared or frightened to report bullies to an appropriate trusted adult. This could be a parent, a school guidance counselor or another trusted adult, for example a youth pastor. Bullies tend to be insecure individuals who may themselves had been bullied in the past or suffered physical abuse or other forms of abuse. Schools must have programs to discourage bullying and encourage victims and other students to report bullies. Websites which adolescents being bullied can turn to include:

> https://pacerteensagainstbullying.org
> https://www.stopbullying.gov/what-is-bullying/index.html
> https://cyberbullying.org/resources/teens

Peer Pressure

Peer Pressure is defined according to the Merriam-Webster on line dictionary as "a feeling that one must do the same things as other people of one's age and social group in order to be liked or respected by them". Peer pressure also known as peer influence can be positive or negative.

Positive peer influence can be:
Joining sports activity, joining clubs or social groups at school, being encouraged to be more assertive, studying hard at school with great goals and aspirations, or trying new positive things because friends are doing them

Negative peer influence can be:
Start being sexually active, joining a gang, breaking the law, drinking, smoking or using drugs at school or in the neighborhood all for acceptance. Negative peer pressure tends to occur in teenagers who feel lonely, have low self-esteem or have some type of a disability and so may be shunned by most kids. They are therefore ready to associate with those who may show some interest in them and start hanging out or spending time with them even though their actions and character may be different from what they believe in

Dealing with Negative Peer Pressure

There are resources for teens who find themselves associating with friends who have ideals or actions contrary to what they believe in. The following are ideas which may help you as a teenager when negative peer pressure is trying to influence you.

- Be prepared and go over in your mind or talk to yourself in front of the mirror practicing what you can say to friends who want you to do something against your will, values or beliefs. Look peers in the eye, stand straight and do not be frightened to calmly resist what they are suggesting which you do not want to do

- Try to avoid friends who want you to do things against your values and what matters to you. Have a prepared plan for when a parent or trusted adult can help you when in sticky situations, e.g. call or text them with a coded message to come and get you
- Be bold to discuss peer influences with a trusted adult like a parent, guardian or other adult. It does not mean you are weak. It takes boldness and it is a sign of maturity and not weakness to talk with them
- Avoid places where you feel uncomfortable because your peers may be up to doing things you may not like to do. Suggest alternative places like the mall or park
- Stick with peers who have the same values as yourself. There is a saying that "birds of the same feather flock together". People who have something in common like to be together and so practice that with other adolescents
- Tough choices may keep you isolated, but be proud of yourself if you make them. You should find new friends who have the same values like you
- You have a right to say "No" and you can walk away from situations that are opposite to your values

These and more tips for young people can be found at: www.cdc.gov/bam/life/tough.html. Parents can also get resources from: www.howtolearn.com/2012/10/how-to-resist-peer-pressure

Sexting

According to the Cyberbullying Research Center, Sexting is defined as – "sexting as the sending or receiving of sexually explicit or sexually-suggestive images or video via a cell phone" (Cyberbullying.org/Sexting-Fact-Sheet). However, according to the center, the term can also be used when teenagers send sexually suggestive pictures of themselves on cell phones and send them to either boyfriends or others. Unfortunately, they can also be distributed via social networking sites, email, instant messaging, and video chat. The research center has an excellent handout giving advice to teenagers about Sexting and how and why they should avoid sending and receiving those pictures. Images which are nude are illegal and against the law, and most kids involved do not realize they are breaking the law. Below is their 10 point advice from their Sexting fact sheet:

Sexting Advice for Teens

Sameer Hinduja, Ph.D. and Justin W. Patchin, Ph.D. | Cyberbullying Research Center, May 2016.

1. Delete any explicit images sent to you. Even having these images on your phone could land you in a heap of trouble
2. Do not distribute explicit images. If someone sends you an explicit image of themselves or someone else, do not pass it on to anyone else. Try to think about how you would feel if someone sent similar pictures of you to someone else that you didn't know or wouldn't want to see
3. Ignore or flat-out reject any requests from others for inappropriate images. It is just not worth it, no matter how much you like the other person— even if you think you can trust them. The potential risk is just too high. If they really care about you, they will understand
4. Block individuals who make you uncomfortable with how they talk to you (or what they send to you)
5. Distract the person requesting inappropriate pictures from you. Engage them in conversation about something else, or direct them to a cool YouTube video you just saw, or an app you think they would like. If they continue to ask about the pics, let them know that they should just chill out
6. Don't support your own objectification. You are not a piece of meat. You don't want people to like you because of your body, but because of your mind and heart. Giving in and sending explicit images just feeds their appetite for more, and continues to devalue your worth
7. Sexting doesn't define a healthy, functional romantic relationship. Sure, it's fun, flirtatious, and risqué, but remember that these images could be seen by a wider audience (including your parents, teachers, or the police)
8. Send images that are suggestive, but not explicit. Keep private parts covered at all times. It's fine to send your partner a picture, just make sure it's PG-13 and not X-rated. Even so, realize that these too may be broadcast to others. If you wouldn't be concerned if your whole school (or grandma!) saw it, it's probably ok
9. If you receive (or someone shows you) an explicit image of someone you know, contact that person to tell them that their images are being circulated. You would want someone to tell you if an image of yours like that was going around
10. Inform an adult you trust if you are concerned about the well-being of the person in the image. If you are worried about the person who is in the picture, whether they are a friend or not, you may need to get help from an adult

(Cyberbullying Research Center. Cyberbullying.org)

Violence

Physical violence may be associated with bullying, sexual abuse and rape, intimate partner violence, and gang violence. Choosing the right friends at school and in the neighborhood helps with prevention of violence, as well as staying away from areas associated with crime and violence. Many communities have After school programs, tutoring classes, girls and boys clubs, sports activities etc. which keep teenagers off the streets and not in the company of gangs.

Sexual Abuse and Rape

The other serious condition that face young people especially girls is sexual abuse or assault. Sexual abuse is treated extensively under the chapter "Sexual violence and Domestic Violence". Sexual abuse is any type of sexual activity that is done against your will (forced) and is termed rape when there is penetration of the vagina or anus. It is never the victim's fault, and unfortunately sexual abuse occurs in all countries – both rich and poor.

In the USA, for example about 300,000 cases of child sexual abuse occur every year and only about a third is reported. It is also estimated that one out of every four girl child is abused, and one out of every seven boys will be a victim of sexual abuse before the age of 18 years. However, professionals think the accurate figures are about 30% of girls and about 14% of boys are victims of sexual abuse (www.healthyplace.com). Unfortunately most abuse is committed not by a stranger but by someone who the child or teen is familiar with.

Types of Sexual Abuse against Teenager girls

When it comes to teenager girls, there are many types of sexual abuse/assault against them. Sexual abuse encompassing all types of nonconsensual sexual contact or behavior, and examples of which are:

- Rape – this is sexual penetration of vagina or anus without consent
- Incest – this is forced sexual contact by a relative, for example, brother, father, uncle, cousin
- Date sexual assault or rape – Drug facilitated sexual assault. It may be drugs and or alcohol which inhibit the victim's ability to resist the sexual assault, or make them forget what happened. It is important to mention that these drugs which are referred to as "date drugs" can be used not only on a date, but by a stranger or even a friend to commit sexual assault because the victim is impaired. It can happen at parties when they are slipped into a drink or when just the two are together
- Intimate partner sexual abuse – Sexual assault committed by a partner who is in a relationship with the victim. It can also occur as a date rape – sexual assault while on a date

Dating Violence

This is more than sexual and is very common. Centers for Disease Control and Prevention (CDC) in the USA defines it as "the physical, sexual, psychological, or emotional violence within a dating relationship, including stalking. It can occur in person or electronically and might occur between (the girl and) a current or former dating partner". A survey among high schoolers in the USA in 2013, reported that about 10% of them had been victims of physical violence and another 10% reported being victims of sexual abuse in the past 12 months from a dating partner (Vagi, K. et al. Findings from the 2013 National Youth Risk Behavior Survey. JAMA Pediatrics, 169, 474–482).

Early Recognition is Important: It is important for girls to recognize the early signs of dating violence like teasing and name calling as indicative of an unhealthy relationship which can lead to more serious consequences like the types of violence described above. It is important to end a relationship if this is happening so that it does not escalate into Dating Violence.

Results of Dating Violence: Teens who go through this may end up with depression and anxiety, thoughts about suicide, unhealthy behaviors, such as tobacco, drug, and alcohol use. (www.cdc.gov/violenceprevention/intimatepartnerviolence/teen_dating). As in many types of abusive relationships, it can result in the victim having a low self-esteem, feeling worthless or even agreeing with the negative things the offender says about them.

Solutions

For all the types of abuse discussed above, it is important for young ladies to realize they are the victims and it is never their fault. It is necessary to discuss concerns with a trusted adult when one is faced with sexual or other types of violence. You are brave and strong when you do that, and do not see yourself as weak by doing so. Parents and guardians should also be in the habit of asking their girls questions about their relationships with boy friends and whether they feel threatened or fearful at times.

Challenging Educational Issues for Girls

Lack of access to education and limited educational opportunities for the Girl Child or Teenager exists in some resource poor nations. Many barriers exist including:

* Girls working to supplement the family income
* Early marriage of young girls and giving birth soon after
* Boys being considered superior to girls
* Poverty in the family and so the girl is denied education which may be expensive

Solutions to Girls Education

Research shows education can improve their livelihood and that of their families and communities as a whole. World organizations like UNICEF and WHO (both are United Nations organizations) have stressed the importance of educating the girl child.

Governments need to address these missed opportunities for girls by

- Removal of barriers created to hinder girl education
- Education of parents and community leaders
- Poverty alleviation
- Enacting relevant laws and regulations are some of the multi-pronged approaches that can improve the education of girls
- Provision of sanitary wear for girls in resource poor countries to use during their menses may be a simple way to improve their attendance at school. This may be unbelievable to many who live in resource rich countries but that is the situation many girls face in poorer areas of the globe

Mothers and Guardians can do protective things or measures to help girls mature into responsible and assertive women who are an asset for societies and countries.

- Ensuring access to education
  Educated girls can make a great contribution to family, community, and country. Any adult lady reading this, and has the means should think about sponsoring a girl child's education in their own country or in a resource poor nation
- Teaching girls at home and school about their bodies
  Adult women can always teach girls about their bodies; from feeling good about how they look, to physical changes they will go through like menstruation, personal hygiene, dating, avoiding sexual abuse, staying safe at home, school and in the neighborhood, cooking, or doing house chores etc. Information available on the internet and in books are good resources. Women in social organizations and churches can make it a point to pour into the lives of adolescent girls they have or can have access to in places like schools, churches, sports, and other clubs girls belong to
- Mentorship programs for girls by social and religious organizations
  These can go a long way to shape a young girl's world view and wellbeing. It makes them articulate, assertive and guide them to achieve their dreams and aspirations

As Women We Can All Invest Time, Resources, and Skills in the Lives of Adolescent Girls

Reproductive Years

....

These are the years during which a woman is capable of getting pregnant and having a child. It is usually between the ages of 12 to 49 years, when she usually is menstruating. The period or menstrual flow stops around the age of 50 years but some may continue into their early 50s. Each woman has a different biological make up and so everyone does not start or end at the same time. Many of the diseases we discussed under pelvic diseases, menstrual irregularities, and conditions associated with the female reproductive organs occur or start during the reproductive years due to the influence of female hormones. Others are due to infections contracted during unprotected sexual intercourse.

Ovulation and Conception

A woman usually has one uterus, two fallopian tubes (tubes) which are attached to the uterus at one end and the other end is funnel shaped and located close to the ovary on either side of the uterus. There may be some anatomical abnormalities in some women e.g. absence of a uterus or fallopian tubes. Each month chemicals or hormones released from the brain act on the ovaries to cause numerous eggs to start developing in fluid sacs known as follicles. One will mature and will release the egg which is directed into the wide end of the fallopian tube and is slowly propelled toward the uterus. Ovulation usually occurs about 14 days after the last menstrual period. During ovulation a developed egg is released from a follicle in an ovary and some women may feel a pain at the side of the body where the egg has been released from. The following month the pain may occur at the other ovary, giving some women the ability to know when they are ovulating.

Fertilization

The released egg travels down the fallopian tube and about the same time, the lining of the uterus under the influence of hormones produced from the remains of the fluid filled sac (this is now known as the corpus luteum) starts to thicken with blood vessels and nutrients, awaiting the arrival of a potential baby. If at this time, sperms are introduced into the vagina through sexual intercourse, or artificial means (artificial insemination), the sperms swim up the cervix, into the uterus and into the tube. The fastest or strongest of the "pack" will meet an egg and when it penetrates the outer wall then fertilization takes place. The fertilized egg moves slowly through the fallopian tube for a few days dividing rapidly and then gets into the uterus and is implanted into the lining of the uterus. If the egg is not fertilized it will be destroyed and will fall apart or disintegrate. Before we continue with what happens after an egg is fertilized, it is important to discuss infertility or inability to conceive, as well as what a woman can do even before she gets pregnant – called Trimester Zero.

Infertility

It is defined as inability to get pregnant after one year of regular sexual intercourse without use of any birth control method. Infertility has many causes and its related to factors from both the man and the woman with male factors contributing about 40–50% . It is often assumed that infertility is only a female problem, but its about the same in both sexes. Worldwide infertility among couples is estimated to be about 8 to 12%.

Causes of Infertility

Female causes:

Related to ovulation
Eating disorders
Age (too old with decreased female hormones)
Infections like STIs and PID leading to blockage of tubes
Anatomical problems like absence of ovary, tubes, and uterus
Cancer
Radiation to the pelvis etc
After chemotherapy treatment
Hormonal Problems – Thyroid, Hyperprolactinemia

Male causes:

Abnormality of sperms or semen
Low sperm count
Abnormal veins like varicose veins in the testes
Undescended testes (they are still present in the abdomen)
Low testosterone
Infections like mumps which affect the testes
Chronic diseases like diabetes, cystic fibrosis
Cancer of male reproductive organs
Radiation
Medications like steroids
Chemotherapy
Illegal drugs like cocaine or marijuana

Combined females and male causes:

Lifestyle issues like smoking, alcohol, obesity, drug abuses and stress
Diseases like Hypothyroid, Diabetes Mellitus, and Anemia

Treatment

Treatment include medications, surgery, or use of assisted reproductive technologies like in vitro fertilization (IVF) etc. details of which are beyond the scope of this book. In the USA, alone there are over 500 fertility centers and many thousands all over. Some patients do Medical tourism for IVF and I know people who have travelled from the USA to Greece for example where the cost of IVF using your own eggs is about $3500. Cost in the USA is about $12,000 per cycle.

Adoption

Many couples who cannot have children of their own can adopt children or use Surrogate mothers who carry a baby produced from their own egg and sperm or from other sources. Just because one cannot carry a baby in one's own body should not deter couples from enjoying parenthood and giving a child an opportunity to be blessed by them.

Pre-conception (Trimester Zero)
What is It?

This is the period before one gets pregnant or conceives. It is also referred to as Trimester Zero and its time for preconception care and counseling. It is often advised to do so about 3 months to one year before one gets pregnant. Seeing a health care provider will allow you to have personalized Trimester zero care. There are some things one has to do in order to increase the chance of having a healthy baby. Some of the plans may include:

- See a healthcare provider to have baseline blood work and examination
- Make sure your blood pressure and blood sugar levels are in good range
- Make sure you are eating healthy adequate fruits and vegetables
- Have a healthy weight, don't be underweight or overweight
- Have a well woman examination so that they check for STIs and do a pap smear/HPV
- Make sure your immunizations are up to date. These may include MMR, Tdap, or Hepatitis
- If you have depression or other mental health discuss with a healthcare provider
- Medications you are on need to be discussed with your doctors, since some can harm the fetus
- Let provider know of your family history and if there are any genetic diseases
- Stop smoking if you smoke, and stop illegal drugs or even alcohol if you drink
- Dad's health is also important, he should stop smoking if he smokes

Vitamins and Other Medicines Needed Before Conception

FOLIC ACID: This is also known as Vitamin B9 and it is important to start taking it before conception. This is needed for cell multiplication and the proper development of the embryo or baby at its earliest stage of development. It helps with the proper development of the spinal cord and prevents NEURAL TUBE DEFECTS. This defect involves the improper closure of the spinal cord or brain due to a defect in the vertebrae or skull. The most common type of birth defect is called "Spina Bifida". Folic acid is also needed to prevent anemia or low blood level. Studies show if folic acid is started at least 4 weeks before conception, the risk of spinal cord defects can be reduced by more than 70%

PRENATAL VITAMINS (PNV): These are special multivitamin and minerals made for pregnant women to take, and it is good to start them before conception. Most of them may contain adequate amounts of folic acid and Omega 3 but these complete ones may be more expensive, and so one can get a PNV with folic acid and then get a script for Omega 3 fish oil

OMEGA 3 FISH OIL: This contains Polyunsaturated Fatty Acids called EPA and DHA and it is important that the developing baby has adequate amounts. EPA helps with the body's heart, immune systems, and also how the body responses to inflammation. DHA on the other hand is more important in supporting developing brain, eyes and nerves. It is important that the developing baby has adequate amounts of DHA and so this has now been included in most prenatal vitamins. However, if a prenatal vitamin does not contain it, then it will be important for an expectant woman to start taking DHA supplement. Although these are found in fish, women are sometimes concerned about high mercury levels in some fish and so the supplements are safer. The fish oil has to provide a minimum of 300mg of DHA

Pregnancy Tests

If one is in the reproductive age group, having regular periods, is having unprotected sex (sex without condom or other birth control means), and misses a period; it is important that they have urine or a blood test to check for pregnancy. These two tests detect the presence of HCG hormone (Human Chorionic Gonadotrophin) which is produced by the placenta and so its presence is an indication of pregnancy. The HCG levels rise quickly doubling about every 2–3 days, and the blood test may be positive about 6 days after fertilization. The blood test is usually done in a doctor's office, but the urine pregnancy test on the other hand can be done in the comfort of your home; and most women may do a urine pregnancy test a week after missing a period which makes it more accurate. Urine pregnancy tests are about 99% accurate but of course it depends on when fertilization took place and how many days its done after missing your period. There are also urine test kits which helps identify the time of ovulation. Both pregnancy and ovulation rapid test kits are sold in pharmacies.

Pregnancy

"The reproduction of mankind is a great marvel and mystery. Had God consulted me in the matter, I should have advised him to continue the generation of the species by fashioning them out of clay"
—Martin Luther leader in Protestant Reformation.

This is a unique experience for women, and it is a result of complex occurrences. Below is a short description of how a normal pregnancy occurs. In this age of great scientific advancements pregnancies can take place outside the body through invitro fertilization etc. but here we are discussing normal pregnancy. Ovulation, Fertilization and Conception have already been discussed above.

Once conception occurs, the result is multiplication of cells containing DNA or genetic material from both the woman and man to form an embryo. The embryo travels from the tube and it takes about a week to ten days to get embedded in the lining of the uterus. It is important that as soon as one misses one's period, one should have urine or a blood test to check if one is pregnant.

Length of Pregnancy

The developing baby is referred to as a fetus or foetus (UK English) after about 9 weeks in the uterus. Pregnancy usually lasts about 40 weeks or just beyond 9 months. It is usually divided into 3 parts called trimesters. So the first trimester is 13 weeks, second between 13 and 26 weeks and the last or third trimester is after 26 weeks to the end of pregnancy.

Prenatal Care

It is important to start regular PRENATAL or ANTENATAL CARE (care before delivery) by a doctor, midwife or other health professional once pregnancy is confirmed. History and physical exam including a pap smear may be done. Blood work checking for anemia, liver and kidney function, and thyroid function are done, as well as testing for sexually transmitted infections.

Keeping Healthy During Pregnancy

Pregnancy is not a disease and so women who are pregnant can have a happy and healthy time. It is important that a pregnant woman eats healthy foods, with lots of fruits, vegetables, protein and calcium-containing foods or supplements. All of these contain important nutrients for the developing baby. Calcium is important for bone and teeth and so if one is not eating enough dairy foods like milk, cheese, yogurt, then non dairy foods rich in calcium like green leafy vegetables, nuts, almonds, sesame seeds, black eye peas, canned salmon with bones, sardines, soybean, tofu, and broccoli, and oranges can be consumed.

Weight Gain During Pregnancy

One does not have to eat for two people during pregnancy, and a weight gain of between 15 to 40 lbs. may be sufficient depending on weight before pregnancy. Over weight and obese women should gain less, while underweight women should gain the higher number. The first trimester is the time to gain more weight and an average of 2 to 4 pounds (lbs.) a week has been suggested. Sometimes it's difficult to gain the weight due to nausea and vomiting (Morning Sickness) which occurs in the first trimester, but may continue up to 20 weeks. After that, during the second and third trimester about 1 lb. a week is usually sufficient to keep the baby growing at a good rate.

Other Supplements During Pregnancy

We have discussed the need to take folic acid and prenatal vitamins. Women may have low calcium during pregnancy and that can affect their teeth, and the bones of the developing baby, so it is important to eat calcium-containing foods like dairy products or take calcium with Vitamin D3 containing supplement for strong bones and teeth. Vitamin D helps calcium be absorbed or pushed into the bones to build strong bones. It is important that your health care provider knows what you are taking as supplements or if you are on any other medicines.

Morning Sickness (Hyperemesis gravidarum)

Morning sickness is pregnancy related vomiting and affects about 75% of pregnant women during the first half of pregnancy. Most of the time it is mild and can be treated with dietary changes and over the counter medicines. The cause is not really known but certain women are at increased risk and these include African American women, older women, those carrying multiple babies, those with history of acid reflux, motion sickness and migraines. The baby is not usually affected and it subsides by the 20th week.

Treatment

DIETARY: Dietary changes which may help include eating small frequent meals, avoid fatty foods, eat dry foods, low fiber and bland foods like crackers, fruits and vegetables, lean meats, eggs, clear fluids like ginger ale, sprite, ginger tea, and soups. These should be taken in small amounts at a time. Avoid strong scents like spicy foods or even perfumes etc. which can bring on a wave of nausea

Medications

Over the counter – Medicines over the counter include Vitamin B6 (10 to 25mg 3 times daily), alone or combined with Doxylamine (Unisom sleeping aid), Diphenhydramine (Benadryl), Dimenhydrinate (Dramamine), or ginger extract capsules 125 to 250 mg, 3 to 4 times daily

Prescription medicines – Prescribed medicines for more severe cases may include Promethazine, Hydroxyzine, Ondansetron, and Metoclopramide

Only a small number of pregnant women have severe vomiting resulting in dehydration or inability to keep foods down. These would require hospital admission for intravenous fluids and medicines.

Medication Use for Common Problems During Pregnancy

It is important that any medicine a pregnant woman takes is safe for the baby. These include both prescribed medicines and over the counter (OTC), nonprescription medications. All medicines which are prescribed and some OTC ones have been categorized in terms of their safety for pregnant women and their developing baby. That is why it is important for a pregnant woman to let her doctor know what medications she is on, because not all medications are safe. Most medicines are labeled on the packaging to indicate whether they are safe for pregnant or breastfeeding women and it is important to check the packaging of OTC medicines for these.

Most obstetricians or doctors who attend to a pregnant woman may give her a list of medicines she can take for certain common illnesses that are treated with OTC medicines. A few of the ones which are safe to take during pregnancy are listed below, however, it is not an exhaustive list. As with other medicines, check with your own provider, and the lowest dose which will work is what should be taken.

Medicines Which are Safe to Take During Pregnancy

Pain medications: Acetaminophen (Tylenol, paracetamol, Panadol). For non-steroidal (NSAIDS) like ibuprofen, and naproxen although they are safe to take during the 1st and 2nd trimesters, they are best avoided in the 3rd trimester of pregnancy. Use acetaminophen first.

Cold medications: Pseudoephedrine, Cough syrups with Dextromethorphan and Guaifenesin

Antihistamines (for allergies and colds): Cetirizine (Zyrtec) or Loratidine (Claritin), Chlorpheniramine, Diphenhydramine (Benadryl)

Constipation: Fiber medicines like Metamucil, Fibercon, and stool softeners – Colace, (docusate) Dulcolax

Heart Burn: Mylanta, Pepcid, Tums, Rolaids, Maalox, Gas-X, Ranitidine, Zantac

Hemorrhoids: Preparation HC, Anusol HC cream, any hemorrhoid cream, and Tucks

Back Pain: Heating pads, several times a day, Warm baths (temperature should be less than 101F or 38.3C), avoid lifting heavy things, use a firm mattress, and one can use a maternity belt. Avoid high heel shoes and wear flat comfortable shoes well-padded or with some insoles

Swelling of the legs (edema): Keep legs elevated when sitting or lying down. Sleep with pillows under your legs. Wear comfortable support hoses or socks, and decrease salt intake

Leg cramps: Tums can supply calcium, potassium from bananas and take OTC Magnesium oxide 400mg at bedtime. Magnesium also helps with constipation

Varicose veins: These can be troublesome. Use of support hoses or socks, and keeping legs elevated when sitting or lying by putting pillows under legs may help

Lightheadedness: This may occur especially with change in position or after standing in same position for a long time. To remedy this, drink more liquids, and increase salt in your diet. Change positions slowly, and avoid standing in the same place for a long time by shifting weight from one leg to another

Reminders on Your Radar

Pregnancy is not a disease; most women worldwide have a normal delivery of a full term baby. However, maternal factors can affect the baby, and some lifestyle changes prior to pregnancy may increase the chances of a first-time mother having a normal pregnancy according to a British study in 2013. These include normal pre-pregnancy body weight, increasing consumption of fruits, reducing blood pressure, and avoid use of illegal drugs. Smoking should be stopped as it affects the birth weight. Certain common problems associated with pregnancy are easily treated even by yourself, but you should let your healthcare provider know of any medicines you take.

Family Planning or Birth Control

....

What is It?

Family planning is the process by which a couple deliberately adopts various methods to prevent a pregnancy.

Why Family Planning?

"The Lord God said "be fruitful and multiple", but that mandate was not given to just one couple; it was a collective mandate, so couples can relax and not strive to carry out the task alone. Family planning may be useful for individual couples for limiting and spacing births, so children can be well taken care of"

—Dr. Barbara Entsuah, MD.

It is important that couples have a good discussion on how they plan to prevent a pregnancy, and to have kids when they want to. Most pregnancies worldwide are not planned and just happen because no birth control method was being used. By practicing family planning or birth control the couple exercise choice. In a study in 2014 by the Guttmacher Institute, they found that worldwide, 40% of all pregnancies (85 million), were unintended in 2012. Of these, 50% ended in abortion, 13% ended in miscarriage, and 38% resulted in an unplanned birth (Studies in Family Planning 2014; 45[3]: 301–314).

Some Advantages of Family Planning are:

- Couples can decide when they want to have a child
- Makes it possible to plan when one wants to get pregnant and have a baby
- A younger child can be weaned first before another baby is conceived
- Couples can space their children adequately, and this gives the mother time to recover fully between pregnancies
- It prevents unintended pregnancies and subsequent abortions which may occur
- It enables a couple to get to know each other a bit more and work on their relationship etc. before the babies start arriving
- It helps a woman who desires to pursue things like attend school, start or continue a career, be able to do so and not be worried about getting pregnant immediately
- Helps the couple space the ages of their children
- Helps couple not to have another child if they do not want any more children

Forms of Contraception

There are several methods used to prevent pregnancy and couples have to discuss the choices with each other and then with their health care provider. The methods can be divided into two broad groups:

- Permanent or temporary forms of birth control or contraception
- Hormones and those without hormones

All of them work either to:

- Prevent sperms from meeting an egg to cause fertilization
- Alter the chemical environment in the woman's body by varying the female hormones so that ovulation does not take place

Permanent Forms of Birth Control

These are considered non reversable and are available for both women and men.

1. Sterilization

This is when sperms and eggs are prevented from meeting by methods which:

- Block the fallopian tubes of women
- Cut or block the tubes through which sperms travel in the testes of men

In WOMEN the process is called BILATERAL TUBAL LIGATION. A woman's tubes are burnt, cut or tied surgically so that an egg cannot travel along it to meet sperms swimming up the tube.

In MEN tubes called the VASA DEFERENTIA are tied and cut surgically to prevent the sperms from entering the penis and the surgical procedure is called a VASECTOMY. After the surgery, the man will have to collect ejaculate or semen and take it to the lab for several months for verification that there are no sperms in the semen, which he will continue to produce. In the meantime another form of birth control method like a condom is used.

Both methods are considered irreversible, although both women and men later on have tried to reverse them. Both are almost 100% effective, (98 to 99.8%) in preventing sperms from meeting an egg, although a few pregnancies have been recorded in women who had had tubal ligation.

2. Essure Inserts

Essure is a non-surgical form of birth control which is also permanent. A small tube is inserted into each fallopian tube and the tube works with your body to block the fallopian tube so that sperms are not able to reach an egg that has been released. The inserts are made of material containing metal and do not contain hormones. It is performed in about 20 minutes and one can go home soon after that. After 3 months an Essure confirmation test which involves injection of a dye into the uterus is performed to make sure that the tubes are blocked or sealed. If they are completely blocked then the dye will not spill out of the open end of the fallopian tubes. When this happens sperms do not reach any egg that is released from the ovary. It is important that another form of birth control is used after insertion for the following three months since it takes about that time for the body to work with the insert to form a natural barrier and block the tubes. In the USA many women have reported serious side effects and filed lawsuits against the company and so since 2018, the company has stopped selling them in the USA.

Temporary Methods of Birth Control

These are reversible methods of birth control, which mean after using a particular method for a while, a woman may decide she wants to have a child, or for some other reason wants to quit using the method. After quitting, it is possible to get pregnant within a short time for most of the methods.

Barrier Methods

These methods prevent the sperms and egg from meeting and so pregnancy can-not take place when used properly. These include

- Male condoms – Used alone or with spermicides which are chemicals that can kill sperms. Condoms have the advantage of preventing Sexually Transmitted Infections (STIs). Male condoms have to be put on properly in order to work effectively, however, they sometimes can break or slip off. Oil based lubricants can make latex condoms break easily, so should be avoided with condoms. Some may contain spermicides but those are not common
- Female condoms – This is a long sheath with a closed part on one end which goes near the cervix. Lubricant is applied to the outside and inserted. It does not need a prescription to buy it
- Diaphragm – It is a flexible dome-shaped plastic device which a woman has to place inside her vagina to cover the mouth of the cervix. A woman has to be fitted with the right size by a health professional, after that she learns how to put it in before sex. It has to be used with spermicides, and has to stay in place for a few hours after sex before it is removed. After removal it is washed and dried and used again as needed

- Cervical caps and vaginal sponges – These are also barrier methods which prevent the sperms from entering the cervix or neck of the uterus or womb. They are usually used with spermicides

Natural Family Planning

This is when sex is avoided around the time the woman is fertile (ovulation period). Using the time of the menstrual cycle and the consistency of the cervical mucus a woman will avoid sex during that time. Some women may know when they ovulate because of pain during their mid cycle associated with ovulation. However, one must remember that sperms can live up to 72 hours after they enter the vagina. Natural family planning is an unreliable method of birth control, and it requires vigilance and a lot of determination to practice it.

Abstinence

This is saying "No to Sex". This is when vaginal sex does not occur, so semen is not introduced into the vagina. It is the only 100% effective method. It is the most reliable form of birth control.

Breast Feeding or Lactational Amenorrhea Method (LAM)

In the first six months after delivery, breast feeding may be used as a form of birth control only if the mother exclusively breast feeds and does not use formula or other food supplements. It is also known as Lactational (breast feeding) Amenorrhea (lack of periods/menses). It is very effective if no other source of feeding is used for the baby, and may be up to 98% effective. The woman will not have periods during this time.

Withdrawal Method

This is when a man will pull out or withdraw his penis from a woman's vagina during intercourse and ejaculate outside of the vagina. This is very unreliable and is not considered a formal method of birth control.

Many people practice it without realizing that pregnancy can occur readily. During sexual intercourse, part of a man's semen may be introduced into a woman's vagina prior to the process of ejaculation. The sperms in the semen may swim up the cervix into the uterus just like occurs with ejaculation. The sperm numbers may be smaller, however; it takes just one sperm to fertilize an egg. Use of a condom will be a better method and adding a spermicide cream or gel inside the vagina makes it even more effective against unintended pregnancy.

Hormonal Birth Control Methods

This is made up of a variety of delivery methods including pills, patches, vaginal rings, injections and Intrauterine Device (IUD) also known as the Loop. These contain both estrogen and progestin or progestin alone. These are hormones similar to what women produce naturally to control their menses, female characteristics, and pregnancy etc. When used for birth control, they work by thickening the mucus produced at the cervix and so inhibit sperms, and more importantly they prevent the ovaries from releasing eggs each month. If no eggs are released then if sperms are introduced into the vagina, they will not meet any released eggs so no pregnancy occurs.

Combined Oral Contraceptive Pills

Combined oral contraceptive pill known as "The Pill" or "Birth Control Pill" is a pill which is taken daily by a woman to prevent pregnancy. It is made up of two female hormones – estrogen and a progestin. Usually the monthly packet of pills has four or seven days toward the end of the month which do not have active medicine in them. These are called "sugar pills" or placebo pills. When the woman takes these ones then she will usually have a period and will then start a new pack. Typically the pills may come in packets of 28 or 21 pills. The 28 type pills have 21 active pills (contain hormones), and 7 sugar pills for the last week. The 21 type pills have 21 active pills and after those are taken, a woman will then have her period and after 7 days starts a second packet. In some of them the last seven days may contain iron pills or folic acid.

Advantages of the Birth Control Pill

- They are very effective in preventing pregnancy if used correctly
- They make the periods lighter
- They prevent cramps or pain during menstruation
- They also have other effects like helping acne or pimples get better
- They protect against ovarian and endometrial cancers
- They help against formation of ovarian cysts

Disadvantages of the Pill (BCP)

- Immediate side effects after starting the birth control pill may include nausea, weight gain, spotting, breast tenderness and headaches, but not all women experience these
- A woman may have a slight increased risk of heart attacks, stroke, and blood clots in the legs or lungs with use of birth control pills especially if she is a smoker above the age of 35 years. Certain antibiotics may decrease the effectiveness of the Pill so it is important to let health care providers know you are

on the pill if they are prescribing antibiotics. A condom may be needed until the next period
- There is also a slight increased risk of breast cancer among current or recent users compared to non uses of BCPs
- They do not protect again sexually transmitted infections, and so condoms may have to be used along with BCPs to prevent STIs

Tips for Taking Birth Control Pills

If a woman forgets and does not remember to take the pills daily, then the pill is not the right type of contraceptive for her. The pills are safe and effective in preventing pregnancy when taken correctly as prescribed. To be effective it has to be taken every day. Missing some of the days increases the risk of getting pregnant. Tips for better compliance include:
- Taking them the same time each day helps you remember to take them daily
- Putting the packet near your toothbrush helps one remember to take your pills when one goes to brush your teeth
- One may also take it at the time you are doing something routinely, e.g. taking it when you take other medicines or after breakfast every morning
- It does not matter what time of the day it is taken. Taking it at the same time is what matters
- Carrying them with you at all times may be a good way of not forgetting them
- Try and pick them up from the drug store or pharmacy the same day of the month, then you will not forget to get them and take them
- Do not miss any pills even when something unusual happens like spotting or bleeding during the middle of your cycle or when your period does not come as expected. It is important to follow up with your health care provider to discuss any issues which may come up
- When you miss a pill, take it as soon as you remember and continue the pack as you are supposed to. If you remember the next day, take 2 pills and continue as usual. You will need a back-up or second alternative method for example, a condom for the rest of that month
- When you miss two days, take 2 on that day (day 3) and 2 the next day, and you will be back on schedule. You have to use a backup method like a condom for the rest of that month
- Use a reminder on your phone to help you remember to take it. There are apps available for that

Vaginal Ring (NuvaRing)

This is an estrogen – and progestin-containing flexible ring which is placed high in the vagina and left there for three weeks. At the end of the third week, it is removed and the woman will have a period. A new one is then inserted. If used as prescribed, it is very effective in preventing pregnancy. Reported side effects include breast tenderness, weight gain, headaches, and vaginal irritation. Women who have a history of blood clots, stroke, breast cancer, and smokers over the age of 35 years should not use it because the risk of getting blood clots in the lungs and stroke is higher in those who use NuvaRing than those using the pill which has other types of progestins in them.

Hormonal Patch (Ortho Evra)

This is a small patch containing both Estrogen and Progestin and it is applied to dry skin e.g. the outer arm, buttocks, or abdomen one patch every week for three weeks. The fourth week is patch free and a woman will have her period during that time. It contains the same hormones as the combined birth control pill and the vaginal ring and so it has similar side effects, however, it delivers more estrogen than the pill and so there is an increased risk of blood clots compared to the pill.

Progestin Only Birth Control Methods

There are some women who cannot take birth control containing estrogens, because it is not advised or it is contraindicated. These situations include:

- Women who smoke and are older than 35 years. They are at increased risk of getting blood clots with estrogen containing birth control methods
- Women who have migraines when on estrogen containing birth control pills
- Women who have high blood pressure which is not well controlled
- Women who have had a stroke or heart attack in the past
- Women who have sickle cell disease

These may benefit from progestin only birth control methods, however, other women may also chose to use these. Progestin only birth control methods include pills, implants, Depo Provera shot, and IUD (intrauterine device). We will discuss them next.

Progestin Only Birth Control Pill

This has only progestin (synthetic progesterone) and it is also known as the "mini pill". It acts by preventing ovulation (release of egg from ovary) and thickens the mucus at the cervix and so prevents sperms from entering the uterus. They have to be taken about the same time every day and a woman may have a period in the last or fourth week while taking this type of birth control pill. It is not as effective as the combined pills which contains both estrogen and progestin compounds.

Progestin Hormone Injection

An example is the "Depo Provera" injection or "Depo" shot. A progester-one-containing injection is given once every three months or four times a year. Common side effects with this include irregular periods, spotting, weight gain and decrease in bone density or bone mass. One may stop having periods while on the depo shot. After stopping the shots, it may take a couple of months to a year before one's period starts again on a regular basis. It is good idea to take calcium with Vitamin D supplement while on this, to help build up the bones.

Hormonal Implant "Implanon" or "Nexplanon"

A small rod the size of a match stick filled with progesterone is inserted into a woman's inner arm. It slowly releases the progesterone and is effective for up to three years. Side effects include irregular bleeding, weight gain, acne, and headaches.

Intrauterine Device (IUD, the Loop).

The IUD is a small plastic device which is inserted into the uterus through the cervix by a health care provider in the office. It does not require surgery. It is a very convenient and effective birth control method and they are long term from 3 to 10 years, but temporary and not permanent.

There are 3 types of IUDs that are used and they are:

MIRENA and SKYLA: These two have progestin which is slowly released into the uterus, and they act by thickening the cervical mucus, slow the movement of sperms, reduce how long they live and also thins the lining of the uterus so implantation of a fertilized egg does not take place. A woman will stop having her period while on the progestin IUD. The Mirena can be kept in the uterus for 5 years and the Skyla for 3 years

COPPER T. – Copper T (ParaGard) contains copper and no hormones and it can last for 10 years

IUD – How to Check its in Place

Each of them has a string which hangs inside the vagina after the IUD has been inserted into the uterus by a health care provider. The woman can periodically during a shower, check if the string is still in the vagina by feeling for it.

SIDE EFFECTS: These include irregular bleeding, cramping, vaginal discharge, infection, the IUD falling out, or moving into other parts of the pelvis. The latter is very rare.

Summary of types of Birth Control Methods

METHOD	DOSING FREQUENCY
Pill	Daily
Patch	Once a week
Vaginal Ring (NuvaRing)	Once a month
Depo Shot	Once every 3 months
Condom	When you have sex
Diaphragm	When you have sex
Implanon	Every 2–3 years
Skyla	Every 3 years
Progestin IUD	Every 5 years
Copper IUD	Every 10 years
Sterilization	Permanent

Menopause – Embrace the Change

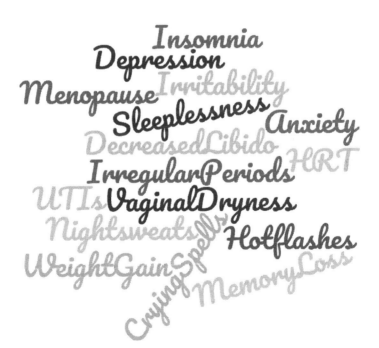

Menopause the Transition

References: North American Menopause Society, www.menopause.org; Family-doctor.org; and others mentioned in the text.

We already have discussed menopause symptoms briefly when we discussed women with breast cancer, but we shall look into more details about what happens and how women can have relief from the symptoms associated with it.

Menopause

"Our mothers were largely silent about what happened to them as they passed through this midlife change. But a new generation of women has already started to break the wall of silence."

—Trisha Posner, British non-fiction writer.

The menopause period is a big part of all women's lives and it is an important topic to cover. Women need to know what happens to their bodies during this time and how it impacts their emotional, and sexual lives as well. Having a good idea of all that may occur during this time will help a woman make the transition from the reproductive stage of her life to this stage smoother and tolerable. Remember Knowledge is Power.

So relax and lets go on THE MENOPAUSE JOURNEY.

There are three stages which merge into each other, however the first two stages have fluctuating levels of female hormones producing the symptoms that women experience during those times

Peri-menopause
Natural menopause or Climacteric
Post-menopause stage

PERIMENOPAUSE (around menopause), MENOPAUSE TRANSITION
What is This?

This is the time between onset of irregular menstrual periods and complete cessation of periods or menses. Most women may have a perimenopause phase lasting from about 4 years up until the period stops completely. The average age when a woman begins this transitional time is about 47 years but some may have a shorter or longer transition time. During the perimenopause and menopause stages, a woman's female hormones get lower in her body because the ovaries which normally produce these start aging and get smaller. They unfortunately do not do so at a steady pace and so the female hormones levels may be up and down resulting in the symptoms a woman experiences. On the contrary, male hormones like testosterone which are usually present in small amounts in a woman's body tend to go up.

Symptoms During the Perimenopause Stage

Symptoms which may occur in the perimenopause time include:

- Irregular periods: This may present as heavy periods, prolonged periods, scanty periods, or no periods at all

- Vaginal and sexual changes: Vaginal dryness, loss of libido or sex drive, and decreased ability to conceive
- Temperature variation: Manifested as hot flashes, chills, and night sweats
- Mental changes: Mood swings, irritability, depression, and poor sleep at night

All these are attributed to the irregular levels of female estrogens which do not decrease steadily but may be going up and down in an erratic manner.

Menopause

....

What is It?

NATURAL MENOPAUSE: A woman is said to have entered natural menopause when she has not had a period for 12 continuous months. This is also known as the Climacteric stage and during this time a woman transitions from the reproductive stage to non reproductive state. Menses stop permanently and a woman is not able to conceive and have children. Menopause normally occurs on average at about the age of 51 years. There is no way to tell when a woman will reach natural menopause; however, it may tend to occur about the same time that one's mother went through natural menopause. The peri-menopause symptoms described above may continue and may even become worse after menopause.

Early Menopause

Some women will experience early menopause at age of 35 years, for example. This may be a result of:

- ARTIFICIAL MENOPAUSE: This is menopause which occurs earlier than is expected because of surgery to remove the ovaries (oophorectomy), destruction by radiation of the pelvic organs, medicines to treat cancer, or other medical treatment which halt the process of release of female hormones. These may cause a sudden drop in female hormone levels and result in sudden onset of menopausal symptoms
- PREMATURE MENOPAUSE: This is cessation of ovarian function before the age of 40 years. Causes include genetics, enzyme deficiencies, infections, autoimmune condition, environmental causes like tobacco abuse and unknown reasons

Symptoms of menopause:

As described above in the perimenopause period but the symptoms may be worse.

- Vaginal and sexual changes: Vaginal dryness, loss of libido or sex drive, and decreased ability to conceive

- Temperature variation: Manifested as hot flashes, chills and night sweats
- Mental changes: Mood swings, irritability, depression, and poor sleep at night
- Short term memory deficits and concentration problems
- Mood swings, irritability, crying spells and has a "short fuse" – easily blows up

Post-Menopause
What is It?

This is the time span after menopause and is the longest time of the three stages (peri-menopause, menopause and post-menopause). Most women if they enter menopause at about 51 years and live until say 85 years for example, would there-fore have lived for 34 years in this stage of their lives. Some women may have menopausal symptoms for a short time e.g. one year, while others unfortunately will have symptoms persisting for up to ten years. Women may experience differ-ences in symptoms and it's thought to be related to genetics. Below are some of the symptoms and the treatments which may help.

Treatment of Menopausal Symptoms
Night Sweats and Hot Flashes (Vasomotor Symptoms)

These symptoms are also known as VASOMOTOR symptoms and are thought to be a result of ways by which the body tries to get rid of heat through sweating and dilation of the blood vessels causing a lot of discomfort for women. At night it disrupts sleep and may cause daytime tiredness or fatigue. These are some of the things you can do or change in your lifestyle to minimize the discomfort when there are mild symptoms like less than 2 hot flashes per day.

- Wear layered clothes so you can easily remove one when the need arises
- Wear cotton or linen night clothes which are breathable materials and can make you feel cooler
- Have a small personal fan at home, at work or even one with a USB port which can be attached to your computer while working
- Take a flask or vacuum insulated mug filled with ice and water to bed so you can sip on it when hot flashes or night sweats occur
- Use layered bed sheets so you can take one off when the need arises
- Keep one leg from under the sheets so that it is cooler than the one under the covers
- Certain foods and beverages may exacerbate or bring about the hot flashes and night sweats. So avoid too much caffeine, spicy foods, alcohol, hot foods and hot baths

- Stress can increase the symptoms so try and de-stress as much as possible. Some de-stress by going for a massage, meditation, acupuncture, tai chi, yoga, stretches or walks
- Go for walks early in the mornings or in the cooler evening time. Walking relaxes you, but should not be done too close to bedtime
- When a hot flash starts you can do conscious or controlled breathing. Take a slow deep breath through your nose, pause and breathe out through your mouth. For example, inhale, pause, and then exhale. Repeat process five times
- Women who are obese or overweight get more symptoms and so weight loss may help
- Low fat diet, with increase intake of fruits and vegetables seem to decrease these symptoms according to studies that have been done
- Cooling pillows, gels, pads, ice packs, are available to freeze and then use inside your pillow or on top of your pillow at night to keep you cool
- One can use a cooling gel memory mattress pad or topper which draws heat away from your body, keeping one cool

Over The Counter (OTC-Non Prescription) Medicines

Several of these have been tried over the years but researchers who have done good studies involving thousands of post-menopausal women think the good results women may get from using OTC medicines are due to placebo effect. This means the same good results of reducing hot flashes will be achieved even if the women are given just "sugar pills" without medicine.

Plant Based Remedies

Some of these include

- Black cohosh
- Soy foods, e.g. soymilk, tofu, soy nuts
- Promensil (this is a soy based pill)
- Remifemin (made from black cohosh)
- Wild yam
- Red clover
- Doug Quai
- Isoflavone supplements

Some of above, including isoflavones are phytoestrogen, or plant based estrogen-like substances are found in many foods, including soybeans, chickpeas, lentils, flaxseed, beans, fruits, and red clover. Most studies do not support their effectiveness. Those with estrogen dependent breast cancer should avoid high doses of plant phytoestrogens due to their estrogen like effects.

Additional Remedies

In studies remedies listed below have not been found to be any better than "sugar pills" (placebo) or are inconclusive in others, but some women claim they help. Please let your doctor know of any supplements you plan to take or are taking.

- Vitamin E 400 iu (small decrease in frequency of hot flashes)
- Acupuncture
- DHEA (may help with decrease libido)
- Evening Primrose oil (may cause bloating, diarrhea and nausea)
- Ginseng Root (may reduce sleep problems)
- Yoga (some practice the physical postures and breathing technics without necessarily adding the spiritual and mental aspect or practice of Hinduism)
- Omega 3 fatty acids (may decrease strength of hot flashes)
- Hypnotherapy and Mindfulness Meditation have been found to be helpful in some studies

Adverse Effects of Supplements

Most of the above will do no harm, however; Black Cohosh has caused liver damage in some women, and Red Clover can affect the clotting of blood. Some may also interfere with other drugs and so your doctor should know what supplements or alternative medicines you are using. If you go to a website like www.drugs.com or webmd.com/interaction-checker and open the drug interactions page you can check the interactions between any two drugs and or between a drug and a supplement.

Prescription Medicines for Hot Flashes and Night Sweats

Women who experience moderate to severe hot flashes (greater than 5/day) may not get relief from the above methods. They can be given HORMONAL or NON HORMONAL prescription medicines to help with the hot flashes.

Non Hormonal Treatment for Hot Flashes

- Antidepressants: Some antidepressants have been found to decrease **hot flashes** in non-depressed patients. Examples are paroxetine, venlafaxine, escitalopram, and citalopram. They may also help with the **mood swings** some women experience at this time
- Gabapentin (Neurontin): This is a medicine usually used for treating epilepsy, migraine and nerve pain. It has been found to help minimize **hot flashes** and **lack of sleep** associated with hot flashes
- Clonidine or methyldopa: These are blood pressure medicines which have been found to reduce **hot flashes and night sweats**. They will be good choices for

treating an affected woman's high blood pressure as well. Clonidine is more popular than methyldopa for this purpose

- Psychological therapy: Cognitive-behavioral therapy (CBT) and, to a lesser extent, clinical hypnosis both have been shown to be effective in reducing symptoms. A Psychotherapist will help with this

Hormonal Treatment for Hot Flashes and Night Sweats

Many studies over the years have shown that ESTROGEN WITH and WITHOUT PROGESTOGEN (progesterone and progestin), are very effective in decreasing these two menopausal symptoms in women. A careful joint decision has to be made by a patient and her doctor regarding the use of hormones. If a woman is post-menopausal and still has her uterus then a combination of estrogen and pro-gestin are used, however, if she is post-menopausal without a uterus then estro-gen alone is used.

Side Effects of Estrogen

The side effects of estrogen include a slight increase in:

- Incidence of breast cancer
- Stroke
- Heart attack
- Blood clots in the legs or lungs (DVT and PE)

Contraindications to Estrogen Use

There are certain contraindications to the use of estrogen. These include:

History of breast cancer
Blood clots in legs (DVT – deep vein thrombosis) and lungs (PE – Pulmonary Embolism)

There are different forms of hormones and these include pills, gels, vaginal rings, and patches. You and your doctor can make the best decision on the type to use, and how long to use; because they are usually used for a short period of time.

Hormones for the Perimenopause Phase

Women who do not smoke and are in the PERIMENOPAUSE phase can be placed on combination birth control pills to control their hot flashes and night sweats, and these also will also help with menstrual irregularities which tend to occur at this time.

Other Hormonal Medications

The combination of conjugated Estrogens and Bazedoxifene (Duavee), was approved by FDA in 2013 to treat moderate to severe hot flashes in women who still had their uterus. Bazedoxifene helps prevent estrogen from causing excess growth of the lining of the uterus (endometrial hyperplasia) as can happen if estrogen is used alone. Analysis of studies done by the North American Menopause Society (NAMS) show that Duavee is able to reduce hot flashes, increase bone density (and so prevent osteoporosis), improve sleep and also decreases symptoms of the genitourinary system in women who had started it either at the beginning of menopause or more than 5 years later after menopause (North American Menopause Society (NAMS) October, 2016 Annual Meeting).

Bioidentical Hormones

(References: North American Menopause society (NAMS), Menopause.org; Harvard Health Publications – Harvard Women's Health Watch)

The term "bioidentical hormones" strictly means hormones that are similar in chemical or molecular structure to those that are naturally produced by the body. There are FDA approved bioidentical hormones produced by pharmaceutical companies, and there are the compounded "bioidentical hormones". We will discuss both of these.

Compounded Bioidentical Hormones
What Are They?

"There is very good reason to beware the inflated promises made by the bioidentical industry and to take better care of yourself during your menopause transition by going to the real experts—licensed medical professionals who have knowledge of the process of menopause and its treatment. Be leery of websites and experts who provide only their own product and recommend only their own tests. If it sounds too good to be true—it probably is. There are better and safer ways to cope with this important life transition, and most women will not require treatment for more than a few years, when risks remain very low. So choose science".

(Nanette Santoro, MD, NAMS Board Member. www.menopause.org. MenoPause Blog. Bioridiculous. April 5th, 2017).

The compounded menopausal bioidentical hormones are produced from plant extracts, for example, soybeans and wild yam, which are altered chemically in a lab to look like female estrogens, and then compounded by pharmacists. They have become very popular partly through media and celebrity endorsements, and they are prescribed by health care providers, for women with menopausal symptoms – mainly hot flashes and night sweats.

The two most common available compounded estrogens

are Biest which contains two Estrogens – 20% Estradiol + 80% Estriol (a milder Estrogen about 1/10th to 1/100th strength of Estradiol); and Triest which has three estrogens – 10% estradiol, 10% estrone and 80% estriol. Estrone is also a weak form of estrogen. A physician may require Biest in a specific ratio of estriol to estradiol and so it can be customized for the patient's use. They are available as capsules, sublingual compounds, transdermal patch, cream, troche or gel.

Other compounded hormones are:

- Testosterone and DHEA which are used to increase libido
- Viagra 1% vaginal suppository is used to increase blood flow to the vagina and to increase sensation
- Progesterone vaginal suppository

How Common Are They?

In a consumer survey in 2015, by North American Menopause Society (NAMS), on use of compounded hormones, It examined the use of US Food and Drug Administration (FDA) approved menopausal hormone therapy Versus compounded bioidentical hormones for treatment of menopause symptoms. They found that about 31% of responders between age of 40 to 84 years were ever users of compounded hormones, and also formed 34% of current users.

Why Are They So Popular?

The popularity of it skyrocketed when the results of Women's Health Initiative (WHI) study in 2002 was published. It concluded that women who took a specific FDA prescribed hormone Prempro (this is a combined estrogen and progesterone – Premarin and Provera used in the study) had slightly higher rates of death, heart disease, blood clots, and strokes than matched women who were not on the medicine (controls). It is not known whether if another hormone combination was used – one in which another estrogen replaced premarin – the similar result would be achieved or not. As a result, most women stopped FDA approved HRT of all kinds and because they needed something for hot flashes etc. they turned to compounded bioidentical hormones which were marketed as "Natural". However, there is more to these compounds as discussed below.

Problems With Compounded Bioidentical Hormones

Unregulated and not FDA approved:

The compounded ones are not regulated by the FDA, and have not been found to be safer, more effective, or have fewer health risks than standard FDA approved hormones. Analysis of some of these custom compounded hormones show that they are not even chemically identical to those produced naturally in the body; and besides, to produce them in the lab extensive chemical reactions are used and so the term "Natural" is misleading. These custom compounded hormones are not FDA approved and have not undergone the rigorous study pharmaceutical products go through. For example, compounded preparations of Biest and Triest, have not been found to be safer or more effective than other FDA approved bioidentical hormones

Quality Assurance of Compounded Hormones

Though they may contain the same ingredients as the FDA approved ones, their effectiveness and quality have not been tested. As a result, different batches may contain different amounts of the active hormones. A concerning factor is that most compounded hormones that require progestogen use topical progesterone as the accompanying progestogen to the compounded estrogen, and research has shown that this route of delivery of progesterone does not produce adequate blood levels to prevent buildup of the lining of the endometrium referred to as "Endometrial Hyperplasia". This has resulted in bleeding and endometrial cancer in some women using these. Some also advocate use of yam extract creams but the body is unable to convert this into progesterone.

Salivary Tests – Are They Reliable?

Some providers of unregulated compounded bioidentical hormones may also measure salivary levels of the hormones, but there is no scientific evidence that these measurements are useful in determining the composition of individualized or custom compounded bioidentical hormones.

Side Effects of Compounded Hormones

The same NAMS study mentioned above found that reported side effects like acne, vaginal bleeding and endometrial cancer rates were higher in women who used or had used compounded hormones.

What Is the Bottom Line Concerning Compounded Hormones?

The bottom line is that if you desire menopausal hormone therapy, do your research, talk to your health care provider and weigh the pros and cons of which type you would like to use. Looking at safety, regulation, and rigorous studies done, I would advice women to use FDA approved menopausal hormones if they want to use hormone therapy for troublesome menopausal symptoms. For urogenital symptoms like decreased desire, low libido, and difficulty in arousal some of the male hormones which are compounded may be useful and could be tried, however; the creams and gels would be recommended rather than forms like pellets which are inserted under the skin for periods up to three months. Side effects of these include itching, skin rash, pain at insertion site, tender breasts, redness of skin, acne, and headaches.

FDA Approved Hormones

After the initial scare from the results of the large women's study, careful further analysis showed that the results were different for various women depending on age and other factors.

What Does Further Analysis of the Study Show?

Further analysis according to age, when during menopause was hormone therapy started, and whether a woman had a uterus or not, revealed that the increased adverse effects affected only a certain group of women. These were those who were:

- Ten or more years post-menopausal before starting hormone therapy
- Women starting hormone therapy after the age of 60 years.

What About Younger Women or Those Who Took Estrogen Alone?

In the study, younger women 60 years and below, had better benefits and less adverse effects on hormone therapy, and those on estrogen alone (because they had had a hysterectomy) had reduced risk of breast cancer.

Examples of FDA Approved Bioidentical Hormones

You may be wondering if there are there FDA approved Bioidentical Estrogens? Yes, there are !!!!, and these are approved plant based estrogens made from soy and wild yam which are safe and effective in treating menopausal symptoms. There are 3 types of FDA Bioidentical Estrogens: 17 Beta-Estradiol, Estrone, and Estriol. These are also "Natural" but are not in capsule form or sold over the counter. Progesterone comes micronized (particles are made smaller) in a capsule or as a vaginal gel. This is made from plants like Yam.

HORMONE	BRAND NAME	FORM	BIOIDENTICAL
17 Beta-Estradiol/ plants (micronized)*	Estrace, others	Pill	Yes**
	Alora, Climara, Esclim, Estraderm, Vivelle, others	Patch	Yes
	Estrogel	Transdermal gel	Yes

HORMONE	BRAND NAME	FORM	BIOIDENTICAL
	Estrasorb	Topical cream	Yes
	Estrace	Vaginal cream+	Yes
	Estring	Vaginal ring+	Yes
Estradiol Acetate	Femring	Vaginal ring	Yes
Estradiol Hemihydrate	Vagifem	Vaginal tablet+	Yes

PROGESTERONE	BRAND NAME	FORM	BIOIDENTICAL
Micronized* Progesterone USP	Prometrium/ Utrogestan	Pill	Yes
	Prochieve 4%	Vaginal gel	Yes

Combined Estrogen/Progestin

17 Beta-Estradiol and Norgestimate	Prefest	Pill	No++
17 Beta-Estradiol and Levonorgestrel	Climara Pro	Patch	No++
17 Beta-Estradiol and Norethindrone Acetate	Combipatch	Patch	No++

*Particles are made smaller for better absorption.

**Bioidentical estradiol until ingested and converted in the liver to estrone.

+For vaginal symptoms only. ++The estradiol is bioidentical but not the progestin.

Adapted: (Harvard Women's Health Watch "What are Bioidentical Hormones? Aug. 2006)

The extensive discussion on treatment of hot flashes and night sweats; including the use of Bioidentical Hormones is to help you to make an informed decision regarding whether you will use non hormonal or hormonal means to help your symptoms. Secondly, if you chose hormonal therapy, would it be an FDA approved hormone or a compounded "bioidentical hormone"? With information provided above, you and your doctor can decide what is best for you.

Vaginal and Urinary Symptoms

Genitourinary Symptom of Menopause (GSM)
What is This?

"It's too hot! Nobody told me it's going to last as long as it feels like it's lasting. And sneezing is a new experience".

Whoopie Goldberg during her menopause journey. HuffPost Julie Dargan, Contributor 2016.

This is also referred to as ATROPHIC VAGINITIS, but GSM is a new and better term because the vagina is not the only tissue affected by menopause. As a result of the decrease in Estrogen, the lining of the genital and urinary structures lose the tissue that keeps them lubricated and thick, and these become thinner and less elastic. These changes occur in the labia majora and minora (major and minor lips of the vagina), clitoris, vulva, vaginal opening (introitus), vagina, urethra, and bladder. These genital and urinary symptoms can also be very troubling after menopause; however, women tend to complain more about the hot flashes and night sweats than these. More than 50% of women may experience some of these symptoms. These symptoms (GSM) unfortunately tend to increase with time, unlike the hot flashes and night sweats which get better with time.

GENITAL CHANGES – These and their presentations include the following:

- Vaginal dryness due to decrease in the usual lubrication and flow blood
- Burning and itching of vulva and vagina due to dryness and thinning of the lining
- Decreased suppleness or stretching ability of the vagina
- Constriction or narrowing of the vaginal opening
- Thinning of the walls of the vagina leading to easy bleeding and pain during sex
- Decreased desire for sex, decreased frequency of orgasm or longer time to reach orgasm
- Vaginal length is shortened and the width becomes narrower, leading to pain with penetration during sexual intercourse
- Pain may lead to decreased frequency of sexual intercourse by some women and can subsequently lead to marital problems
- Changes in the acidity of the vagina, (pH increases to above 4.5) lead to vaginal infections like yeast infections and Bacterial vaginosis (BV) presenting as vaginal itching, irritation, discharge and fishy odor

URINARY CHANGES – These and their presentations include the following:

- The decrease in estrogen causes the urethra to be narrower and the lining gets thinner
- Easy invasion by bacteria leading to frequent urinary tract infections (UTIs)
- There is dryness and irritation leading to urinary symptoms like frequency, urgency, and pain with urination
- Bladder control problems like urgency and frequency
- Urge and stress incontinence (loss of urine)
- The weakened top vaginal wall affects its ability to hold up the bladder which is above it, and results in prolapse of the bladder, or pressing of the bladder into the vagina space from above. This may cause urinary retention, increased UTIs, and pelvic or intercourse pain

Treatment of Vaginal Symptoms

VAGINAL DRYNESS: There are several over the counter (non-prescription) medicines which can be used and they include:

Lubricants

These help with the dryness and also friction during intercourse. Water soluble ones are non-staining and cause less irritation. Silicone based ones are also available, but avoid oil based ones which may cause irritation and may cause latex condoms to break. Examples include Astroglide, K-Y jelly, K-Y Silk-E, Just like Me, Slippery stuff, etc. and these are used during intercourse. Warming lubricants may contain menthol or capsaicin and these may cause vaginal irritation or sting when used.

Vaginal Moisturizers

These are used every one to three days and not just during intercourse. They may help women who feel vaginal irritation most of the time and not just during intercourse. They keep the walls of the vagina moist, maintain vaginal acidity and help relieve the dryness. They also help control easy bleeding of vaginal walls and cervix associated with dryness. Examples are Replens, Luvena, Allation, Gentle Moisture, Vitamin E oil, KY liquibeads, Moist Again, Fresh Start, etc.

Compounded Moisturizers Or Lubricants

There are compounded moisturizers and lubricants containing Vitamin E and Hyaluronic acid. The latter can come as a suppository inserted into the vagina, which is supposed to retain water and keep vagina moist. Examples are RepaGyn and Hyalo GYN and both are vaginal moisturizers made from Sodium Hyaluronate and used to treat vaginal dryness in breast cancer patients on Tamoxifen or peri or menopausal women who need non hormonal treatment. Besides these, others used include: Aloe gel, coconut oil, olive oil or canola oil.

Regular Sexual Intercourse

Regular sexual intercourse helps keep the vaginal tissues moist. Intercourse increases blood flow to the vagina tissues and this may help with the dryness and so frequent sex is encouraged to minimize vaginal dryness. It also helps keep the opening of the vagina wide, and not constricted.

Laser Treatment for Vaginal Dryness (Vaginal Atrophy)
Mona Lisa Touch

A laser therapy called MONA LISA TOUCH, developed in Italy was approved by the US FDA (Federal Drug and Food Administration) in 2012 to be used to treat vaginal dryness in post-menopausal women. It is already approved for use in Europe, Asia, South America, and Australia. Similarly to post-menopausal women, those women who have had breast cancer and are put on anti-estrogen drugs, or have had removal of ovaries (oophorectomy) to decrease recurrence of the cancer also experience symptoms of GSM because of low Estrogen levels.

How It Works

- The treatment uses three sessions of laser treatment six weeks apart, each lasting about 3 to 5 minutes
- It stimulates the vaginal lining wall to produce more collagen and other supporting tissues
- It increases the thickness of the lining and increase lubrication or wetness resulting in healthier vaginal tissue and increase blood flow to the vagina
- The results are less dryness, less pain, and vaginal bleeding associated with sex
- It is a painless procedure done in a doctor's office. Clients who have had the treatment testify that they are less dry and have little or no pain during intercourse, making their sex life more enjoyable

It is however, not a cheap procedure, but those who testify of its success in their lives say it has been "life changing" and they are willing to pay for it. (http://www.smilemonalisa.com).

Vaginal Dilators

As part of the changes of GSM, the vaginal opening, its width and length all become smaller and so, a woman can use special lubricated vaginal dilators each night to stretch the vaginal walls. These are sold in pharmacy and medical equipment shops. A woman can also wash her two fingers and insert two lubricated fingers from each hand into the vagina to stretch the walls while in the shower. That sometimes helps stretch out the vagina making penetration during sex less painful.

Hormonal Therapy for GSM

Hormone therapy in the form of estrogen or combination of estrogen and progesterone can relieve not just hot flashes but genitourinary syndrome of menopause as well. A careful joint decision has to be made by a patient and her doctor regarding the use of hormones.

Vaginal Hormones

If a woman is peri or post-menopausal and her symptoms are mostly GSM related, and not hot flashes or generalized symptoms, then a vaginal estrogen in the form of a pill, cream or ring can be used whether the woman still has her uterus or not. Estrogen vaginal creams when used, produce about a fourth of oral estrogen's blood levels, but are about four times more potent in relieving vaginal symptoms. As a result of low blood levels, progestin is not required except in the case of the vaginal ring Femring, which releases significant amounts of estrogen into the blood and so progesterone has to be used in those with a uterus to prevent buildup of the uterine lining (termed endometrial hyperplasia). Femring is indicated for hot flashes and night sweats (vasomotor symptoms) as well as for GSM.

Estrogen Products

- Vaginal creams – Estrace, Premarin, and Estragyn
- Vaginal rings – 2 types are available and do not have to be removed during intercourse
- Estring – Soft ring inserted into vagina and it can remain there for 90 days. Effects will be seen after about 2–3 weeks of use
- Femring – described above
- Vaginal tablet – Vagifem – inserted into the vagina initially for 2 weeks and then 2 times a week.

Non Estrogen Product

Ospemifene (Osphena) is an FDA approved drug which belongs to a group of drugs which work on estrogen receptors (but it does not contain estrogen), and in the uterus helps with pain associated with intercourse and other symptoms of GSM like dryness and thinning of lining. It helps with bone loss, but may cause hot flashes and sweats. More useful if no hot flashes present.

Vaginal Pain During Sexual Intercourse (Dyspareunia)

Also known as Dyspareunia (dis-pa-ry-nea) it can cause discomfort, dissuading a woman from having sex. This symptom may be a result of GSM described above and so the other treatments mentioned above for GSM may help this.
    Treatments include:

- Moisturizers and lubricants
- Vaginal dilators

- OSPEMIFENE (Osphena) which affects vaginal tissue like estrogen does, but it is non hormonal
- Estrogen in the various forms described above under GSM

Insomnia (Sleeplessness)

Perimenopausal and post-menopausal women may suffer from sleeplessness or insomnia at bedtime. This is partly due to hot flashes and night sweats, and so usually when hot flashes and night sweats improve with treatment, sleep also gets better.

Treatment

- Treat any accompanying hot flashes and night sweats as described above, and this will improve insomnia
- Sleep Hygiene

Sleep Hygiene: These are non drug measures one takes to get a good and restful sleep. It is discussed in details in the chapter where Insomnia is discussed under "Brain and Nerve conditions". Some of the tips include:

- Try to go to bed and also wake up the same time each night
- Don't exercise too close to bedtime (make interval greater than two hours)
- Bed should only be for sleep, sex, and resting; not reading, watching TV etc.
- Avoid caffeine, alcohol, and nicotine too close to bedtime
- If you lie down and cannot sleep get up and read or do something not too stressful, then go back to lie down when you feel sleepy
- Do not eat a large meal just before bedtime
- Keep the bedroom quiet and the light soft. Use of a bedside lamp helps
- Sometimes soft background music may help you fall sleep
- If something is bothering you, get up and write it down, and go back to bed
- Try not to sleep or take a nap in the afternoon. Keep busy during the daytime
- Practice relaxation technics like mindfulness meditation and deep breathing

OTC Supplements and Oils

Supplements: Melatonin, Valerian root, or herbal teas like chamomile may help with sleep

Essential Oils: these include Neroli, Lavender, Valarian, Clary Sage and Roman Chamomile. These may be sprayed on the pillow or on tissue near the pillow and may promote sleep

Prescription Medicines

If other treatments fail, these can be used, however, it is best to use on a short time basis only, since some of them can lead to serious side effects and addiction problems. They include:

Z DRUGS FOR SLEEP: Zolpidem (Ambien) and Eszolpiclone(Lunesta) and Zaleplon (Sonata). The first two can help you fall asleep and stay asleep, but Zaleplon only helps you fall asleep

GABAPENTIN and CLONIDINE mentioned earlier can help with both hot flashes and sleep.

BENZODIAZEPINES: Include diazepam (valium), lorazepam (Ativan), temazepam (Restoril) and alprazolam (Xanax). They are all controlled substances and have the potential to be addictive and so are not to be used on a long term basis. They can cause drowsiness and even falls in the elderly, and so it is best to avoid these

Warning: Avoid using Tylenol PM or Advil PM on a regular basis. These contain Diphenhydramine (Benadryl) which can cause memory problems and drowsiness if used too frequently.

Mood Swings

Some women may complain about being, teary, irritable, and "cranky" or "short tempered" with everyone and they have family members and friends commenting about their tempers or moods. It has not been verified that this is due to the hormonal changes per say, however, with hot flashes, night sweats, and sleeplessness; women may feel emotional or snappy.

Treatment: Treating these individual symptoms mentioned above may help, however;, if not, use of antidepressants like PAROXETINE, VELANFAXINE or SERTRALINE may help not only with hot flashes but mood changes as well. Even if your moods are fine they still work for hot flashes and night sweats if these are present.

Body Changes

These include deposition of fat in the mid-section, weight gain, and swollen ankles and feet.

•   WEIGHT GAIN:
    There are many factors which may contribute to these changes. These include the changing levels of female hormones, usual decrease in body protein and increase in fat deposits associated with aging and genetics (if it runs in the family). To help

with the weight gain associated with menopause in general, one should eat healthy by trying to eat less high carbohydrate, junk, and fatty foods, and increase fruits and vegetables. Regular exercise may help decrease the weight

- SWOLLEN ANKLES:
Swollen ankles and feet in particular may bother a lot of women. It has been suggested that this may be caused by increased water retention associated with the hormonal changes. The weight gain may also cause blood flow from the legs to be sluggish and cause pooling in the ankles. Swollen ankles attributed to menopause is usually painless, no redness and is found to be an isolated symptom

Serious causes like heart failure, blood clots in the legs, anemia, liver or kidney diseases, pelvic tumors, and varicose veins will have to been eliminated. These if present, may be associated with pain, redness, shortness of breath, chest pain, difficulty in breathing and other abnormalities noted in blood work or chest x-ray.

Medicines can also cause swollen ankles and these include: steroids, female hormone replacement medicines (HRT), amlodipine (a blood pressure medicine) and even gabapentin used for seizures, hot flashes and sleeplessness. Changing these or reducing their dosages may help eliminate the swollen ankles.

Treatment of Swollen Ankles Caused By Menopause

The following may help:

- Keeping legs elevated above the heart (if possible) when sitting or lying down
- Wearing support or compression stockings or socks during long sitting hours
- During the day, get up and move, or walk periodically to keep the leg muscles pumping
- Use of a pillow under the legs while sleeping may also help by moving fluid up toward the heart
- Decrease salt intake in one's diet, especially if one has high blood pressure
- If one has hypertension or high normal blood pressure, a diuretic (anti-hypertension medicine) also called a "water pill" in layman terms, may be used regularly or on an "as needed" basis to treat the swollen ankles or legs

24

Bone and Skeletal Conditions

There are several types of bone and skeletal conditions or diseases, but we will deal with a few common ones in this chapter. These include:

Osteoarthritis
Rheumatoid Arthritis
Fibromyalgia
Muscle Strain
Ligament Sprain
Carpal Tunnel Syndrome
Gout
Plantar Fasciitis (back of heel pain)
Osteoporosis (decreased bone density)

Low back pain
Back muscle strain
Degenerative disc disease
Sciatica
Spondylosis (spine arthritis)
Facet Joint Arthritis
Spinal Stenosis
Sacroiliac joint dysfunction
Use of narcotics for low back pain

Arthritis

. . . .

This refers to conditions affecting joints. The body has different types of joints, but the commonest one is the synovial joint made up of two bones with cartilage at their ends, enclosed in a fibrous capsule which is lined by a tissue called the synovium. The capsule encloses a cavity or space containing fluid called synovial fluid which is produced by the cells of the synovium. The fluid lubricates the joints, acts as a shock absorber and nourishes the joint. There are severe types of arthritis and may be up to 100. Osteoarthritis is the commonest, but others include Rheumatoid, Psoriatic, Lyme, and Gouty arthritis. These have certain specific abnormal blood work and presentations which help identity them. We will discuss just a few of these.

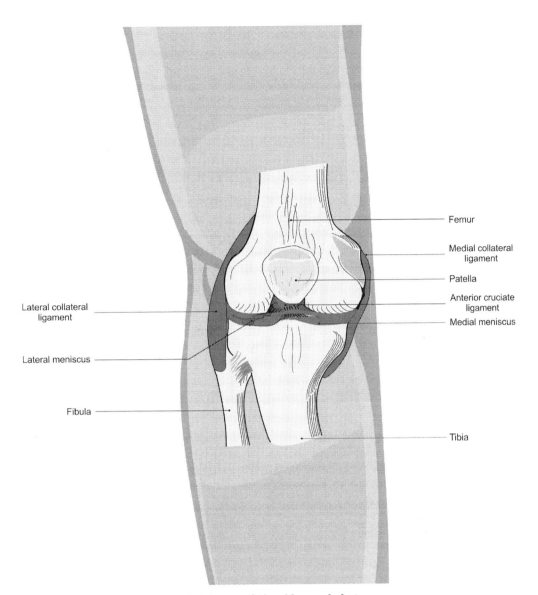

Picture of the Knee Joint

Osteoarthritis

....

What is It?

"My message is - keep moving. If you do, you'll keep arthritis at bay".

—Donna Mills. American Actress. www. brainyquote.com/authors/donna_mills

Osteoarthritis is the most common type of arthritis and is also known as "Arthritis" or "wear and tear" of the joints. In the USA according to the CDC, it affects over 30 million people. It affects mostly weight bearing joints, and they include the knee, hip, shoulder, spine and smaller joints like fingers, toes, and wrists. There is wearing down of the cartilage at the ends of the bone, and the bone itself changes. The loss of the cushion or cartilage leads to bone resting on bone, resulting in pain when the joint is moved. The synovium (thin membrane producing fluid which nourishes and lubricates the joint) lines the knee and other joints, and together with surrounding ligaments may get inflamed when osteoarthritis is present.

Who Does It Affect?

It tends to affect older people and women are affected more than men especially after the age of 50 years. It may develop early in younger people whose joints have been injured in the past, for example in athletes, or people who use a particular joint repetitively. It can also run in families because there is a genetic component to its development. Being obese or overweight put a lot of weight on the joints and cause early development of osteoarthritis.

Symptoms

- Pain in the joint especially with repetitive use or when one wakes up
- Stiffness in the morning and especially after sitting
- Swelling of the involved joint
- In the knee joint it becomes "bowlegged" (curved or rounded) if it is severe
- Limitation of movement in activities like walking, running, twisting, opening a jar, or lifting the arm up depending on which joint is affected
- Crackling noises in the joint known as "crepitus" caused either by popping air bubbles in the joint fluid, or cartilage rubbing on the joint surfaces
- Some complain of more pain when the weather is cold and others can "predict" it is going to rain from the pain they feel in their joints when the weather is changing or rain is on the way
- It is a progressive illness (gets worse with time) and does not go away once it has started

Treatment

There are non drug and also medications that are used to lessen the pain and improve movement of the affected joint, thereby slowing its progression or damage to the joint. A health care provider may order X-RAYS of affected joints, or even blood work if the history or symptoms may suggest another type of arthritis. Treatments will not cure it, but will lessen the pain, unless a joint replacement surgery is done.

1. PHYSICAL ACTIVITY: It is important that one keeps moving the joint through physical activity and exercise like walking. If the knees are affected, swimming and using a recumbent bike take some of the pressure off the joint. Control of pain with medications can keep one active. If not, then there is disuse of the muscles around the joint involved and this can result in weakness of the muscles further limiting movement. For the knee joint, resistance exercises to strengthen the thigh muscles (quadriceps) decreases pain

2. HEAT AND COLD: Some people benefit from reduced pain and stiffness by using either heat or cold, or moist heat by way of compresses, pads, or water bottles on the joint

3. PHYSICAL THERAPY: Which is supervised physical activities by a therapist can be ordered to strengthen the involved joint and muscles around it

4. OCCUPATIONAL THERAPY: May also be involved and they provide advice on aids one can use like walking cane, roller walker, joint braces or splints, grab bars in the bathroom etc. all of which help with movement or prevent falls and injuries

5. WEIGHT LOSS: Losing weight if overweight, takes some pressure off the joint when the hip or knees are involved and that will help with pain and also make one more active

6. PAIN MEDICATION: Most people may be able to manage their pain with medicines like Acetaminophen (Tylenol), Non-steroidal anti-Inflammatory Drugs (Ibuprofen, Aleve, Diclofenac, Brufen, Naproxen etc.). Stronger pain pills may be needed but most people do well on the above

7. JOINT INJECTIONS: Depending on which joint is affected, injections of steroids or other medications which act like lubricants can be injected into the joint to improve movement and decrease the pain. However, with the lubricants – called Viscosupplements (for example Hyaluronic acid), large clinical studies have shown they are no better than Placebo (substitutes without any medications). Two other injections are Platelet Rich Plasm and Placenta Tissue Matrix.

8. SURGERY: May be arthroscopy or joint replacement
    a. ARTHROSCOPY: It is a minimal invasive procedure, in which the joint can be examined and treated by "cleaning the inside of the joint" using a type of endoscope and camera which is inserted through a small incision.
    b. JOINT REPLACEMENT: More extensive and involve a partial or complete replacement of the joint with an artificial joint. Common replaced joints are knee, hip and shoulder joints. Most people with replacement joints seem to do a lot better after surgery; they are pain free and can resume physical activities which they could not do before.

9. DIETARY SUPPLEMENTS/MIND AND BODY PRACTICES:
    SUPPLEMENTS: Glucosamine, Chondroitin, Turmeric, Fish oil, Omega 3, Ginger, Dimethyl Sulfoxide (DMSO), and Methylsulfonylmethane (MSM). Local

treatment with arthritic rubs, or creams containing Methol, Camphor, Capsaicin, Eucalyptus oil, and Cinnamon oil may be used to rub the affected joints BODY MANIPULATIONS: Tai Chi, Yoga, Acupuncture, massage, and Magnet therapy; some CAM herbal products may contain hidden drugs like NSAIDS

What the Studies Show

Of these complementary treatments, studies show that **Glucosamine with or without chondroitin** had similar beneficial outcomes as Celecoxib (Celebrex) which is a non-steroidal anti-Inflammatory medicine.

Another review published by Arthritis Research UK in the United Kingdom showed that among many studies done using CAM products, those which were of high quality indicated that Acupuncture and Tai Chi help with Osteoarthritis.

It does not mean others do not work; it is just that some have no studies done, while others do not have good or large studies to support their claims.

Arthritis of the smaller joints like those in the hand can be helped with creams like Capsaicin, Diclofenac cream, warm Paraffin wax bath, and Splinting according to Dr. Mahsa Tehrani, a Rheumatologist (www.everydayhealth.com).

Rheumatoid Arthritis (RA)

What is It?

"Up to 40% of people with RA may develop other conditions during the course of their disease. While RA affects the joints, people with RA may also be more likely to have the following conditions: heart disease, bone loss, anemia, infections, lung disease, rheumatoid nodules, (knots of tissue under skin), Sjogren's syndrome (dry mouth and dry eyes)".

Understanding Rheumatoid Arthritis (www.ra.com).

Rheumatoid Arthritis is a type of chronic autoimmune condition resulting in inflammation of joints and their linings; and more importantly also manifests in other body systems like the Cardiovascular and Respiratory systems. As a result of it being a systemic disease it is now often referred to as "Rheumatoid Disease". It's cause is unknown but its thought to be triggered by infection, injury and environmental factors like cigarette smoking, insecticides, and air pollution. Its believed female hormones and obesity both have a role to play, and also those who carry certain genes. It affects mostly women (70%) and is the second commonest type of Arthritis. According to the Arthritis Foundation about 1.5 million Americans are affected in the USA. The annual incidence is about 200,000 cases per year in the US. World wide the prevalence is between 0.4 to 1.0% according to WHO estimates. It is thought that those who have RA have a shorter life expectancy by as much as 10 to 15 years.

Signs and Symptoms

It normally affects small joints like those of the hands, feet, wrists, elbows, and ankles, however; the knees can also be affected.

It usually affects same joints on both sides of the body, e.g. both hands symmetrically.

Initially there may be fever, malaise, weakness and redness, swelling and pain in the joints.

Morning stiffness and weeks of swelling may occur in joints.

Painful swelling with knots on joints, as well as deformed joints especially of hands and wrists.

Other body systems may be affected and may include lungs, blood vessels, nerves, eyes, skin, and low blood levels causing anemia.

Treatment

Diagnosis is made by the clinical presentation, physical exam, blood work and imaging studies of joints. The treatment has been with Medications, Non Medication methods and surgery.

Non Medications

These range from using orthotic splints for hands and wrists, hot and cold therapies, physical therapy, and occupational therapy which teaches equipment use and adaptation of home gadgets.

Medications

Medicines are used to stop the progression of the disease by blocking or decreasing inflammation and accompanying pain. Anti-inflammatory medicines like Ibuprofen, Naproxen, Celecoxib etc. are used for mild cases, however, treatments have been introduced called Disease-Modifying Anti-Rheumatic Drugs (DMARDS) which are used for severe disease or to stop progression of damage to joints and tissues. There are 2 types of DMARDS:

Non-Biological DMARDS

Hydroxychloroquine (Plaquenil)
Leflunomide (Arava)
Methotrexate (Trexall)
Sulfasalazine (Azulfidine)
Minocycline (Minocin)

Biological DMARDS

These are injections and work by blocking the paths that immune cells use to cause inflammation and subsequent damage to joints. They are used when those listed above do not control the disease well enough. Some of the common ones are:

Abatacept (Orencia)
Rituximab (Rituxan)
Adalimumab (Humira)
Etanercept (Enbrel)
Infliximab (Remicade)

They can make any infections e.g. TB and others present become very serious and so it's important that your Rheumatologist (doctors who treat joint diseases) does regular blood work while you are on any of these DMARDS, and a Tuberculosis test must be done before starting the Biological ones.

(For more information see WebMD.com, www.arthritis.org, cdc.gov/arthritis/basics/rheumatoid-arthritis.html).

Surgery

This may be required for deformed and damaged joints which are causing a lot of disability or pain.

Fibromyalgia (FM)

What is It?

Fibro Quote: Invisible Pain. They just don't understand what they cannot see. This quote about invisible pain says what you wish you could say, "My pain is invisible, so is the pain you inflict when you don't believe me."

fibromyalgianewstoday.com

Fibromyalgia (FM) is a condition in which individuals experience chronic widespread pain in soft tissue and muscles for greater than three months, associated with extreme tenderness when a small amount of pressure is applied. The pain perception experienced with pressure is above and beyond what an ordinary person without the condition will experience. Research shows that many women who suffer from FM, have gone through a lot of psychological stress. In the USA, about 3 to 6 million people suffer from fibromyalgia and generally about 90% of sufferers are women. In the past, doctors (and some still think this way) have thought of the condition as one that was "all in the head" of women when they had complained about pain, and yet no specific inflammation was seen in joints or muscles and blood tests did not reveal any known disease.

What Causes FM?

It is believed to be a result of increased sensitivity to neurochemicals (chemicals produced in the brain and spinal cord – central nervous system) which are associated with production of pain. The pain is in areas where tissues called connective tissue are present and occurs in both upper and lower parts of the body. Connective tissue connects various tissues and organs together, giving them structure. Several new studies have shown it is probably a combination of:

- Increased sensitivity to pain due to abnormalities in the ratio of the different neurochemicals
- Alterations in certain genes that control the perception of pain, making the individuals very sensitive to pain and tenderness at different parts of the body

Symptoms

Chronic pain and stiffness in muscles and sometimes in joints
Fatigue
Sleep disturbances
Mood problems and memory problems especially attention and concentration
Sufferers may have depression and anxiety as a result of the chronic pain
Sufferers may also experience other painful conditions like: Osteoarthritis, Irritable Bowel Syndrome, and Rheumatoid Arthritis in addition to FM

Diagnosis and Treatment

It may take a long time before a diagnosis is made because there are no specific tests and it is a diagnosis of exclusion. This means that all the blood tests, and x-rays done turn up to be negative, and the symptoms cannot be attributed to any other known condition like arthritis. Therefore, it's important that a doctor takes a good history and does a good examination, together with blood work and imaging studies.

Treatment

There are no known cures, however, combining medications and non-drug methods of treatment may help a sufferer manage it with the tools available to them, and live a productive life inspite of the condition.

Treatments target

Pain
Mood disturbances like anxiety and depression
Sleep problems mainly insomnia
Fatigue

Non Medication Treatments

EXERCISE: Aerobic exercises have been found to be very useful for patients with fibromyalgia, but one should pace one's activity with intermittent rests and not overdo it. Aerobic exercises include walking, jogging, swimming, and water walking. The use of massage, acupuncture, yoga, tai chi, and relaxation has also been found to be helpful. Working with a physical therapist may be needed to do exercises, and other things which may help alleviate pain

EDUCATION: Knowing about the disease is important because it helps patients have a realistic expectation of how their therapies can help them. Symptoms especially pain may not go away completely, but knowledge is power, and can help you be involved in your own treatment

SUPPORT GROUPS: Some patients are involved in FM support groups and "attend" meetings on internet chat rooms, face to face meetings or write blogs. This helps connect with others who have the disease and one gets to know what treatments others have found effective

A very useful website developed by the University of Michigan called FIBROGUIDE (http://fibroguide.med.umich.edu) can help an individual know more about the disease and how to cope with it

PSYCHOTHERAPY: This is talk therapy with a trained professional who will help you cope with living with the disease, and also help you with the mood or depression that may accompany the disease. It requires multiple visits or sessions and some guide to this is also found on the University of Michigan FIBROGUIDE website

Medication

Medications used are those which affect the amount and balance of neurochemicals in the brain. These chemicals affect pain levels, fatigue, and moods of affected individuals. It is important that medications be combined with the non-medication treatments mentioned above. There are three drugs approved by US FDA for use in FM. These are Duloxetine, Pregabalin and Milnacipran. Others are also used off label as listed below.

ANTIDEPRESSANTS: For Pain and depression: Amitriptyline, Duloxetine, Sertraline, Paroxetine, Fluoxetine and Milnacipran

MUSCLE RELAXANTS: These help with muscle spasm, sleep and pain control for example Cyclobenzaprine (flexeril). Other muscle relaxants are not very effective

NERVE PAIN DRUGS: Gabapentin, Pregabalin, and Amitriptyline, to treat nerve pain and improve sleep

OTHERS: Tramadol for pain

Treatment for Fatigue

Many patients with fibromyalgia experience fatigue which may be related to both the pain and the lack of deep sleep associated with the condition. A list compiled by an author of the National Pain Report gives a list of 23 treatments including CAM therapies and medications that have helped some sufferers in reported small studies. These include some already used for pain treatment. They include:

Aerobic and strength training exercises

Vibration exercises of the whole body

Balneotherapy (soaking in Epson salt baths or mineral spring waters)

Transcranial Magnetic Stimulation (TMS) and ElectroConvulsive Therapies (ECT) both are used for treating major depression

Low energy laser therapy, Pulsed Ultrasound, and Interferential current

TENS units sold over the counter in pharmacies

Sensory Motor Rhythm treatment and Noninvasive cortical electrostimulation

CAM supplements: Acetyl L-carnitine, an amino acid, and D-ribose

(National Pain Report. 23 Clinically-Proven Ways to Beat Fibromyalgia Fatigue. By Donna Gregory Burch)

Note that most of these are not specifically approved by FDA to treat fatigue in fibromyalgia, however, you together with your doctor can decide on what will best suit you. You may also have to try several until you come up with one or two which work best for you.

Sprains and Strains

Before we discuss what they are, we have to understand the meaning of certain words:

Ligament – Ligament is a fibrous tissue that joins two bones, e.g. the bones that form the knee or ankle joint

Tendons – Muscles are attached to bones by tendons which are also fibrous tissues

What Are Sprains and Strains?

These are terms used to describe stretching or tearing of ligaments (sPrains) and stretching or tearing of muscles and tendons (sTrains).

Sprains

There are a few joints that tend to experience sprains and these are mostly in lower extremities.

ANKLE JOINT: The joint that experiences the most sprain is the ankle joint when one twists or rolls the ankle while walking, running, or tripping; as well as when it is injured during sports or exercising. There may be immediate swelling of the ankle area, bruising, pain with bearing weight or walking, and limitation of movement

KNEE JOINT: The anterior cruciate ligament (ACL) which holds the two bones of the knee joints together can also be sprained or torn and this makes the knee joint unstable. Mild cases involve stretching but severe ones results in tear of the ligament

Treatment

Treatment depends on the ligament involved and the severity of the injury. Immediately a minor sprain occurs, one can use the RICE method of:

- REST: Stay off the joint or leg
- ICE: Apply ice intermittently to decrease pain and swelling
- COMPRESS: Wrap the joint to limit the swelling e.g. with a stretchy or ACE bandage
- ELEVATE: Lift or prop up the involved extremity

Take some Anti-inflammatory medications like Ibuprofen or Naproxen which may help with the pain and swelling.

It is important to see a doctor or health care provider if there is no relief after 48 hours or if the injury is so severe that one cannot bear weight, and pain is severe. The doctor after examination will decide whether other measures like x-ray or MRI are needed and further treatment depends on the extent of the sprain. One may need a splint or brace to keep the part from moving, or crutches may be needed to keep weight off the leg/foot while it heals. Physical therapy may be needed as well.

Surgery

For severe tears surgery may be required.

Treatment for Strains

As mentioned, strains involve muscle or tendons and can affect the extremities or back following a fall, injury or motor vehicle accident. Treatment for strains is similar to sprains; however, muscle relaxants e.g. Cyclobenzaprine, Methocarbamol or Metaxalone may be included in treating muscle spasm of the back for example as well as Physical Therapy, Osteopathic or Chiropractic Manipulations.

Carpal Tunnel Syndrome (CTS)

What is It?

This condition occurs in the palm aspect of the wrist and It is caused by pressure on the median nerve which runs through the middle of the wrist (palm side). Any thing that makes the passage way (carpal tunnel) through which the nerve passes smaller or swollen may lead to this condition. The risk factors for developing CTS include:

- Repetitive hand motion like in typing with hands held lower than wrist
- Medical conditions like Obesity, Hypothyroid and Diabetes
- Osteoarthritis or Rheumatoid Arthritis of the wrist
- Pregnancy due to associated weight gain and fluid retention

Signs and Symptoms

It presents with numbness, tingling, weakness or pain in hands, fingers, arms, and even up into elbows at times. It seems to be worse at night, and may be aggravated when driving with the tingling or numbness mostly in the thumb, index, and middle fingers. If it progresses then there may be weakness of the hand, poor grip and dropping of objects.

Treatment for Carpal Tunnel Syndrome

A health care provider, after taking a history and examination of the hand and arm as well as the median nerve will make the diagnosis. Sometimes blood work, nerve studies, muscle tests, ultrasound or MRI of the wrist may be done to help with the diagnosis. Treatment may include:

- Weight loss if overweight or obese
- Rest, icing the area, anti-inflammatory medicines e.g. Ibuprofen or steroids
- Use of a Wrist Splint at night to keep the wrist in a position so as to open up the space/tunnel
- Do exercises like rotating the wrists and stretching out the palms and fingers
- Avoid sleeping on your hands

- If there is no improvement, physical therapy may be ordered
- Steroid injection into the wrist area may help with pain and inflammation
- If all the above fail, symptoms do not improve, or there is weakness of hand, then surgery is performed to open up the space around the median nerve

Gout

What is It?

"People wish their enemies dead - but I do not; I say give them the gout, give them the stone!"

—Mary Wortley Montagu. Writer.
(May 15, 1689—Aug. 21, 1762).

This is a painful inflammation of a joint as a result of crystals deposited in joints. It usually affects the big toes, and used to be associated with affluence and so was called "the rich man's disease".

Currently, developed countries have a higher prevalence of gout than developing countries. It occurs when there is excess amount of a chemical called URIC ACID in the blood, and when it reaches a certain concentration, it is able to form sharp needlelike crystals which deposit in the joints especially of the extremities. These may cause an acute painful attack, and some individuals they may have several attacks in a year. It can also occur in the ankle, wrist, elbow and knee joints, and repeated attacks can go on to destroy the joint, resulting in arthritis of the joint and deformity which is known as GOUTY ARTHRITIS

Risk Factors

- Males, older people, and obese individuals
- Those with a family history of gout
- People who engage in excessive alcohol intake
- Medications which increase URIC ACID levels in the blood, for example aspirin and hydrochlorothiazide (blood pressure medicine)
- Individuals who have hypertension, diabetes, heart attacks and kidney stones
- Post-menopausal women; (unlike men who get it at an earlier age)

Symptoms of Gout

During an acute attack, there may be:

Sudden onset of redness, and swelling of the involved joint

Pain or throbbing in the joint involved

The big toe is often affected (Podagra) with swelling, redness and pain at base of the toe

Bedsheets touching an affected big toe may not be tolerated due to intense pain

After an attack which may last 3 to 14 days, the pain goes away, the joint gets back to normal unless damaged from recurrent attacks

Attacks become frequent if the uric acid level is high

Chronic Gout

Some patients experience 1 to 2 attacks a year or in their life, however, others have several attacks with shortened interval inbetween attacks. This leads to chronic gout which may present with white growths (uric acid crystals) just under the skin on top of the joints called TOPHI. They cause deformity of the join, destroying bone and cartilage, and they may impair the function of the joint.

Uric acid can also be deposited on the tip of the ear, tip of elbow and in the kidneys forming kidney stones when levels are high.

Treatment

An acute attack may be treated with the following:

Rest, keeping limb raised, and applying ice in a bag wrapped in a towel

Use of anti – inflammation medicines like:

- Ibuprofen, naproxen, indomethacin (NSAIDs) and colchicine
- Steroid injections or pills, e.g. Prednisone

Prevention of Gout Attacks

- Lifestyle changes like weight loss and appropriate diet
- Adequate hydration and limiting or stopping alcohol altogether
- Use of medications that lower uric acid levels
- Well controlled blood sugar in those with diabetes

Medications to Lower Uric Acid Levels

These prevent attacks by lowering uric acid, and stop crystals forming in the joints.

ALLOPURINOL and FEBUXOSTAT block formation of uric acid

PROBENECID increase elimination of uric acid in the urine

COLCHICINE is used for both prevention and treatment of acute attacks

PEGLOTICASE given intravenously. It changes uric acid to a harmless substance which is passed in the urine. Used for severe cases not responding to other treatments

LOSARTAN (for hypertension) and FENOFIBRATE (for cholesterol and tri-glycerides) can also lower it and so they may be the medicines to use if one has gout and those other conditions

It is important to know that one can have an acute attack or flare when one starts prevention medications, and to avoid this, anti-inflammatory medications (e.g. NSAIDS or colchicine) may have to be taken along with prevention medication for the first 3 to 6 months. It is important to be compliant with prevention medications which are taken for a long time. Your health care provider will choose the appropriate medicines for treatment and prevention for you.

Therapeutic Lifestyle Changes
Diet

Foods which may bring on an acute attack include:

- Beer, sugary drinks with high fructose corn syrup used as a sweetener
- Foods like organ meats – kidney, liver, and sweetbread, high intake of beef, pork, lamb, as well as certain sea foods like shellfish and even sardines. These tend to be high in "purines" which eventually break down to form uric acid

Foods which may prevent attacks include:

- Foods which are low in purines like enriched bread, pasta, fruits and vegetables. Some vegetables are high in purine but do not seem to cause frequent gout attacks, e.g. lentils, soy bean, asparagus, cauliflower, spinach, and peas
- Diets high in vegetables, cherries and low fat dairy products are helpful and may lower uric acid levels
- Some studies have shown that Vitamin C, cherries, and coffee (both decaffein-ated and caffeinated) seem to lower levels of uric acid in the blood

PHYSICAL ACTIVITIES: These may help prevent attacks and include:

- Losing some weight
- Physical activities
- Exercising helps the joints and also may decrease pain and increase mobility

Plantar Fasciitis (PF)

The PLANTAR FASCIA (FAR-SHIA) is a thick band or connective (supportive) tis-sue that stretches or fans out from the bottom of the heel bone of your foot (at the back) to the ball of your foot where the toes are. It provides support to the muscles, creates the arch of the foot, and helps the foot with weight bearing.

What is It?

Plantar fasciitis is pain and inflammation of the plantar fascia especially in the inner or medial aspect of where it attaches to the heel bone. This results from tiny tears in the heel attachment.

Signs and Symptoms

- Include sharp pain when one steps on the foot first thing in the morning, and it eases off as one continues to walk
- Walking to the bathroom in the middle of the night can bring about the pain
- Pain at the end of the day after one has been on their feet for a long time
- When one presses the bottom of the heel especially the inner part, the same pain is elicited
- The pain may be on for some weeks and then go away (recurrent episodes of intermittent pain), however, those with severe PF may have daily pain
- X-RAY of the foot may show a bone spur. Not everyone with plantar fasciitis has a bone spur

BONE SPUR: When PF has existed for a while, a reaction to the inflammation will be the formation of a small piece of bone on the heel bone. The tiny curved bone may be seen jutting from the heel like a "spike" on an x-ray and is called a Bone Spur.

Treatment of Plantar Fasciitis

Foot Stretches

Do foot stretches and prevent the sudden flexion (movement of forefoot backwards toward the leg) of the foot. Before one gets out of bed, one has to gently stretch the forefoot backwards (toward your body) and hold it for a count of five, and then release it. This controlled stretching is done about 5 times before you step out of the bed. This minimizes the sudden impact of the foot on the floor that causes pain.

Cold Treatment

You can also freeze a bottle of water, wrap it in a towel and roll it under your foot. The cold helps with the pain. This can be done two to three times a day as needed.

Wear A Plantar Fascia Splint to Bed

This is an L shaped splint called a Posterior Splint which can be worn at night to bed. It keeps the foot at a 90 degree angle while asleep and so when one wakes up and steps on the floor there is no sudden jerk of foot from an extended to a flexed position resulting in a sharp pain. They are found at pharmacies or stores that sell medical devices.

Use of A Heel Cup

These are molded with gel or special cushion and fit into one's shoes at the heel area or generic gel heel pads can also be used. They act as "shock absorbers" so that pain from contact of the foot with the ground is minimized.

Use of Tennis Shoes With Good Arch Support

Laced up tennis or running shoes with good orthotic arch supports are able to help absorb the impact on the ground and help minimize the pain.

Taping the Foot

Firmly wrapping the foot with an elastic ACE wrap or taping the heel with athletic tape.

Wearing A Walking Boot

An orthotic walking long or short boot is also used when pain is severe. It takes away some of the pressure on the heel.

Anti-Inflammatory Medications

Any of the Non-Steroidal Anti-Inflammatory Drugs (NSAIDS) e.g. Ibuprofen or Naproxen can be used to help with pain and inflammation. To be effective they need to be taken as prescribed.

Steroids

Oral steroid tablets may be given for a few days to help with the inflammation. They need to be taken with food and are not for long term use. Steroid combined with lidocaine (numbing or local anesthetic medicine) may be injected into the heel at the area of greatest pain.

Physical Therapy

Physical therapy by a therapist utilizing ultrasound treatment and other modalities may help relieve the pain, together with ongoing prescribed home exercises.

Amniofix Injection

This is an injection derived from the amniotic membrane which surrounds a developing fetus (it is NOT obtained from an aborted fetus, but during a cesarean birth).

It is used to treat plantar fasciitis and tendonitis (inflammation of tendons, e.g. Achilles tendonitis) when surgery is not desired. It is given by a Podiatrist (foot doctor) or Orthopedic surgeon.

Surgery

Surgery by a podiatrist may be needed when all else fails. It will require some down time off the foot as it heals. Crutches or a walking boot are used during healing.

Osteoporosis (low bone density)

What is It?

"It does seem incredible that a disease that can be diagnosed and can be successfully treated is not a major health issue. We must do all we can to prevent, treat and ultimately cure this painful and life restricting disease."

—Baroness Julia Cumberlege, Former UK health minister 2006

This is a condition in which the bones have decreased in mass, as a result of bone loss, and results in weakness and decreased strength; making one susceptible to bone breaks or fractures.

It occurs frequently with aging because the bone mass tends to decrease with age. Women mostly suffer from osteoporosis, especially after menopause because estrogens which protect against osteoporosis are low. It can also affect men, but at an older age, since their bone loss start later and it progresses at a slower rate than in women. Both estrogen and testosterone protect bones.

Prevalence

It is common with about 3 million cases diagnosed in the USA each year, and it is estimated that one in every two women above the age of 50 years will have an osteoporotic fracture in their lifetime. in the USA about 10 million people mainly women are affected. Osteopenia which is a milder form of the disease affects another 18 million. World wide, about 200 million people are affected, and so It is an important disease with serious debilitating complications that can happen. It can be described as either primary or secondary.

Primary Osteoporosis

Osteoporosis can be primary when no specific cause is found, other than age related.

Secondary Osteoporosis

When it is caused by disease, deficiency, medicines, or immobility. These include:

- Low Estrogen states/diseases like premature menopause

- Female athletes of intense sports
- Endocrine problems like Hyperthyroidism and Diabetes
- Deficiencies of minerals like calcium and Vitamin D
- Intestinal problems like post gastric bypass, celiac disease, malaborption, and chronic diarrhea
- Inflammatory diseases like rheumatoid arthritis, inflammatory bowel diseases and Lupus
- Medicines like long term steroids, chemotherapy (may cause ovarian failure), a diuretic like furosemide (however, other diuretics called thiazides increase bone density) and anticonvulsants like phenobarbtial and phenytoin
- Breast cancer medicines which decrease Estrogens like Anastrozole, diabetes medicine called Pioglitazone, Heparin (blood thinner), and even Antacids containing aluminum like Aludrox

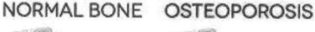

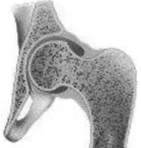 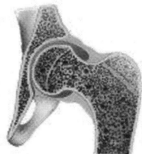

Diagram; Herbert S. Diamond. Fast Five Quiz: Do You Know Best Practices for Osteoporosis? - Medscape - Oct 05, 2015.

Signs and Symptoms

- There may be no symptoms until a fracture occurs as a result of a small fall
- A history of a fracture of the wrist, hip, or spine after a small fall or minor injury in a post-menopausal woman or elderly man high endurance female Athlete signifies a high probability of osteoporosis
- Presentation of pain and deformity in a post-menopausal woman following a fall on the outstretched hand, may signify a fracture and osteoporosis
- Women may also have fractures of the vertebrae or spinal bones in the back, causing a "hump" (kyphosis) to be formed and this is called "Dowager's hump". This will result in pain and inability to straighten the spine

Osteopenia

This is when there is low bone mass or density but not severe enough to be labeled as osteoporosis. There are measurements to distinguish between the two.

Diagnosis of Osteoporosis

Screening for osteoporosis or osteopenia is available. It helps you and your doctor know if you have the condition or whether one is at risk of developing osteoporosis or breaking a bone. Special x-rays or Ultrasound techniques are used for screening and diagnosing.

DEXA SCAN

This is done by measuring bone mineral density at the hip and in the spine by a special X-RAY scan known as a DEXA SCAN or BONE DENSITOMETRY. A calculation of your risk of fracturing a bone at the hip or spine is made using the measurements taken by the machine. This is a simple painless test done with you lying down on a table. This measurement can be used for screening, diagnosis and even for ongoing monitoring of people who are being treated for osteoporosis.

Heel Test for Osteoporosis

A quick and simple measurement of the heel, forearm or finger using a smaller mobile machine is used for screening as well, but it is not as accurate as the DEXA SCAN. If such a screen is positive, then a Dexa scan will have to be done to confirm the diagnosis.

X-ray

Osteoporosis if severe may be seen on x-rays as an incidental (accidental) finding, but by then, the condition will be quite advanced. X-ray is not a screening method.

Risk Factors for Developing Osteoporosis

"Such lifestyle factors such as cigarette smoking, excessive alcohol consumption, little physical activity and low dietary calcium intake are risk factors for osteoporosis as well as for many other non-communicable diseases".

—Gro Harlem Brundtland Director-General of the WHO from 1998 to 2003. (https://www.azquotes.com/author/2074-Gro_Harlem_Brundtland)

These include some which are modifiable (changeable), but others are not (non-modifiable).

Modifiable ones include:

Smoking
Poor health or bed ridden
Lack of exercise or physical activity
Low intake of calcium and Vitamin D
Excessive Alcohol consumption
Malabsorption after gastric bypass

Non Modifiable ones include:

Female sex
Advanced age
White or Asian ancestry
History of fracture as an adult
Family history of Osteoporosis
Loss of height greater than 4cm or 1.6 inches
Surgery to remove uterus (hysterectomy) and ovaries (oophorectomy) leading
   to loss of estrogen
Early menopause or low estrogen state
Dementia
Immobility due to sickness
History of hyperthyroid or overactive thyroid
Individuals on medications like long term steroids, and thyroid replacement
   medications used to treat hypothyroid like Synthroid, Levothyroxine, or
   Armour thyroid.

Complications of Osteoporosis

- Could lead to fractures especially of the hip and spine. Ankle and upper arm also occur
- A hip fracture causes inability to walk, resulting in complications like pneumonia or lung infection due to prolonged lying in bed by a frail woman
- All the above may prevent affected women from going back to independent living, and they may end up in a nursing home or assisted living facility
- Bed sores may result from prolonged immobilization
- There are psychological effects on patients given their sudden change in living conditions from active mobile to possible immobility
- Fracture of the vertebra of the spine results in compression of the anterior part of vertebra, this is called kyphosis resulting in hump in upper back – "Dowager's hump"
- The kyphosis results in decrease in height and curved spine with possible pain
- Hump on the back and inability to stand straight up, may cause decreased mobility
- Chronic back pain resulting from fracture of vertebrae may occur
- Apart from physical disability, it also has economic, social and psychological consequences on the patient and their families

Prevention of Osteoporosis

"Given the serious public health burden of fractures associated with osteoporosis, it is important to learn as much as possible about ways to prevent and treat bone loss".

—Joan McGowan, MD. Director of the Division of Musculoskeletal Diseases, NIH. USA.

There are things one can do to prevent or delay the development of osteoporosis. These include:

- Regular exercise and physical activity like walking help strengthen the bones
- Stop smoking cigarettes if you smoke
- Decrease alcohol use to one serving or less per day
- Be exposed to sunlight though one has to be careful of consequences like skin cancer
- Strength training and balance to prevent falls
- Taking Vitamin D3 supplement is important to help absorb calcium from the gut. It is more potent than VIT D2 which is got from plants
- Eat foods fortified with Vit. D and fatty fish like salmon, mackerel which contain Vit. D. Milk cheese are also fortified with it.
- Outside activities in the sun, will help with Vitamin D production by the skin.
- If on thyroid medicines like levothyroxine, avoid taking excess medicine since this may cause bone loss. Regular blood tests are needed to make sure your levels are not in overdose range.
- Women with breast cancer being treated with Aromatase Inhibitors like Anastrozole (Arimidex) which inhibit Estrogens, are at increased risk, so will need bone density scans, and if affected be treated for Osteoporosis

Treatment of Osteoporosis

Once the diagnosis is made by a bone density scan, your health provider and you can make the decision to start medications which halt the process and can reverse the bone loss or decrease fracture risk in those with Osteoporosis.

Medications Used to Treat Osteoporosis

There are several medications that are available and some are oral or injected.

- Bisphosphonates are oral tablets taken daily, weekly or monthly, and examples are Alendronate (Fosamax), Ibandronate (Boniva), and Actonel (risedronate)
- Raloxifene (Evista) which acts like estrogen, causing increased bone density
- Injectable ones include those given subcutaneously (under the skin) every 6 months (denosumab – Prolia), into the vein every 3 months (Ibandronate – Boniva), or once every year in a doctor's office (Zoledronic acid-Reclast)
- These medicines may be taken for three to five years, and have been found to continue to work for years after one stops taking them

- For all these medicines to work, the body has to have adequate amounts of calcium and Vitamin D present. Therefore one may also need to be on these supplements
- To check or monitor the effectiveness of treatment, periodic BONE DENSITY scans will have to be done

Your doctor will prescribe which medicine is the right one for you after discussions with you.

The Human Spine
What is It?

The upright human spine is a remarkable part of the body and stretches from just below the skull to the buttocks area. It is made up of 33 interlocking bone structures known as vertebrae which encase the spinal cord. A vertebra has a solid disk like body with side wings toward the back known as transverse processes and a back wing or protrusion called a spinal process. These 3 bones encircle the central canal through which the spinal cord runs from the bottom of the brain. From the sides of the spinal cord, nerves exit through side holes of the vertebrae. Bundles of the exiting nerves join together to form major nerves, and these supply the different parts of the body. To give the spine flexibility, and also to act as "shock absorbers", adjacent pairs of the vertebral bones have cushions or paddings between them known as intervertebral DISKS or DISCS. These are made of fibrous material on the outside and the inner part is made up of a gel like protein which has a consistency like toothpaste. The spine is divided into roughly five parts based on location and each has a specific number of Vertebrae:

Cervical or neck (7)
Thoracic with ribs attached to most of them. (12)
Lumbar or lower back (5)
Sacral or base of spine. Vertebrae are fused and forms back part of pelvis (5)
Coccyx or tailbone (3 to 5 tiny bones)

Low Back Pain (Lumbago) (LBP)
What is It?

Low back pain (LBP) is pain in the lower part of the back and if it is from the spine and its surrounding structures, it can be acute or chronic pain. Acute LBP may last up to 12 weeks and it may be due to muscle spasm or strain, herniated or bulging discs pressing a nerve. It is chronic if it has lasted more than 3 months. LBP can be further divided into mechanical and non mechanical. It is a very serious and common condition, and in the USA about 20–30% may suffer from it at any given time; and in about 80% of people at some time of their lives according to studies. It tends to increase with age and occurs in both men and women. It results in loss of work, unemployment, depression, addiction to narcotics or pain-killers and disability in sufferers. Chronic low back pain causes more disability than any other condition worldwide.

Mechanical LBP

This is originating from the spine and surrounding tissues like discs, muscles, tendons ligaments, vertebrae and facet joints.

Non Mechanical LBP

This may be due to other things outside of the spine and surroundings. There are 3 main types:

- Referred Pain: This can be pain from other parts of the body, e.g. from cancer with bony metastasis, other infections or inflammation of organs like kidney or abdomen
- Neurological: Present in conditions like Diabetes, Autoimmune diseases (diseases where body is attacking itself), Cauda Equina Syndrome (compression of spinal nerves leading to new urinary retention or overflow), Progressive motor or sensory loss
- Other bone and muscle diseases: For example, Fibromyalgia, Osteoporosis, and Rheumatoid Arthritis, Osteomyelitis (infection of the bone of the spine)

The individual will have other symptoms pointing towards a non mechanical cause of the back pain, or history of fever, recent cancer, and other specific medical conditions.

Causes of Low Back Pain

It may be a result of strain of muscles, injury during sports or by a motor vehicle accident, prolonged standing or sitting, lifting heavy objects, and even a mattress which is too soft or too old.

It may be related to the spine and nearby structures which are the following:

Bones (vertebrae)
Discs
Muscles
Ligaments
Interlocking side joints known as facet joints
Nerves

Other Conditions Causing Low Back Pain

Conditions affecting the abdomen, pelvis and urinary system, may also cause low back pain however; with these, other symptoms may be present which helps recognize them. Examples are pregnancy, during menses, or even a urinary tract infection.

Signs and Symptoms for Low Back Pain Related to The Spine

The pain can be anywhere from the area of the spine beneath the rib cage to the buttocks area

Pain may be dull, sharp, stabbing, annoying, or intense

It may also radiate into the thighs and legs

There may be curvature of the back or scoliosis

Numbness and tingling may be present

Bad posture may be obvious

Obesity

Limping may be present

Low Back Pain in Females Above 50 Years

Among the causes of Low Back Pain in females above the age of 50 years the following occur frequently:

Lumbar Degenerative Disk Disease

Facet Joint Arthritis

Lumbar Disk Herniation

Lumbar Spinal Stenosis

Sacroiliac Joint Dysfunction

Younger people may not experience many of the above, however; we will discuss these and other causes of low back pain.

Back Muscle Strain

This is due to acute injury from bending the wrong way, vigorous working out, exercise, or involvement in a motor vehicle accident. The muscles around the spine are inflamed or stretched resulting in muscle spasm and pain.

Treatment

This may take a week or two to resolve. Treatment is with anti-inflammatory medicines like Ibuprofen, muscle relaxants, arthritic rubs, ice, use of a heating pad and rest; however too many rest days are not advised. Exercises are available to help muscles relax and be strengthened.

Disorders Associated With The Disk (Disc)
The Disc and Its Function

The discs serve many purposes including acting like shock absorbers to absorb any pressure on the spine, e.g. when we walk or run; and they cause flexibility of the spine so we can bend and twist. The oval-shaped disc is made up of connective tissue (a type of supporting tissue present throughout the body) which has a softer gel-like central part (like a jelly filled donut).

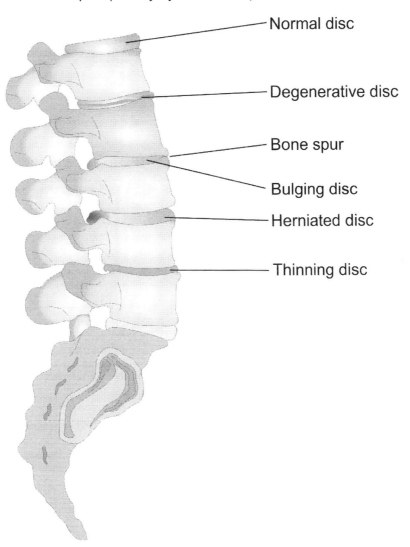

Normal disc

Degenerative disc

Bone spur

Bulging disc

Herniated disc

Thinning disc

The Spine With Different Types of DISC Disorders

Degenerative Disc Disease (DDD)
What is It?

This is also referred to as "wear and tear" of the discs (disks may be used inter-changeably) and this increases with age. There may be drying out of the supple disc as a result of loss of water, so it becomes stiff and the disc height is reduced; causing the adjacent vertebrae to be closer together resulting in pinching of the spinal nerves and or spinal cord.

Bulging or Herniated DISCS

Both acute and chronic conditions may cause one or several discs to BULGE, RUPTURE or HERNIATE backwards or sideways and sometimes press on the spinal cord or a nerve as it exits through the side of the vertebra. This can lead to intense pain at that part of the back and if the nerve roots which form the sciatic nerve are involved then Sciatica results.

Sciatica (Sciatic Nerve Pain)
What is It?

Sciatica is pain felt from the buttock and down the back of the leg and sometimes to the toes due to irritation of the roots of the nerves which form the sciatic nerve. The nerve courses down the buttock, hip and back of the leg. Pain is usually on one side. It may be caused by many factors but the most common ones are:

- Herniated or bulging disk pressing on the roots of the spinal nerves
- Forward slipping of one vertebra over the one immediately close to it
- Spinal stenosis (when the canal is narrowed pressing on the spinal cord within it)
- Bone spur on a vertebra (from osteoarthritis) projects into part of the nerve
- Osteoarthritis of the vertebrae, the side canals and posterior small joints called the facet joints
- Injury to the back following a car accident

Other less common causes are:

- A pregnant uterus sitting on the roots of the sciatic nerve
- Tumors inside or outside of the spinal canal
- Piriformis muscle syndrome – which is when this muscle which lies above the sciatic nerve presses on it. Even a fat wallet in the back pocket can press on the piriformis muscle and cause sciatic nerve pain

Signs and Symptoms

Pain which radiates from the lower back on one side and goes into the buttock
and down the thigh into the calf muscles of the back of the leg
Pain may be burning, sharp, achy, or very severe especially on sitting down
Pain may be accompanied by numbness and tingling down the involved leg
Pain is worse with sitting and standing up may relieve some of the pain
If it is SEVERE there may be leg weakness, or bowel and bladder problems

Treatment

A careful history and examination by a health care provider is needed. Most will
resolve after a week or two if its mild. Treatment may include:

Rest, pain medications, steroids, Anti-inflammatory medications, Muscle relaxants, Physical Therapy, Manipulation therapy, heating pads, and medications that
help nerve pain.

It may take up to six weeks to recover. If there is no improvement, or there are
"red flags" or unusual accompanying symptoms like urine or stool incontinence,
urine retention or progressive motor or sensory loss, then the health provider may
order imaging studies like X-ray, CT scan or MRI scans to have a more careful look
at the bones, nerves, discs and muscles.

Steroid Shots

Epidural steroid injections may also be used and injected near the irritated spinal
nerves to help with pain and inflammation. This injection is placed outside the
casing or covering of the spinal cord but within the canal and is done under the
guidance of an X-ray called a fluoroscope.

Surgery

Surgery is rare, but occurs if there is associated weakness of that limb, chronic
pain not relieved by above or problems with bowel movements and/or bladder.

Spinal Arthritis (Spondylosis)
What is It?

This is a broad term to describe the wear and tear of the spine. Since there are
joints in the spine, there can be Osteoarthritis of the joints between the Vertebrae
or at the joints formed by the interlocking wing like bones of adjacent Vertebrae
(facet joints). This condition is known as spinal arthritis or SPONDYLOSIS and in
effect it is degeneration which increases with age, and can affect discs, vertebrae
and facet joints of the spine.

Symptoms

Sometimes there are no symptoms and it will be discovered by chance on an x-ray. For others it can cause pain and stiffness just like Osteoarthritis in other parts of the body. Pain is usually at the part of the back involved, and it mostly affects the neck and lower back. More severe degeneration may cause narrowing of the spinal canal and therefore affect the spinal cord resulting in weakness of legs, numbness and tingling and even loss of bladder and bowel control.

Treatment

X-rays of the back will show that the bones are affected, or the disc space is narrowed because the disc has lost its height or shape. Treatment is by anti-inflammatory drugs, physical therapy, movement, heat, ice, arthritic creams etc. Sometimes pain management doctors may give Facet Joint injections when those joints are affected. Surgery is indicated when there are bowel and bladder problems or pain is so severe it affects one's daily activities.

Lumbar Facet Joint Arthritis

What is a Facet Joint

This is the joint formed by posterior parts of two adjacent vertebrae and are present just below the posterior wings of the vertebrae causing one vertebra to link to the next one. They allow the back to be flexible allowing bending and twisting especially of the neck and low back. Just like any joint in the body it can be affected by Osteoarthritis, Gout, Psoriasis, and Rheumatoid Arthritis. Osteoarthritis is the commonest Arthritis affecting these joints in the lumbar area.

Osteoarthritis of Facet Joint

It is found in over two thirds of adults aged 45 to 65 years. It is often accompanied or preceded by Degenerative Disc Disease, which tends to put more stress on the facet joints. Risk factors for developing this include: age, increased weight, being female, and caucasian.

Symptoms

It presents with pain in the side of the lumbar area involved and pain may go into the buttocks, hips, groin, and upper thigh areas. The pain is worse with extension of the spine, and with palpation of the facet joint involved.

Treatment

Tests done include X-rays, CT or MRI of the spine. Treatment include Physical Therapy, medicines like Anti-inflammatory, weight loss if obese, and injections known as Facet Joint injections using steroids and numbing or local anesthetic medicine(Lidocaine). Another procedure call radiofrequency ablation can destroy the nerve which serves the particular Facet Joint and so eliminate the pain.

Spinal Stenosis

This is mostly seen in older people and it is usually due to compression of the spinal canal in which the spinal cord or nerves that exit from the sides of the cord are located. Spinal stenosis of the lumbar region is the common reason for spinal surgery in people older than 65 years. It usually occurs in the lower back (lumbar) or neck (cervical) area of the spine. There are several causes resulting in this narrowing and these include:

- Bulging and herniated discs
- Arthritis of the facet joints
- Thickened of ligaments within the canal
- Slipping of a vertebra
- Arthritis of the vertebra causing bone spurs to push on the cord or nerves within the canal
- Damage to the vertebrae from accidents in younger individuals
- Tumors
- Fracture of the vertebra from osteoporosis

Symptoms

It usually presents as buttocks or lower leg pain with or without back pain, numbness, and tingling, weakness of the legs if lumbar area is involved or symptoms in the arms if the neck area of spine is involved.

In lumbar area, there is usually pain with standing, walking and extension; while it is relieved by sitting, flexion of the spine, or lying down. Walking up a hill with flexed back relieves the pain and walking down a hill with extended back makes it worse.

Flexion tends to open up the space around the cord, relieving the compression. It can affect both nerves and blood vessels within the canal.

If very severe it may result in loss of control of bladder and bowels (incontinence).

Treatment

After a careful history and physical exam by a health care provider she may request X-ray, or MRI of the involved part of the spine. Treatments are non-surgical and surgical.

Non surgical

These include non-steroidal anti-inflammatory drugs, other pain and nerve medications (Gabapentin, Duloxetine, Pregabalin), physical therapy, and steroid injections. Some patients will improve over time, while others do not.

Surgery

When above fail or the symptoms are very severe, surgery called Spinal Decompression is done to release pressure on the involved nerve or spine by removing the bone or other structures compressing it.

CAM Treatment For Low Back Pain (Alternative methods)

A. The American College of Physicians (ACP) gave a strong recommendation for using non pharmacological methods for treating chronic back pain along with exercise

Moderate quality evidence: These include exercise, multidisciplinary rehabilitation, acupuncture, mindfulness-based stress reduction

Low quality evidence: Tai chi, Yoga, motor control exercise, progressive relaxation, electromyography biofeedback, low-level laser therapy, operant therapy, Cognitive Behavioral Therapy, or spinal manipulation

(Non-invasive Treatments for Acute, Subacute, and Chronic Low Back Pain: A Clinical Practice Guideline From the ACP, Annals of Internal Medicine. April 4th 2017)

B. According to the National Center for Complementary and Integrative Health (NCCIH)

Spinal Manipulation – either Osteopathic, Physical Therapy or Chiropractic – **moderately effective for chronic low-back pain**

Acupuncture – **fair evidence that it is helpful in relieving chronic back pain**

Yoga – **carefully adapted set of yoga poses may reduce low-back pain and improve function**

Massage – **fair evidence that massage is helpful in relieving chronic low back pain**

Body Mind Therapy

In a recent study reported in the Journal of American Medical Association, two mind and body practices – mindfulness based stress reduction (MBSR – which combined mindfulness meditation and yoga) and cognitive-behavioral therapy (CBT – training to change pain-related thoughts and behaviors) – resulted in greater improvement in pain and functional limitation compared to usual care for up to a year. (Cherkin DC, Sherman KJ *JAMA*. 2016; 315(12):1240–1249).

If you plan to use a CAM method, make sure you first discuss it with your health care provider.

Sacroiliac (SI) Joint Dysfunction

The sacrum is the lower part of the spine and its vertebrae are fused together. At both of its sides it forms the SI joint with the second pelvic bone called the ilium. The joint has a cartilage between the bones and so arthritis can affect it. However, many other conditions can lead to dysfunction of the SI joint. It is believed to be a cause of pain in up to one third of individuals who present with low back pain and this number is even higher in pregnant women.

Dysfunction of this joint may be due to many factors including:

Osteoarthritis
Injury
Gout, Psoriasis and Rheumatoid Arthritis
Stress fracture of the sacrum
Pregnancy
Unequal leg lengths
Pain in hip and knee

Symptoms

It can present with pain over the joint on the affected side and this can radiate down to the buttocks, thighs, and lower legs.

Treatment

Diagnosis is by physical exam and doing a diagnostic joint injection with numbing medicine like lidocaine. Relief from this gives the diagnosis. Treatment includes: Physical therapy, Taping, use of a brace, medications (anti-inflammatory), steroid injection into the joint, and destruction of the nerve supplying the joint (radio-frequency ablation). Surgery is a last option, but its success rate is low.

Narcotics and Low Back Pain

Many individuals have become addicted to narcotics which had been initially prescribed for low back pain. In a recent report by the American College of Physicians (2017), non-drug therapy like heat, massage, spinal manipulation, physical therapy, acupuncture is recommended for acute or subacute low back pain. Most would improve over time. If non drug methods fail, they can be combined with non narcotics. Medications recommended include non-steroidal anti-inflammatories, tramadol or duloxetine (this is an anti-depressant with helps nerve pain even in the non-depressed patient). Evidence was insufficient about helpfulness of acetaminophen, systemic corticosteroids, or antiseizure medications on chronic low back pain. Narcotics and opioids are to be avoided due to their addictive potential, and potential for abuse. Many have died in the USA from Opioid overdose and it has been termed an "Opioid Epidemic".

Opioid Overdose Deaths in the USA

According to the CDC, the deaths from opioid overdose in the USA during 2017, (including prescription opioids and illegal opioids like heroin and illicitly manufactured fentanyl) was 6 times higher than in 1999. Around 68% of the more than 70,200 drug overdose deaths in 2017 involved an opioid, and currently, about 130 people die every day from opioid overdose and so they have to be avoided (www.cdc.gov/drugoverdose/epidemic/index.html). It is such a big problem that overdose reversal drug Naloxone (Narcan) is being sold OTC and addicts or their families can purchase them. Police Officers, Fire service officers and Ambulances all carry them to use when needed. It is given either intranasally or as an intramuscular injection. It will not reverse overdose from non-opioid drugs, like cocaine, benzodiazepines, or alcohol.

25

Blood Conditions

There are many diseases associated with blood that flows through our blood vessels, however; we will discuss some of the common conditions which affect the blood cells and lymphatic system of the body. These include:

Anemia
Sickle Cell Disease
Leukemia
Multiple Myeloma
Hodgkin's Lymphoma
Non Hodgkin Lymphoma

Diseases of the Blood Cells

The blood is made up of fluid called plasma (PLAS-MA) and several different cells. The three main types of cells are red cells, white cells, and platelets and each of these performs specific functions in the body. Diseases can affect each set of cells, depending on whether there is underproduction or excessive production of the cells. Blood is a vital component of our bodies and this is even mentioned as the life of the body in many religious books including the Bible.

Blood Cells and Their Functions

"For the life of the flesh is in the blood, and I have given it to you upon the altar to make atonement for your souls; for it is the blood that makes atonement for the soul".
—Bible, Leviticus 17v11 NKJV.

All these cells are produced in the bone marrow of bones and each type has a certain number of days it circulates in the blood, and then it is removed and broken down

RED CELLS: The red cells give blood its color and they carry oxygen from the lungs and supply all the different organs and tissues of the body with oxygen and nutrients. They also remove carbon dioxide from the cells and carry it to the lungs to be expelled from the body when we breathe out.

WHITE CELLS: The white cells are subdivided into different types of cells but the main ones are neutrophils and lymphocytes. The white blood cells help in fighting infections when the body is attacked by viruses, bacteria or other organisms. The average life span for a white blood cell is two to three weeks.

PLATELETS: The platelets help in clotting to prevent further blood loss when there is bleeding from a cut or wound. Both low or high platelet counts can cause disease.

Red Cell Production

The red cells carry oxygen and carbon dioxide in a protein and iron complex called HEMOGLOBIN (Hee-mo-glow-bin). Certain chemicals are needed to produce the hemoglobin and the most important ones are: Iron, Folic Acid, Vitamin B12, Protein and a hormone produced in the kidney called Erythropoietin. If there is deficiency of any of these, then there is decreased production of hemoglobin and a condition called Anemia is the result. The average life span of a red cell is 120 days and it is then removed from the blood by special cells mostly in the spleen and liver, and then the contained iron is recycled.

The Lymphatic System

One also needs to know about the lymphatic system which is related to the blood circulation, and it is an important part of the body's defense system. The lymphatic system is made up of vessels, fluid, and cells and the whole system is part of the body's immune system.

Vessels – Carry lymph and transport white blood cells from bone marrow to lymph nodes

Lymph – Fluid containing white blood cells mainly lymphocytes

Lymph nodes – Small oval structures that make immune fighting cells and trap foreign cells including cancer cells.

Organs – Tonsils, Adenoids, Spleen and thymus

How the Lymphatic System Works

- The special white blood cells called lymphocytes can remove viruses, dead cells, and cancer cells
- The body has lymph nodes in several areas and there are about 600 of them present with some being found in front of the ear, in the neck area, back of the

head, under the chin, under the arm pit (axilla) and in the groin. Others form chains in the abdomen and pelvic area of the body
- Cancer cells can be trapped in lymph nodes near the origin of the cancer. For example, cancer of the breast can spread to the lymph nodes under the armpit or axilla
- Cancer can also originate from the lymphocytes themselves and is called Lymphoma (lim fo ma). A common type of lymphoma is Hodgkin disease where a tumor starts in the lymph node
- When lymph fluid is prevented from flowing well, as in the case when the regional lymph nodes in the axilla are removed during surgery for breast cancer, then a woman may develop lymphedema of the arm which was discussed under breast cancer

Conditions Affecting Blood Cells

We will discuss a few common conditions affecting all these different blood cells.

Anemia
What is It?

Anemia occurs when there are low numbers of circulating red blood cells in the body and results in low hemoglobin, leading to low supply of oxygen and nutrients to the cells. Anemia can also be described as acute when it occurs quickly like rapid loss of blood during surgery, or in a car accident, or chronic when it develops over a period of time.

What Causes Anemia?

There are many causes of anemia but they can be classified according to whether there is:

Decreased production of red cells
Excessive destruction of red cells
Loss of red cells
Presence of abnormal red cells

Signs and Symptoms

Anemia or low blood results in:

Tiredness and fatigue
Shortness of breath, dizziness, palpitations
Listlessness and excessive sleep
Some women will crave to eat ice, clay, or chalk and this is called PICA

In acute or rapid loss of blood the signs may also include:

Low blood pressure
Palpitations and fast pulse
Shock (blood not supplying the organs so they fail)
Heart complications like heart attack and heart failure

Tests

In anemia the tests measure mainly the number of red cells, concentration of HEMOGLOBIN as well as another entity called HEMATOCRIT (this is the volume of red blood cells in the blood), and all these can decrease when anemia is present. Tests measuring the other chemicals mentioned above e.g. Iron, Vitamin B12, folic acid etc. are done to pinpoint the cause of the anemia.

Iron-deficiency Anemia
What is It?

This is anemia caused by low blood IRON. There are several causes and they include:

Excessive menstrual bleeding in women of reproductive age
Lack of adequate intake of iron rich foods
Bleeding hemorrhoids
Bleeding stomach or peptic ulcers
Bleeding from cancer of the large bowels, bladder, and uterus
Parasitic infections of the intestines like hookworm, or of the bladder
Loss of blood from other sources
Decreased absorption following gastric bypass

Treatment

After a history and physical exam, various tests apart from the ones mentioned above will be done to identify the cause of the anemia. These may include:

For excessive menstrual flow – A pelvic ultrasound or hysteroscopy (using a lighted tube to look in the uterus) may identify causes of excessive menstrual flow like fibroids

Bleeding from the intestines – Special stool cards (called fecal occult blood cards) on which stool is placed is an easy test done to look for minute blood in the stool. Upper and lower endoscopies (small lighted magnifying tube with a camera is used to look into the stomach and large intestines) may be performed to look for sites of bleeding in those places. Hemorrhoids may be identified if bleeding

In unreachable places like the small bowel, one may swallow a small camera in a capsule called Capsule Endoscopy and this can produce pictures showing possible bleeding spots

Bleeding from the bladder – Urine tests and cystoscopy – putting a lighted tube with a camera into the bladder to view the lining, and ultrasound of the kidney system may be done

Once the cause is identified and corrected, the anemia can be treated by:

- Oral iron tablets or intravenous infusion of iron. Some people get constipation with iron, and this can be corrected by increasing fiber in the diet or taking a stool softener. Absorption is increased with vitamin C.
- Eating more iron rich foods like meats, liver, poultry, fish, oysters, mussels, and leafy green vegetables like spinach, as well as legumes like beans, soy and lentils will also help build up the low hemoglobin

Vitamin B12 Deficiency
What is It?

Vitamin B12 deficiency is when one has low vitamin B12 level in the blood. It is a very important vitamin needed to produce red blood cells and DNA which is the hereditary material found in all your cells. It is also needed for myelin (tissue covering nerves) and nerve functions. Our bodies are not able to produce it and so it has to be absorbed in the stomach from foods we eat or Vitamin B12 supplements we take. Vitamin B12 is found mostly in animal products, fortified foods and yeast and it is absorbed in the stomach with the aid of acid present there.

CAUSES OF VIT B12 DEFICIENCY:

Low levels or deficiencies may be found in:

Inadequate intake in the diet

Strict vegetarians who do not eat any meat (vegans)

Diabetics and others who are on a medicine called Metformin for a long time

People who have had gastric bypass surgery

Surgery removing part of the stomach where Vitamin B12 is absorbed from

People taking acid blocking medicines for acid reflux (called proton pump inhibitors – PPI) for a long time. Examples of these medicines are Omeprazole, Lansoprazole, and Pantoprazole

Tape worm infection of the intestine

Vegans not using Vitamin B12 supplements

Signs and Symptoms

Low levels or deficiency of Vitamin B12 may cause:

Anemia: one will have the symptoms mentioned above
Mental changes: depression, memory issues
Numbness or tingling of the lips, hand, legs, or feet (neuropathy)
Fatigue, shortness of breath, weakness
Diarrhea, loss of appetite
Paleness or jaundiced skin

Treatment

To find out if one is deficient, the blood levels of both Vitamin B12 and folic acid will need to be tested as well as blood tests mentioned under anemia tests. Vitamin B12 deficiency may be treated with:

Grain fortified with vitamin B12 for vegetarians
Vitamin B12 injections every 3 to 4 weeks
Oral or under the tongue (sublingual) vitamin B12 supplements

Foods rich in vitamin B12 include meat, poultry, eggs, dairy products, nutritional yeast, some types of Tempeh, mushrooms, and almond milk.

Sickle Cell Disease (SCD)

What is It?

"My sole aim, and I mean this, my sole aim is to tell those like my brothers and one sister who inherited an abnormal haemoglobin from both father and mother to give them sickle cell disease – to tell them that they have inherited other genes from the same parents that can produce great achievement in their lives"

—Professor Felix I D Konotey-Ahulu, Sickle Cell physician/researcher July, 2017. blog.sicklecell.md/sicklecell/world-sickle-cell-disease-patient-week.

This is an inherited chronic blood disorder due to alteration of the gene which is responsible for red blood cell formation. It results in abnormal elongated and sickle shaped red blood cells which are rigid and easily destroyed. When under stress, e.g. in the presence of decreased oxygen the red cells get more sickled, sticky and block the vessels, leading to decreased oxygen to the organs. There is rapid destruction of the sickled red cells due to shortened life span of 10 to 20 days, resulting in anemia. All these result in the symptoms sufferers present with. It is found predominately in areas where malaria has been endemic in the past and so it is often seen in people with African, Indian, Arab and Mediterranean ancestry, and is also in countries where people from these places have migrated to. It is found in the USA, African countries, South and Central America, Caribbean Islands, Greece, Italy, some Asian and Middle Eastern countries.

The Genetics of Sickle Cell Disease (SCD)

About 100,000 people in the USA suffer from Sickle Cell Disease or Anemia, with 3 million people and 10% of African Americans carrying the Trait. In Canada about 5,000 have the disease; and in Ghana for example, about 2% of the population have the disease. About 75% of sufferers live in Sub-saharan Africa, however, as mentioned above it's not a "blackman's disease". If an individual inherits the sickle cell gene from each parent they will have SS disease; or if they inherit a C gene from one and a sickle cell S gene they will have SC disease. Both of these diseases cause sickling of red cells and severe disease and both are regarded as types of Sickle Cell Disease. However, if the sickle cell gene is inherited from just one parent then the person has sickle cell trait (AS) and such persons tend to live normal lives without typically having the bone pain and other complications. Further discussion of AS is seen below

Thalassemia

There are other gene defects which affect the red cells shape and there are other gene abnormalities resulting in a blood disease caused by inadequate production of normal hemoglobin called Thalassemia. The gene defects cause decrease production of the alpha or beta globin chains which make up the adult hemoglobin molecule, resulting in anemia, stunted growth, decrease carriage of oxygen, and frequent destruction of the red cells. It may be inherited as a trait or as full blown symptomatic disease when different abnormal genes combine in an offspring of two individuals with abnormal genes. There are different types of Thalassemia depending on what genes are affected, and the commonest ones are Beta Thalassemia and Alpha Thalassemia. Thalassemia disease is common in individuals from the Mediterranean region like Greece and Italy, as well as in Asian countries like India and Pakistan. There are fewer than 200,000 cases per year in US.

Signs and Symptoms of SCD

- The rapid destruction of the abnormal red cells (hemolysis) lead to severe anemia
- Recurrent bone pain known as "sickle cell crisis", due to the sickled cells blocking blood vessels as a result of released chemicals causing the cells to stick together
- Stunted growth and shortened life expectancy results in those who are not well managed

- Persons with SCD may be small in stature and may have jaw bones that protrude out and give them a certain facial characteristic if they are not well treated as in resource poor countries
- The anemia which is from rapid destruction of the abnormal red cells may result in difficulty in breathing, frequent hospitalizations, and frequent blood transfusions

Results of Vaso-Occlusion and Anemia

The results of rigid sticky sickled cells blocking arteries (vaso-occlusive), hemolysis and anemia affect many organs in the body. The following can occur:

In the brain it leads to strokes

In the lungs causing lung problems and difficulty in breathing (chest syndrome)

In the legs causing leg ulcers

In the eyes vision may be affected

In the heart anemia may lead to heart failure

In the kidneys it leads to kidney failure

In the gallbladder stones may be formed

In the bones causing chronic bone pain

In the hip joint death or destruction of the head of the hip bone due to poor blood and oxygen supply to it (avascular necrosis)

Complications of Repeated blood Transfusions

Sufferers who have had several blood transfusions over the years can also experience an overload of iron and this deposits in several organs especially the liver.

All these conditions end up interfering with a sufferer's education, career, work or school attendance. However, there is hope due to advances in research and new medications and treatments.

Testing for Sickle Cell Disease

Usually done on blood and is expensive for low resource countries, however; recently a new test called HemoTypeSC is an accurate that costs less than $2, and requires only a small drop of blood can be used for screening children. Already some of these countries are also doing newborn screening to identify kids with sickle cell earlier, so they can be followed up for preventative treatment, ongoing care, and prevention or early treatment of complications so as to increase life expectancy.

Treatment

In this century, the life expectancy of people with sickle cell disease has increased due to recent advances. Some measures in treatment include:

- Early diagnosis (newborn screening) and appropriate childhood vaccinations
- Preventive antibiotics to prevent infections in childhood
- Medications called HYDROXYUREA, Hydroxycarbamide (hydrea), are used to prevent crisis
- Early treatment of complications like chest syndrome, bone crises etc
- Blood transfusion to prevent recurrent stroke, sickle cell crises, and chest complications
- Endari (L-glutamine oral powder) recently approved in some countries including USA in 2017, is used for decreasing bone pain and chest syndrome.
- For patients requiring chronic blood transfusion to prevent crises and strokes, stem cell transplant from bone marrow of a suitable donor has resulted in cure of patients
- Non sickler Sibling donor stem cell transplantation to children with sickle cell has led to cure of sickle cell disease for those children and is being used in some countries like USA and France
- Ongoing research into Gene Therapy using stem cells from the patient to produce a gene which makes a non sickling form of hemoglobin

There are other exciting new research in treatment of sickle cell disease with new medicines to help prevent crisis and anemia in the pipeline. The US FDA has recently approved two drugs: Crizanlizumab which is by infusion every 2–4 weeks, and is used to reduce frequency of crisis due to blocked vessels (vasoocclusive). The second one is Voxelotor which is an oral medication and it inhibits the red cell from forming the sickle shape and being destroyed. Therefore anemia is prevented.

Self Care Management in SCD

There are several things one can do to improve one's health when you have Sickle Cell Disease. This list by the Centers for Disease Control (CDC) USA, is very useful to follow. These include:

- Regular follow up with your doctor or health provider who is taking care of you
- Know about your disease and things which may trigger a "crisis". Some sufferers identify lack of rest, not drinking enough fluids, cold weather, infection etc. as common causes of triggering a crisis
- Adequate rest and sleep are important to stay healthy. One has to learn to listen to your body. When tired, cut down on your activities and rest

- Eat a healthy diet, fruits, vegetables, grains with high fiber, and not too much red meat which has a lot of iron in it
- Take your medicines as prescribed. Some may be on daily Hydroxyurea or Glutamine to prevent crisis and keep hemoglobin at a relatively high level, folic acid, and pain medications.
- Using pain medications appropriately to relieve pain is necessary and may enable one to stay out of the emergency room or hospital.
- Iron overload in the body may occur from frequent blood transfusions and rapid breakdown of red cells. It may have to be treated when it becomes excessive, affecting the liver, spleen or heart. The treatment is known as "IRON CHELATION" therapy and it removes excess iron from the blood and organs.
- Have emotional support through family and friends. Talk to a professional if one feels overwhelmed, depressed, or anxious. You may need treatment for depression or anxiety.
- Know basic things about your disease, like your baseline (normal) hemoglobin level. Most sickle cell patients have low hemoglobin and their bodies have adjusted to that level. Their "normal" levels may be 7gm/dl, while someone with normal red cells will have normal hemoglobin of 13gm/dl.
(cdc.gov, living well with sickle cell self-care kit).

All the above are part of effective self-care management of the disease. It keeps you in better health and helps avoid complications that result from inadequate care. YOU HAVE A ROLE TO PLAY IN YOUR CARE.

Prevention of Sickle Cell Disease

Genetic counseling and even testing for sickle cell trait or other abnormal hemoglobin, in would be couples with family history of sickle cell disease is advocated by some, so that they get the facts about the possibility of having children with sickle cell disease, or make informed decision as to whether they would have biological kids at all.

New Born Screening for Sickle Cell Disease

"Our biggest challenge is that we simply don't make the diagnosis early enough. Ghana is one of the few African countries that has a new-born screening program. But there's not a single country that tests all their children for SCD".

Prof. Kwaku Ohene-Frempong, President of the Sickle Cell Foundation of Ghana and Program Coordinator of the New-born Screening Program for Sickle Cell Disease. January, 2019.

In the USA, Canada, France, England, and Brazil, there are established New-born screening programs for sickle cell disease. Babies are screened with a heel pick soon after birth, so if they are affected, they can be identified and followed up more closely with parental education and enrollment in clinics which care for patients with sickle cell disease. In Ghana, West Africa, a new born screening program which had previously been piloted in a few centers, would soon be on a national scale in the not too distant future. Newborn screening is a program that needs to be introduced by sub-Saharan African countries and those in Asia with large SCD populations so that prevention of childhood deaths from SCD can be curtailed by introduction of immunizations, antibiotics (Penicillin) to prevent bacterial infections, early treatment of diseases like malaria, and prevention and treatment of crisis.

Sickle Cell Trait
What is It?

This is when one inherits a normal hemoglobin gene from one parent and an abnormal S or C hemoglobin from the other parent ending up with AS or AC or sickle cell trait. Now a child can inherit SCD if parents who are healthy carriers (AS or AC) each pass an abnormal gene to the child who can end up with SCD SS or SCD SC. In the USA, the trait affects about 1 in every 12 African-Americans and in Ghana (West Africa) for example, one in every 4 people −25% of population has the trait.

A person with a trait may not have any symptoms and such a person tends to live a normal life without having the bone pain and crises seen in those with the full blown sickle cell disease. The presence of the normal hemoglobin tends to negate the effects of the S hemoglobin due to less sickling involved. However, some of the red cells can become more sickled and sticky in situations of low oxygen, dehydration, and high temperatures. Most of the time, individuals with sickle cell trait may not know they have the condition and it may be an incidental finding.

Signs and Symptoms

Most times there no symptoms, however, when performing as an athlete, during intense exercise, or when performing at a high altitude, they may have symptoms which may include shortness of breath, fatigue, muscle pain, and weakness. A few US college football athletes have died in the past during training.

Prevention of Complications

To prevent this, students or individuals have to let their coaches know they have sickle cell trait and pay attention to any symptoms which may develop during training. They should rest often, cool down when it is hot and humid, and drink plenty of fluids.

Treatment

If symptoms develop, the activity should be stopped, pulse or heart rate checked, and individual should be cooled down. If there is no improvement, one has to go to the hospital for further treatment with oxygen and intravenous fluids. Severe symptoms can lead to muscle breakdown with kidney failure and heart rhythm abnormalities which have caused some athletes to die suddenly on the sports field.

Reminders on Your Radar

Sickle cell disease is a genetic hemoglobin disorder inherited from one's parents, and it is associated with recurrent chronic bone pain, anemia, and crisis due to sickling of red blood cells, blocking vessels in different organs including brain, lungs, skin, kidneys. It affects many races and It is not a "black person's disease". Self care management is important and each patient needs to know about their disease. New medicines and treatments have led to better quality of life for sufferers especially in rich countries, but resource poor nations are also developing better strategies for care. New born screening is crucial for early disease identification and management to improve length of life and quality of life. SC trait individuals may have exercise related collapse and death.

Cancers Involving the Blood Cells

....

There are several blood cells as discussed previously and to recap, these are red cells, white blood cells, and platelets. All these are produced in the bone marrow, which is present in the center of most of the long bones and hip bones in our bodies. The blood cells develop from immature bone marrow cells called Myeloid STEM CELLS which give rise to red, white cells and platelets. Examples of white cells include neutrophils, monocytes, and basophils. These stem cells normally develop into the mature cells. Each of these cells can have abnormalities occurring, resulting in many diseases including cancers. Leukemia is cancer involving lymphocytes or myeloid type cells, and Multiple Myeloma is cancer of plasma cells which are cells that develop from blood cells known as B lymphocytes.

Leukemias
What are They?

Leukemias are cancers of white blood cells and can develop from abnormal cells (produced through mutated or genetic errors in cells) produced in the bone marrow, which multiple rapidly and soon take over the bone marrow. They are named according to what cells they develop from as well as how fast the disease progresses. For example:

Leukemia from Lymphocyte type cells are called Lymphocytic Leukemia
Those from Neutrophils, red cells or platelets are called Myelogenous Leukemias

Acute and Chronic Leukemia

They can also be grouped as acute or chronic depending on how fast the disease progresses.

ACUTE: A person can be very sick quickly and may present with anemia, bruising, pain and swelling of lymph nodes, fever, infection and bleeding
CHRONIC: Chronic leukemias develop slowly and symptoms are not so intense
TREATMENT: After the diagnosis is made from blood lab results, doctors may treat patients with chemotherapy and radiation if needed. Sometimes, bone marrow transplant is required

Multiple Myeloma
What is It?

When bacteria or viruses invade the body, the body's defenses respond by causing special types of lymphocytes called B-lymphocytes to be changed into cells called PLASMA CELLS. The plasma cells produce antibodies called Immunoglobulins which then fight these invaders. However, in MULTIPLE MYELOMA, the plasma cells become abnormal or cancerous, multiply excessively in the bone marrow and form tumor cells in many bones. They may literally take over the bone marrow resulting in the decreased production of other cells like red cells, white cells and platelets. They also produce abnormal proteins instead of the usual antibodies. Also present in the blood and urine is an increased amount of proteins called monoclonal proteins and these can damage the kidneys. The disease tends to develop in older people.

Symptoms

It may not cause any symptoms initially, but may also present with weakness, fatigue, anemia, bone pain, fracture of bone, spinal cord compression, numbness, easy bruising, bleeding, and infections.

Treatment

After blood, bone marrow biopsy and urine tests are done and a diagnosis is made, then treatment may be started. Treatment kills cancer cells and may include chemotherapy, targeted therapy which destroys cancer cells only and corticosteroids which help with inflammation. Some individuals may have a mild form which does not necessarily need medications initially, but careful and regular monitoring is done by an ONCOLOGIST who is a doctor who specializes in treating people with various forms of cancers.

Cancers of The Lymphatic System

As mentioned before, the lymphatic system is made up of lymph, cells, vessels and organs and it is part of the immune or defense system of the body. The organs include lymph nodes, tonsils, thymus, and the spleen.

Lymphomas
What are They?

Lymphomas are due to excess production of abnormal lymphocytes in the lymphatic system and this leads to swelling of lymph nodes in various parts of the body. They affect the body's ability to fight infections which is what normal lymphocytes do. The two most common cancers affecting the lymphatic system are Hodgkin and Non-Hodgkin lymphomas, and the most common type is Non Hodgkin Lymphoma. The main difference between the two lymphomas is the presence of a particular type of abnormal cell called a Reed Sternberg cell which is present in Hodgkin but not in the non-Hodgkin lymphoma. There are different types of Non-Hodgkin lymphomas depending on the type of lymphocyte that is affected.

Symptoms and Signs

All the lymphomas present with similar symptoms, and include:

Fever, chills, fatigue and weight loss
Increased itching of the skin and night sweats
Enlarged lymph nodes in the axillae, groin and neck area, which become painful after drinking alcohol

Treatment

Once a diagnosis is made the type or types of treatment which is best for you will be suggested by your oncologist. Treatments include chemotherapy, radiation or stem cell transplant, and this will depend on the extent of the disease and the type of lymphoma. Some Non-Hodgkin lymphomas are slow growing and the oncologist may suggest no treatment, however regular follow up and tests are done to make sure it has not changed. Some are fast growing and need to be treated aggressively.

Reminders on Your Radar

There are several cancers affecting all the blood cells and these may be acute which cause rapid onset of symptoms and deterioration if not treated immediately; while some are slow growing and may not require immediate treatment. A Hematologist/ Oncologist specializes in treating blood cancers.

Part Four

Mental Health

26

Common Psychiatric Conditions

Topics discussed here are the common mental health problems and diseases, which occur in many individuals, but unfortunately many remain undiagnosed or do not go for treatment due to the stigma associated with many mental illnesses. Michelle Obama, former first lady of the United States said it precisely in the quote below when she was giving a speech on Mental Health during her time at the White House.

How Big A Problem Are Mental Health Diseases?

....

"At the root of this dilemma is the way we view mental health in this country. When it comes to mental health conditions, we often treat them differently from other diseases like cancer, diabetes or asthma. And that makes no sense. Whether an illness affects your heart, your leg or your brain, it's still an illness, and there should be no distinction. Because we know that mental health is just as important to our overall well-being as our physical health".

Remarks by The former First lady Michelle Obama at "Change Direction" Mental Health Event. March 04, 2015. Washington DC.

On a global scale, it is estimated that about 120 million people suffer from depression and 24 million from schizophrenia, and so mental health conditions are a huge public health problem (www.globalmentalhealth.org). According to WHO reports about 20% of children and teens worldwide experience mental illnesses, so they are not just adult diseases.

Both resource rich and resource limited nations, lack enough resources and public health policies to help patients with mental health problems. There are not enough trained staff and even until recently, most Health Insurance companies in the USA did not adequately cover mental health counseling for patients with mental health problems. The lack of adequately trained mental health workers, Psychologists, and Psychiatrists (doctors trained to treat mental health problems) also compounds the situation and prevents adequate treatment of those who want to be treated. Training Primary Care Providers and Mental Health nurses and other staff so they can be comfortable treating patients with mental health conditions in all countries is one solution to the problem. This is because there are not enough Psychiatrists or even Psychologists (they do counseling) in all countries to treat individuals with these problems.

Introduction

. . . .

"When our emotional health is in a bad state, so is our level of self-esteem. We have to slow down and deal with what is troubling us, so that we can enjoy the simple joy of being happy and at peace with ourselves."

— Jess C. Scott. Writer. AZQuotes.com

Mental health has to do with the health of your mind — emotions, thoughts, feelings, thinking, and intellect. The mind is under the influence of the brain which is the center of our nervous system. The brain's actions through a complex system of cells and tissues, as well as electrical signals and neurotransmitters (chemicals released from nerve endings) control our thoughts behavior and emotions as well as how we function physically — whether it is moving, talking, eating etc.

Neurotransmitters
What are They?

Chemicals called Neurotransmitters are involved in the brain's ability to transmit information or messages to different parts of the body, and also how we function mentally. Nerve cells are not joined together and in order for a message to be sent from one to another, these chemicals are released from one cell into the gap between two cells. The chemicals are then taken up by the receiving nerve cell and the message is conducted on.

There are over one hundred different types of Neurotransmitters and a few of them have been identified as helping with our emotions, mood, behavior, alertness, focus etc. Examples of these are Serotonin, Norepinephrine, Epinephrine, and Dopamine. For example, it has been found that:

*   Depressed people have low serotonin levels in their brain
*   Parkinson's disease (a movement disorder) patients have low levels of dopamine
*   Schizophrenia patients may have excessive dopamine

Therefore, treatment of each of these is based on the ability to alter levels of these Neurotransmitters.

Stigma of Mental Illnesses

It is important for all to understand that mental illnesses, just like physical illnesses are treatable and once treated, an individual can function well in society. Unfortunately, there is a lot of stigma attached to mental illnesses and because of that, some sufferers are not willing to discuss their symptoms and receive the help they need. There is no need to be afraid or feel ashamed when one needs help with a mental problem. It is always suggested to people that when someone has Hypertension (high BP), they take medicine daily to keep the blood pressure down. Similarly, if someone has depression, they can be treated with counseling and or medicines in order for them to feel better and live a normal fulfilled life.

Screening Questionnaires

There are screening tools administered as questionnaires to screen one for a number of these mental illnesses. These should be answered as accurately or truthfully as possible. These can be scored by the health provider, and can indicate the presence and or severity of an illness. Examples are PHQ 2 and PHQ 9 for depression, GAD 7 for anxiety, and MDQ for bipolar.

Types of Mental Illnesses

Most mental illnesses are grouped under a particular disorder and some are discussed here (Others can be found on the internet).

Anxiety Disorders
Depressive Disorders
Psychotic Disorder – Schizophrenia

Other Mental States

Chronic stress
Taking time to smell the Roses

Anxiety Disorders

There are different types of anxiety disorders and these include:

General Anxiety Disorder (GAD)
Post-Traumatic Stress Disorder (PTSD)
Obsessive Compulsive Disorder (OCD)
Phobias (fear of different things)

Anxiety caused by certain medical conditions

Medical Conditions Presenting As Anxiety

Certain medical conditions may result in anxiety-like symptoms and these include:

Thyroid conditions: Hyperthyroidism or overactive thyroid (palpitations, rapid heart rate)

Respiratory illnesses: Asthma and emphysema (shortness of breathe, difficulty in breathing)

Heart conditions: Irregular heartbeat, Coronary heart disease, Angina (chest pain and chest pressure)

Your health care provider may refer you for blood work or other tests to make sure those conditions are not the cause of your anxiety, depending on how you describe your symptoms

Generalized Anxiety Disorder (GAD)

What is It?

"Anxiety in the heart of man causes depression, but a good word makes it glad".
—Proverbs 12v25: (NKJV – BIBLE)

People have excessive and uncontrollable worry and anxiety, and they tend to worry about everything, with the worry being out of proportion with reaction associated with that particular circumstance. This ends up affecting their everyday life negatively. It is believed to be a result of genetics, environmental stressors, and neuro-biological influences. Environmental stressors include overcrowding, excessive noise or sound, or natural disasters.

Symptoms

Fear, tension headache, neck pain, worry, sleep problems, irritability, trembling, palpitations, and lack of concentration and focus, always on edge, and muscle tension are some of the common symptoms.

Treatment

A health care provider after taking a history and examination, may do blood work, administer a questionnaire and will make the diagnosis. This can be treated with medications and or psychological counseling (therapy).

NON DRUG METHODS: These help to minimize GAD and include:

Identifying and minimizing triggers like stress, caffeine (coffee, chocolate, and tea) and alcohol

Avoiding foods containing monosodium glutamate (MSG)

Avoid illegal drugs which may act as stimulants e.g. marijuana and methamphetamine

Improved sleep (practice sleep hygiene discussed under insomnia)

Smoking cessation

Physical activity may take your mind off your symptoms

Relaxation techniques, like deep breathing, prayer, meditation or yoga

Medications

There are a few different classes of medicines which can be used, but those that are frequently used are known as Selective Serotonin Receptor Inhibitors (SSRI). Examples are Fluoxetine, Sertraline, and Paroxetine and these can treat all the different types of anxiety and depression. Others that may help but are not SSRIs are Bupropion, Venlafaxine, Amitriptyline (Elavil), Sinequan (doxepin), and Nortriptyline. This is not an exhaustive List of Medicines. Some people are prescribed Benzodiazepines like Alprazolam (Xanax), Lorazepam, Diazepam etc. but these are usually avoided since they are habit forming and may have side effects like drowsiness. Your doctor will make a choice depending on additional symptoms that may be present.

Counseling (Psychotherapy or 'talk therapy")

Done by a professional counselor or therapist, this can help people uncover the source of their problems, identify them, understand their problems, and develop ways to work on them. A type called Cognitive Behavioral Therapy (CBT) helps individuals by challenging their behavior, thoughts and attitudes and helping them change through personal strategies. A recent study showed that Guided CBT done on line has helped improve mental health quality of life for patients with anxiety and depression (Rollman et al. JAMA Psychiatry. 2018;75(1): 56–64).

Post-Traumatic Stress Disorder (PTSD)

What is It?

"Unlike simple stress, trauma changes your view of your life and yourself. It shatters your most basic assumptions about yourself and your world – "Life is good," "I'm safe," "People are kind," "I can trust others," "The future is likely to be good" – and replaces them with feelings like "The world is dangerous," "I can't win," "I can't trust other people," or "There's no hope."

— Mark Goulston MD, Psychiatrist.
Post-Traumatic Stress Disorder For Dummies

PTSD used to be considered an anxiety disorder problem and classified as such, but this has been changed recently, to being a type of stressful and trauma related disorder brought on after one has experienced a serious traumatic event; or when one sees such a thing happening to someone else. It is also thought to be a condition involving the interplay of the brain, nerves and endocrine systems. It affects individuals who have survived events such as:

Sexual abuse, physical abuse, domestic violence, sex trafficking
War, civil war, and torture
Natural disasters like Tsunamis or earthquakes
Serious vehicle accidents or a plane crash

It has become more prominent in recent years due to the vast number of United States army veterans from the wars in Iraq and Afghanistan who returned home and are suffering from this problem. However, it was always present, and it is more common in women who have suffered Intimate Partner Violence and sexual abuse; and in other parts of the world, it is also rampant where women have been raped and abused due to civil wars and tribal conflicts.

Symptoms

Symptoms usually occur within 3 months of the event, but may occur later. All the emotions listed above under generalized anxiety disorder may occur, but major ones are:

Re-experiencing the events
Nightmares or vivid dreams of the events
Insomnia – inability to sleep
Avoidance of people and places
Refusing to speak about the event
Negative thoughts and negative emotions like hopelessness
Hypersensitivity in certain areas like getting angry easily
Lack of focus and concentration
Suspicious of others (paranoid)
Not enjoying activities one used to enjoy
Engaging in self-destructive and harmful behavior like excessive drinking or
    drug abuse
Depression and suicidal thoughts
Some affected individuals may even commit suicide

Although one may experience some of the above emotions immediately after the event, one does not necessarily have PTSD unless the symptoms occur for more than a month, or your life does not get better after the experience.

Treatment

It is important that one talks to a trusted person after an experience like sexual abuse or serious car accident and one continues to have flash backs and other mental and physical changes in one's life. Only a trained medical person can make the diagnosis of PTSD. Treatment consist of several non-drug treatments and medications

Non drug treatments: These include:

Talk therapy (counseling by a trained psychologist or psychiatrist)
Support from others who are going through the same thing (group therapy)
Support from family and friends (social support)
Pet therapy has also helped some war veterans who experience PTSD
Getting involved in athletics and competitive sports
Adopting or training dogs may be helpful
In children, art therapy, and play therapy have been found to be helpful

Recently the Veterans Affairs which treat military veterans in the USA have started using a novel method known as Stellate Ganglion Nerve Block were a group of nerves in the neck is injected with Lidocaine (numbing medicine) for cases which are resistant to medications. It's found to be very effective in reducing symptoms and helping individuals.

Medications

Medications like the SSRIs (e.g Fluoxetine) discussed above, Benzodiazepines (for example, Lorazepam, Alprazolam), beta blockers e.g. Propranolol, and an alpha-adrenergic blocker called Prazosin are used for those who suffer from easy arousal or hypersensitivity.
Antipsychotics help with depression and paranoid behavior.
Anticonvulsants for those whose emotions or moods fluctuate a great deal.

Panic Disorder
What is It?

This is a type of anxiety attack, and often presents suddenly and repeatedly as an intense or strong feeling of fear, discomfort or impending doom associated with certain physical symptoms. Statistics show that for US adult, about 4.7% experience panic disorder in their lives, and it is higher in females than males. Some individuals who suffer from this may initially think they are having a heart attack, however all heart tests done are usually negative. There may be repeated visits to the Emergency Department but all tests turn out alright.

Symptoms

Those above feelings may be accompanied within a few minutes by rapid heart-beat, palpitations, sweating, chest pain, shortness of breath, or difficulty in breathing, dizziness, and intense thoughts that one is going to die. It may be prompted by being in crowded places or enclosed spaces for some people.

Treatment

After a history and examination is done by a doctor, there may be tests done like a EKG and other heart tests, chest x-ray and blood work to rule out any medical conditions, like thyroid or heart diseases. Treatments available include medications and counseling which tend to decrease the frequency or intensity of attacks. Combining the two achieves better results for most individuals. Non drug treatment for individuals have been found to be helpful.

Non-Drug treatment

Counseling by a trained therapist
Meditation e.g. mindfulness meditation or christian meditation
Relaxation techniques (e.g. breathing techniques)
Biofeedback, (e.g. EMG biofeedback which measures muscle relaxation and
    teaches people to control their own level of muscle relaxation)

Medications

SSRIs (e.g. Fluoxetine and Sertraline) discussed above are used to treat this type of anxiety. To quickly calm those who are having an acute panic attack Benzodiazepines (e.g. Lorazepam, Alprazolam) or Hydroxyzine (which belongs to another class) may be given. Patients may carry a couple of these tablets on their person or purse at all times, and just carrying them gives some people reassurance and calms them because they know it is readily available to use when needed.

Obsessive Compulsive Disorder (OCD)
What is It?

This is a type of chronic anxiety disorder in which the individual's mind is constantly bombarded with preoccupied unwanted thoughts (obsessions) and to try to get rid of them, the individual would perform compulsive or uncontrollable actions/behaviors over and over again. For example, the obsession or preoccupation may be in the areas of cleanliness, fear of germs, aggressive thoughts toward others, or unwanted thoughts in the area of sex, and religion. People may have obsessions or compulsions or both. The lifetime prevalence of OCD is about 2.3% and it is higher in females than in males. These thoughts and or actions are so intense they affect the individual's day-to-day life, taking a lot of the person's time, and affecting social relationships with others, work or school life. Scientists are not sure why certain people have them, but it may be due to lack of the chemical messenger (neurotransmitter) in the brain called Serotonin.

Symptoms

The thoughts may bring about fear, worry or anxiety and the action is done to get rid of them.

Obsessions:
These may include fears of germs and infections, fear of harming oneself or others, arranging things symmetrical and fear of losing things

Compulsions:
Repeatedly cleaning the counter tops and washing hands, repeatedly checking if the door is locked, hoarding unnecessary things, and ordering and arranging things in a certain order. For example if the preoccupation is about germs being everywhere, a person to try to get rid of these thoughts, would constantly wash her hands, or clean their kitchen continuously with bleach

Treatment

OCD is treated by medications which will increase the Serotonin levels in the brain, and by Psychological counseling or "talk therapy". The medicines used to treat or minimize the condition are also the same used to treat Depression and Anxiety disorders and examples are; Paroxetine (Paxil), Fluoxetine (Prozac) to name a few. Talk to a healthcare provider if you think you may have such a problem, you do not have to be embarrassed about it.

Phobias

What are These?

These are anxiety disorders which are a result of FEAR of something. The fear is out of proportion to what most people will have or experience when encountered with that same situation. It may be fear of:

Being in an enclosed space, e.g. in an elevator/lift or plane (CLAUSTROPHO-BIA)
Being in public or open spaces (AGORAPHOBIA)
Being among people (SOCIAL PHOBIA)
A specific thing or animal, e.g. extreme fear of spiders (ARACHNOPHOBIA)

Symptoms

These include those seen in anxiety and include increased heart rate (palpitations), perspiration, Diarrhea, elevated blood pressure, fear of impending doom, shortness of breath, tingling of hands and feet, shaking, chest pain and dizziness.

If one experiences any of these and it greatly affects where one goes, how one socializes with other people, one's day-to-day life, school or work, then it is important one talks to a Health Care Provider.

Treatment

Treatments include psychological counseling and medications.

- Counseling:
  By a trained therapist will help one know how to cope with one's phobia
- Exposure therapy: This is when the individual confronts the situation in a graduated manner either by themselves, with the help of the counselor or through computer-generated programs
- Breathing techniques and Relaxation techniques: Have been used to help individuals

There are also self-help manuals or techniques on the internet one may use if the condition is not severe and does not require professional help.

Certain things like excessive Caffeine, certain illegal and even legal drugs, and alcohol abuse may cause or influence an individual's response to a particular phobia, so one must avoid too much Caffeine and limit alcohol intake.

Medications

Most of the ones used are the SSRIs (e.g Paroxetine and Fluoxetine) which are discussed above.

Dietary Supplements Used to Treat Anxiety

Many individuals prefer to use supplements or botanicals to treat anxiety. Most lack scientific evidence for successfully treating anxiety and need more studies, however people still use them and some people find them useful. These include:

Kava extract which seems to work but has adverse effects on the liver, and should be avoided

Tryptophan, St John's Wort, and SAMe; these should not be used if taking the SSRIs because they have similar effects like the SSRIs (e.g Fluoxetine)

Passion flower, Valerian, L-Theanine, and Vitamin B complex pills

Depression

What is It?

"Mental pain is less dramatic than physical pain, but it is more common and also more hard to bear. The frequent attempt to conceal mental pain increases the burden: it is easier to say "My tooth is aching" than to say "My heart is broken."

— C.S. Lewis, Theologian, British writer
The Problem of Pain

This is a mental condition in which there is a feeling of sadness, and loss of interest which lasts more than two weeks accompanied by other symptoms affecting one's mind and body. It is not the same as feeling sad for a few days, and it is not the same as "feeling the blues" which is when one feels stressed and sad for a few days, but snaps out of it soon afterwards.

Incidence

In the USA, about 19 million adults suffer from depression, and the incidence which is about 20% in women and about 12% in men seems to have increased in recent years. Worldwide severe depression affects 350 million individuals and WHO considers it the leading cause of disability. It also is a leading cause of suicide. It affects adolescents and children as well.

What Causes Depression?

Medical people and scientists do not know all the reasons why some individuals end up with depression, however; it has been related to:

Chemical imbalance in the brain (the neurochemicals described above)
Family history of depression (some genetic basis)
Stressful events like rape, domestic violence, and distressful social issues etc

Other Causes of Depression

There are several other types of depression which are associated with medical illness or reaction to certain medications.

Medical Illnesses Associated with Depression

There are medical illnesses which are associated with depression and up to a third of people with medical illnesses may have depression. These illnesses include chronic medical conditions like:

Stroke and Parkinson's Disease
Heart Attack (Myocardial Infarction)

Vitamin deficiencies e.g. Vitamin B12 and Vitamin D
Cancers
HIV infection
Hypothyroidism
Diabetes
Hepatitis infections

Medicines and Depression

Some drugs deplete some of the chemicals associated with mood in the brain and can also cause depression. Note that not all people on these medicines or have above medical conditions have depressive illnesses. The medicines include:

Interferon-alpha, Corticosteroids, Reserpine (blood pressure medicine)
Accutane for treating severe acne, Oral Contraceptive pills
Statins for high cholesterol and Digoxin for heart problems
Other blood pressure medicines have been thought to also cause depression
but research is not clear on these. These include Clonidine, and Beta blockers like Metoprolol

Symptoms of Depression

Apart from sadness and loss of interest or pleasure in things one usually enjoys, other depressive symptoms, may include:

- Change in diet – may be excessive eating or decreased eating
- Weight gain or loss
- Sleeping problems, e.g. not sleeping enough or sleeping too much
- Not able to concentrate or focus on things
- Restlessness and inability to sit still
- Sudden slowness in doing things or becoming agitated
- Feelings of worthlessness, hopelessness or guilt
- Having thoughts that people will be better off without you being around
- Thoughts or plans of harming oneself or someone else (suicide or homicide)

If someone has the first two SADNESS and LOSS OF INTEREST and at least three of the others for some or most of the days for two or more weeks, then they may be suffering from depression and have to see a health professional.

There are other symptoms which can occur in depression and these include:

Feeling weepy with frequent crying without cause
Memory problems

Feeling pessimistic

Aches and pains in joints

No interest in sex

Uncontrolled anger

Drug or alcohol abuse to cover it up

Withdrawal from family and friends

Very sensitive to things that are said by others etc

Psychotic symptoms like hearing voices, paranoid

Why Is Treatment Important?

It is important to get treatment because depression not only affects the individual psychologically or physically, but it has led to death by suicide when individuals feel hopeless and helpless, but fail to realize that they can get help if they let people know what is happening to them. Research shows that people function better when treated for it. Often some refuse medications because they think being treated is a sign of weakness, or the stigma of a mental illness stops them from getting help.

Diagnosis

Talk to one's health care provider if one has been experiencing a number of the symptoms described above. The healthcare provider may be a Psychiatrist (doctor who specializes in treating people with mental problems), trained Psychiatric nurse, physician assistant or a medical doctor like a Family Medicine specialist or Internist (adult medicine specialist). She will take a careful history, do an exam and may do some blood work. They may also administer one of the depression screening questionnaires mentioned above and make a diagnosis of whether one's depression is

Mild

Moderate

Severe

Treatment of Major Depression

The important message is that depression is treatable. Depression can either be treated with medications or psychological therapy (counseling). In those with resistant severe depression or psychotic symptoms of depression (hearing voices, delusional, paranoid), Electroconvulsive Therapy (ECT) and other types of medications called Psychotrophics may be added to the regular medications. Recent research shows that certain foods and lifestyle changes (Self Care) may help in depression and these will be discussed below.

The Treatment of depression caused by medications or medical diseases

These have to have treatment either by withdrawal of the offending medication or treating the depression associated with the medical condition with antidepressants, e.g. after a stroke. Counseling may help with some.

Mild and Moderate Depression

Psychotherapy (talk therapy) may be all that is needed, however, lifestyle changes and dietary measures should also be incorporated. If these fail, then medication, mainly the SSRIs like Fluoxetine, Sertraline or Paroxetine etc. may be used. Some others have preferred using the herbal supplements mentioned under treatment of anxiety with CAM products and medicines.

Treatment of severe Depression

Many may benefit from both medicines and counseling. The SSRIs and other medications belonging to other classes are also used. Examples of some of the medicines used include Fluoxetine, Paroxetine, Sertraline, Escitalopram, Venlafaxine, Amitriptyline, Bupropion, Duloxetine and Remeron. Your health care provider will make the best choice of medicine for you. One has to follow up for review to check if there are any adverse effects and whether the dose is adequate or not. It may take a few weeks to see improvement in mood and sleep.

Severe Depression Unresponsive to Optimal Medications

In some people, despite optimum doses of a particular medication they may not respond to the treatment. In this case counseling will be included and they may also be changed to a different antidepressant or dose may be increased. If there is still no improvement then they will be offered "Augmented treatment".

AUGMENTED TREATMENT: This is when a second antidepressant or medication is added to the first. In such cases a psychiatrist, doctor or healthcare provider with experience in treating mental illnesses should be consulted. Examples of these medicines are Bupropion, antipsychotic medications Respiridone, Apipramazole, and thyroid replacement medication like Levothyroxine. Other psychiatrists may use ECT or TMS mentioned below.

Electroconvulsive Therapy (ECT)

This is also known as "Shock Therapy", and it involves a small electrical current passed through the individual's brain after they are sedated and their muscles have been relaxed. Patients who benefit most are those who have severe depression, those who are not responding to medications, or have suicidal thoughts or attempts. Only trained Psychiatrists do this.

Transcranial Magnetic Stimulation (TMS)

This is a non invasive procedure used to treat resistant depression. It involves use of magnetic pulses from a coil which delivers magnetic fields to areas of the brain thought to be under active and so contribute to depression. It is performed in a doctor's office while the patient is awake. It lasts about 20–30 minutes and it's given 5 days a week for 4–6 weeks. It is painless and is said to not affect memory or alertness. People can go back to work soon after a treatment session.

How Foods May Help With Depression

Recent research has focused on how what we eat affects our brain health, and a number of foods have been labeled BRAIN HEALTH FOODS and these include sea foods and plant foods.

Brain Health Foods

Seafood rich in Omega 3 fatty acids (e.g. oysters)
Greens, nuts, beans (e.g. red beans and lentils)
Some occasional dark chocolate

These when incorporated in the diet may help with depression, however the Paleo diet (meat, berries and nuts) which has also been suggested needs more research.

Brain Essential Nutrients (BEN)

In a recent American Psychiatric Association meeting (American Psychiatric Association (APA) 2016 Annual Meeting), researchers at Columbia University in New York headed by Dr. Drew Ramsey who study food and psychiatry reviewed how certain foods affect and help with depression, and they have compiled a list of "Brain Essential Nutrients" (BEN) which include:

Long-chain Omega 3 fatty acids
Magnesium
Calcium
Fiber
Vitamins B1, B9, (thiamine and folate) and B12
Vitamins D and E

"Brain Food Scale Scores" have been assigned to different foods depending on their content of BEN. Plant and sea foods rich in Omega 3 fatty acids but low in mercury content like octopus, squid, salmon, and sardines score high on the scale.

Vitamin B12 is a very essential nutrient for brain cells, mood, memory, proper cell function, and red cell production. This is found mainly in animal products; and so they emphasize one should include grass fed animal meat, organ meat and wild game in one's diet.

(Pauline Anderson. Medscape medical news. "New 'Brain Food' Scale Flags Best Nutrients for Depression," May 26, 2016).

A new book on brain healthy recipes featuring the 21 Brain Power Nutrients has been produced by Dr. Drew Ramsey called "Eat Complete."

Post Partum Depression

What is It?

"Postpartum depression is a very real and very serious problem for many mothers. It can happen to a first time mom or a veteran mother. It can occur a few days... or a few months after childbirth".

—Richard J. Codey former Governor of New Jersey

This is a type of depression that occurs within the first six months after delivering a baby. About 85% of mothers may experience some mood changes which are temporary, however, about 10% to 15% may have more persistent symptoms. It tends to occur after birth of the first child and may be due to a combination of genetic, changing female hormonal levels and stress. Women who experience family strife, financial problems and lack of social support are more prone to it, as well as those with previous history of depression or family history of depression. This is different from the "baby blues" which occurs soon after giving birth when a new mother feels sad or tearful, or overwhelmed; however, in postpartum depression, there are more severe symptoms which are present for several weeks.

Symptoms

These include severe and prolonged symptoms in addition to some of the normal depression symptoms. These include extreme sadness, worry, irritability, anger, trouble eating or sleeping, tiredness, feeling worthless and thoughts of harming the baby or one's self.

Treatment

If untreated, it places both mother and child at risk. The good news is that it is treatable. This, like regular depression can be treated with medicines and talk therapy either individually or in a group session. Support groups may be useful and a strong family or social support will be helpful for recovery. The SSRIs are often used. If breastfeeding the safest antidepressants to use include: Sertraline, Paroxetine, Nortriptyline and Imipramine. The levels tend to be low or undetectable in the infant's blood. One must talk to their doctor if after delivering a baby one experiences the above symptoms. One must not be shy about bringing it up.

Prevention

It is important that all pregnant women and new mothers be screened for depression by just two simple questions administered by a health professional during antenatal and postpartum visits, and this is known as the PHQ 2 depression screening questionnaire. It asks:

Over the past two weeks, how often have you been bothered by any of the following problems:

Little interest or pleasure in doing things
Feeling down, depressed, or hopeless

There are other questionnaires which are longer and have also been used for screening. It is important that health care workers broach the topic when seeing patients in the postpartum visits.

"When you study postpartum depression, there is a very clear understanding that in communities where you see more support, there is less depression."

—Ariel Gore, writer

It is important that spouses, family and friends watch out for new mothers and give them help in caring for the new baby as well as look out for signs of postpartum depression. Remember it can occur up to six months after delivery.

Seasonal Affective Disorder (SAD)
What is It?

This is a form of depression that is recurrent and tends to occur with specific seasons and so is thought to relate to season changes. It tends to occur in the late fall and early winter seasons and goes away in spring and summer; but a few people experience it in spring or early summer. The depression has to recur for at least two years and the symptoms have to coincide with that season.

Exact reason is not known but the following may play a role:

The decreased light causes adjustment of the body's internal wake-sleep clock
Decreased light may decrease the level of Serotonin in the body which affects moods. It is used to produce Melatonin

The change in season may disrupt Melatonin levels whose production is triggered by darkness and inhibited by light. Melatonin is involved in the wake-sleep cycle, and it is related to Serotonin. It is thought abnormal Serotonin regulation, overproduction of Melatonin and decreased levels of Vitamin D all contribute to SAD.

Symptoms

Individuals may present with depressive moods but they get better during the spring or summer months for the winter type of SAD. Symptoms are the same as seen in Major Depression and include feeling depressed or down, loss of interest in activities, sluggish or low energy, sadness, irritation, agitation, over eating, weight gain, lack of sleep, and even suicidal thoughts.

Treatment

- It can be treated with light therapy (Phototherapy) during which the person is exposed to light for some hours during the winter months. Some shops sell special light machines which deliver the light during the daytime
- Moving to states like Florida with lots of sunshine has improved the condition for some individuals who have the disorder
- Antidepressants like Fluoxetine (SSRIs) and Bupropion have been effective
- If Vitamin D levels are low they should be replenished since it's found to be low in persons with SAD. Studies have shown mixed results whether it is effective by itself
- Talk therapy (psychotherapy) by a trained therapist

Complementary and Alternative (CAM) Therapies
Mind Body Techniques

These may be helpful for SAD as well as for other depressive disorders discussed above

Relaxation techniques such as Yoga or Tai chi
Meditation
Guided imagery
Music or art therapy

Other things which may be helpful are:

Exercising
Eating brain foods
Exposure to the outside even on a cloudy day

Bipolar Depression (Bipolar Disorder – Manic Depressive Disorder)
What is It?

"Which of my feelings are real? Which of the me's is me? The wild, impulsive, chaotic, energetic, and crazy one? Or the shy, withdrawn, desperate, suicidal, doomed, and tired one? Probably a bit of both, hopefully much that is neither."

— Kay Redfield Jamison, An Unquiet Mind:
A Memoir of Moods and Madness. Professor in Mood Disorders and Psychiatry at Johns Hopkins, School of Medicine

This is also known as Manic Depressive Disorder, and when present, the individual has periods of mania/hypomania (highs) alternating with depression (lows).

The characteristics are:

Manic state – an individual is in an excited or overdrive state, has rapidly changing ideas and thoughts, with little need for sleep or rest. The person may not feel tired, is always on the go and may feel invincible with impulsive and irresponsible behavior. They may engage in alcohol and drug abuse or binges, excessive and careless sexual behavior, and go on reckless money spending sprees or gambling. There may be encounters with law enforcement or police

Depressive state – is similar to that which was described above under depression and this is the "down" part of the illness. This may include sadness, feeling depressed, no interest in usual activities, excessive sleep, change in eating habits, weight gain, and suicidal thoughts

There are two main types of Bipolar disorders known as Type1 (more severe manic episodes), and Type 11 which has a milder manic phase (Hypomania), but tends to have more depressive bouts. Many famous artists, entertainers and stars suffer from the disorder or have relatives who have Bipolar, and have publicly advocated for mental health awareness and treatment.

Treatment

"Bipolar robs you of that which is you. It can take from you the very core of your being and replace it with something that is completely opposite of who and what you truly are. Because my bipolar went untreated for so long, I spent many years looking in the mirror and seeing a person I did not recognize or understand---".

—Alyssa Reyans, Letters from a Bipolar Mother.
www.goodreads.com/quotes/tag/mental-illness

This illness is treatable and an individual may be put on different medications to treat both conditions that exist in this disease. However the manic treatment is what is important, and not treating this and using only antidepressants is not advised because it can cause the individual to quickly cycle between the two mood states. Medicines used include: antidepressants, mood stabilizers like Lithium, Valproate, carbamazepine and Lamotrigine Counseling by a Psychologist is also important since it gives one insight into the disease and helps an individual develop better coping skills and social interactions.

Schizophrenia
What is It?

This is a chronic mental illness which is characterized by changes in:

- Thinking
- Behavior
- Feelings

It may start between the ages of 16 and 30 years and occurs in all races. The prevalence worldwide is 1%, and in the US, about 3 million are affected in any given year. The symptoms must be present for at least 6 months before a diagnosis can be made. Many mental health patients who are seen on the streets, talking to themselves, unkempt, homeless, or sometimes even acting violently have Schizophrenia. However, there are sufferers who are on medicines and live a normal life.

It is characterized by:

- Psychosis – thinking and emotions which signify individual has lost touch with external reality
- Delusions – strong beliefs that are held despite evidence to the contrary
- Hallucinations – individual may hear voices or see objects that others do not see
- Abnormal behavior – withdrawal into self
- Unpredictable behavior and unrealistic thoughts and ideas
- Disorganized speech – may not make sense and may ramble on or make up pretend language

Symptoms

There is gradual deterioration of social interaction and behavior.

Delusions may be of self-importance (grandiose) or paranoid (suspicious and distrustful) and these false beliefs are fixed and one cannot reason with the individual.

Depression.

Deterioration in school and work.

Unkempt appearance and isolation.

Treatment

A psychiatrist or doctor who deals with mental illness will need to take a careful history, do blood work, and make the diagnosis. The individual will be treated with medications called Antipsychotics. If an individual takes their medications, Schizophrenia can be stabilized and sufferers can lead stable lives especially if they have insight into their illness and accept the fact that they suffer from it. A depiction of this medical condition and one man's struggles with it is portrayed in a brilliant Academy Award Best Picture called "A Beautiful Mind" which is the film based on the biography of a brilliant mathematical genius called John Nash Jr. who was diagnosed with this condition. He went on to win a Nobel Prize in Economic Sciences in 1994. Another one is a novel by Robert Kolker 'Hidden Valley Road' 2020 a true story about an American family which had 6 out of 12 kids diagnosed with it.

Chronic Stress

People are under a lot of chronic stress. The demands of life, be it family, job, school, finances, deadlines, traffic jams, kids education, etc. can lead to stress reactions in the body and of the mind. However, if stress is not relieved or decreased it becomes chronic with release and persistence of certain stress hormones and their effects.

What is It?

Stress is an overwhelming, pressuring, worrisome, negative emotional experience resulting in psychological, emotional and physical illnesses. It is defined as an "emotional experience accompanied by predictable biochemical, physiological and behavioral changes" (Baum, Andrew. Health Psychology, Vol 9(6), 1990, 653–675). Stress affects both males and females, adults and children and according to a survey by the American Psychological Association, over 40% of adult Americans report staying awake at night because of stress (www.apa.org/helpcenter/understanding-chronic-stress).

What Happens During Chronic Stress?

Among other things, it leads to the release of stress hormones mainly Cortisol and Adrenaline (the fight and flight hormone) which trigger the symptoms one experiences when stressed, and prepares a person to fight a perceived danger or flee from it. So in the latter case, it can be positive and save an individual being chased by an enemy from being devoured; with the return of these hormones to their normal lower levels once the danger is over. However, if one is in a constant or prolonged state of stress, the hormones stay elevated, and disrupt the body's normal systems and functions including the cardiovascular, nervous, immune and endocrine systems.

Diseases and Conditions Linked with Stress

High stress has been linked to:

Physical medical conditions like Hypertension, Stroke, Heart Attacks, Asthma, skin problems like Eczema, and obesity from overeating

Psychological conditions like Anxiety, Depression, Insomnia, and Post Traumatic Stress Disorder

Unhealthy lifestyle choices like excessive eating and drinking, use of illegal drugs, or even uncontrolled shopping (excessive retail therapy)

Signs and Symptoms

Physical symptoms of stress may include: Tension headache, Migraines, clenched muscles, palpitations, lack of sleep, abdominal pain, Diarrhea, shaking, and tremors, Itching of the skin, hives, overeating and weight gain.

Signs include increased blood pressure, and blood sugar; and decrease in one's immune response leading to susceptibility to infections like shingles.

Emotional or psychological symptoms include: anxiety, depression, irritability, memory problems and lack of focus or concentration.

Stress Management

Although stress is inevitable, it is possible to manage it and curtail the triggers. Some people have chronic stress because they think and act like a "super woman" and take too much load or burdens on themselves.

Taking time to Smell the Roses

This means one makes a deliberate effort to slow down at times to relax and chill. When sick it is okay to take time off from work to recover. People who fuss about work when sick and do not want to take time off, must remember the saying that "your bosses will always find someone else to do your work when you die because of self neglect".

Some practical things one can do to minimize or deal with stress include:

Set realistic goals that are achievable

Make lifestyle changes and behavior choices which reduce stress

Learn to delegate work or chores to other people

Sometimes insecurity leads to not trusting others to do a job so one takes it on and does too much

Build healthy relationships in which there is mutual trust and respect

Discuss problems with trusted individuals – family member, mentor, coworker, or friend

Practice activities like paced breathing, prayer, Tai Chi, guided imagery meditation, Yoga

Learn relaxation techniques like controlled breathing, listening to soothing music, laughing out loud, sitting in a quiet dimly lit room with low nature tunes (ocean, rainfall, forest etc.) playing

Get a pet e.g. a dog, they help people relax and calm down

Make time for oneself and learn to do something fun which one enjoys

Try doing adult coloring books, painting or beading

Start a new hobby like gardening or scrapbooking

Engage in exercise. This causes the brain to release good endorphins – the feel good chemicals

If stress involves one's job, and it does not improve, consider changing jobs

Make sure one takes vacations, to travel in country or outside the country or region where you live, exploring new places and cultures

Excessive overtime work has led to deaths of people, and in Japan the phenomenon is called "Karoshi" or "death from overwork"

Seek professional help from a psychologist or counselor to help deal with stressors

Have a support system of family, friends etc.

A recent study by Dr. Hirshberg of the Center for Healthy Minds University of Wisconsin (PLoS ONE 13(12): e0207765) showed that contemplative practices like "loving-kindness meditations" and "breath awareness" help to tackle stressors and also prepare one for stress. See below on meditations.

Contemplative Practices

These are used more and more by individuals and have been said to increase attention, help with physical issues like pain, social interactions like improving relationships, and mental health like stress reduction, anxiety, depression, substance abuse among others. Some of these include the following:

Christian Meditations

Christian meditation was discussed under Mind Body practices in an earlier chapter of the book.

Mindfulness Based Interventions (MBI)

MINDFULNESS has been defined as "simply a way to pay attention on purpose, in the present moment, and nonjudgementally" (Dr. Jon Kabat-Zinn Prof. emeritus, Univ. of Mass. Med. School). He has made Mindfulness-Based Interventions (MBI) famous and has a course called Mindfulness-Based stress Reduction (MBSR). It is said to be supported by scientific research, and individuals and companies send employees to learn the techniques. The Interventions resulted from Yoga and Buddhist meditative techniques, but this is secular, and one does not have to practice these religions in order to engage in contemplative practices.

MBSR Program

In a gist its an eight week evidence based program that offers secular, intensive mindfulness training and contains a number of techniques:

Awareness of breath
Awareness of body sensations
Walking meditation
Mindful movement
Loving kindness practice

There are certified teachers all over the world and online trainings some of which are free. Dr. Kabat-Zinn denies it is a new age practice, but "there are a lot of different ways to talk about mindfulness, but what it really means is awareness" (www.cbsnews.com/news/mindfulness-anderson-cooper-60-minutes). It is practiced in over 100 countries, and used in over 700 hospitals worldwide.

Other Mindfulness Practices

Another resource for mindfulness and self care practices is the Greater Good Science Center at UC Berkeley. Their Greater Good online magazine defines mindfulness as "maintaining a moment-by-moment awareness of our thoughts, feelings, bodily sensations, and surrounding environment, through a gentle, nurturing lens". Several topics on mind and body can be found on their website (https://greatergood. berkeley.edu/mind_body).

Gratitude

What is It?

"Gratitude unlocks the fullness of life. It turns what we have into enough, and more. It turns denial into acceptance, chaos to order, confusion to clarity. It can turn a meal into a feast, a house into a home, a stranger into a friend".
—Melody Beattie, American Author. www.azquotes.com/author

Just like how "our words frame our world", our attitude also affects our physical, mental and spiritual health. An attitude of gratitude does a lot for our health as noted below.

Definition

According to the Merriam-Webster dictionary, gratitude is the state of being grateful, thankfulness. It comes from the Latin word gratus 'pleasing, thankful'. Robert Emmons, a leading researcher of gratitude, defines gratitude "as a recognition of the gifts that others give us, a recognition of the source of those gifts, and an appreciation of those gifts". Sometimes we forget to be grateful for our lives and things in our lives, not appreciating how blessed we are compared to others. Gratitude is an attitude we have to develop because it has a lot of benefits.

Why is it important?

Over the last few years, research has shown that there are benefits for being grateful or appreciative for the small and big things in one's life. Studies show benefits like:

Decreased materialism
People are more generous
Better sleep
Improvement in interpersonal relationship
Lowered stress (National Public Radio Health News, Dec. 24th, 2018)

Other research studies have shown that for those with Mental Health issues, practicing gratitude by writing or journaling about gratitude resulted in:

- Improved mental health
- Changes in the brain giving a distinct brain activity
- Participants became more attentive to how they expressed gratitude

(Wong, J, Brown, J.; June 6, 2017. How Gratitude Changes You and Your Brain. (Greatergood. berkeley.edu/article/item)

Biblical View

The Bible, a Book very dear to me teaches a lot about being grateful and expressing gratitude. For example, Jesus after healing ten lepers, found that only one came back to give thanks – "And fell down on his face at his feet, giving thanks . . . . And Jesus answering said, "were there not ten cleansed? . . . arise, go thy way: thy faith hath made thee whole" Luke 17v16-19. I believe the wholeness here was more than physical healing – it was body, soul and spirit.

Practicing Gratitude

To practice gratitude and reap its benefits, one can do the following:

1) Recognize the Gifts others give you
2) Recognize "Gifters" (givers of gifts) in your life
3) Appreciate the many gifts in your life
4) Be a "Gifter" to someone else
5) One can start by keeping a Gratitude Journal and write down things one is grateful for

There are people who are "gratitude bloggers" and there are gratitude journals used for journaling. Some people journal once daily, once a week or once a month.

27

Social Transitions in A Woman's Life

What are They?

These are the many social changes that can happen in a woman's social life and I have termed these "Social Transitions" and are included under "Mental Health" because they involve emotional and psychological issues at each stage. These include:

- Singleness
- Marriage
- Parenting
- Divorce and Separation
- Widowhood
- Bereavement and Grieving
- Remarriage
- Death and Dying

Life is A Journey

Life is a journey and one may move through transitions of life facing the challenges that come with each one. Some transitions come with great joy and not all of them are challenging events. As one seeks direction, I personally recommend a GPS to give one direction. For me, I consider the most reliable GPS as one called "God's Positioning System", in which God is involved in giving one direction. I have personally used this for many years and found it credible.

Everyone starts as a child and grows to become a teenager or adolescent and then a young adult who either ends up single, in a relationship but not married, or married. Others along the journey may encounter situations like break ups, separation and or divorce, remarriage, or widowhood. Finally, we will all die and return to the dust. (from dust we came and to dust we shall return).

In my discussions of these transitions in life and some of the challenges that one may face, I refer to the Bible, because it is a guidebook that has helped and continues to help me and countless others in our lives' journeys.

I highly recommend the Bible to everyone, because it:

- Connects you to your Creator
- Tells you how important you are to Him
- Tells you how He wants to have a relationship with you
- Guides you to live the way He wants you to, in order to fulfill His plans and destiny for you
- It is a true and tested guide for living life

Everyone is Important to God

I believe God puts everyone here on earth for a purpose, and the purpose may change at different times in one's life, however, each one's path is unique; and relying on God makes the journey exciting and fulfilling, because He is there to help you. You do not have to walk alone.

Living As A Fulfilled Single Woman

It's possible for a woman to be single and satisfied, as she lives life to the fullest, enjoying her life and purpose at this time. First of all, I detest the word "spinster" which according to Wikipedia means "an unmarried woman who is past the usual age for marrying and is considered unlikely to marry". With many women entering the workforce and opting to pursue a career first, many are choosing not to get married early and are postponing that next phase of their lives until later. Some individuals also may not want to get married at all. Not everyone falls into that category, because there are some who would like to get married and start a family but have not found the 'right man' yet. To those I would say, do not just sit and wait for "Mr. Right" to show up, but pursue other passions, hobbies and friendships, as these will enable you to be single and satisfied until you meet and settle down with a "Mr. Right". For those who chose not to get married, that is also fine, enjoy your life and fulfill your God given Purpose.

Things One Can Do

During this time of being or staying single, you have a purpose in life and should discover that while living life to the fullest. I believe the full life applies to all areas of your life: spiritual, physical, financial, social, relational and mental. Enjoy the company of friends, pursue a career, serve others through volunteerism, pursue your dreams and aspirations, pursue higher education, join civil or social groups, school alumni groups or non-profit organizations or start one. With social media, one can get much accomplished and get others to join your "cause". Getting involved with social organizations, clubs, churches which have men involved will introduce you to men who may have the same interests as you do.

Below are other ways to meet guys.

- Young adult groups like school alumni groups, and political parties' groups
- Churches and other religious organizations have different groups like young adults and singles ministries which one can get involved in
- Non-Traditional Dating: Some people go on blind dates, speed dating, or meet men online through dating sites or singles social groups etc. If single, be careful about online dating since there are many who have been duped and defrauded of money by internet fraudsters and scammers who pose as single men looking for love; they take advantage of vulnerable, lonely single women who are looking for meaningful relationships

If you are young, use the time while single as preparation, self-development and maturation time. It is possible to be single and be satisfied with life. This preparation time allows you to be ready, so that when you eventually meet the right person and get married, you will be able to deal with the challenges which may arise (as they do) in your marriage.

On the spiritual front, explore a deeper relationship with your God. If you have a relationship with God, allow Him to help you mature in every area of your life; physically, financially, socially, mentally, relationally, emotionally and spiritually. Your love for Him is demonstrated by your obedience to Him and your service to others. One has to not only talk, but one has to walk the talk.

Finally, being single is NOT a Sit and Wait time, for those wishing to get married. It should be an active and purpose driven time to get engaged in all areas of your life and be happy. Have Fun and enjoy life with family and other single people. Travel, engage in sports or exercise, volunteering and pursuing a hobby are just a few things that can bring you satisfaction.

Finding Fulfillment In Marriage

....

What is Marriage?

" 'For this reason a man shall leave his father and mother and be joined to his wife, and the two shall become one flesh'; so then they are no longer two, but one flesh. Therefore what God has joined together, let not man separate"

—Jesus Christ. (The Bible, Mark 10v5-9. NKJV).

Marriage is an agreement, pact or covenant between a man and a woman which is to be entered into with care and due consideration, and not lightly. Most times it is based on love or affection for one another and common ideals, however, a woman should look beyond that physical attraction and emotional affection and look at what qualities the man has.

There are some basic or fundamental qualities a Man should have and it's important for a Woman to have the right answers to questions below.

- Does he respect you and treat you like a lady?
- Does he have a job? Either a full or part time job is fine
- Is he sleeping on the couch the whole day watching TV or playing video games?
- Is he pursuing an education, if he is unemployed?
- Does he tear you down and shame you in private or in public?

These are important questions a woman should ask herself and answer, because if he is not "pulling his weight" or treating you with respect before the marriage, it is unlikely he will change afterwards. Marriage is intended to be a lifelong commitment, however, in these times it is unfortunately not considered so by many for a variety of reasons. It seems to be regarded by many as a contract a couple may enter into without much thought, and that it can be dissolved easily, when problems arise (microwave mentality). For some, when challenges are encountered, there is little or no attempt to deal with or solve the problem because divorce is considered the only solution. This so called "microwave" mentality is applied to this important institution ordained by God Himself. There are of course other reasons which can lead to marriage dissolution and may include infidelity (adultery), abandonment, and abuse which are valid reasons.

No One is Perfect

Marriage is a "give and take" (giving and receiving) relationship. No one is perfect, and everyone has faults and so once a couple starts living under the same roof, they will start discovering things about their spouse and THEIR OWN SELF which they did not know existed previously. However, some individuals find it very easy to overlook their own faults and mistakes, but readily see their spouse's errors and short comings. Jesus rightly said in Matthew 7v5: "Hypocrite! First remove the plank from your own eye, and then you will see clearly to remove the speck from your brother's eye" (https://www.bible.com).

Now individuals have different personalities, likes and dislikes, upbringing, family background, and values, so initially, there will be quite a steep "learning curve" regarding living with another individual under the same roof and sleeping in the same bed. A newly married couple will have to go through a rapid learning experience in the first few years together and this is expected, since even couples who have been married for longer periods will from time to time discover something new about their spouse which they did not know before.

Making One's Marriage Work

Below are some tips which may help one's marriage, and it is by no means exhaustive.

- BEFORE MARRIAGE, it is important that couples go for pre-marriage counseling and hold each other accountable in a loving way
- SOON AFTER MARRIAGE, maybe in the first 4 to 6 months, arrange to meet with your marriage counselor since the honeymoon is over and reality sets in. A counselor may be able to help iron things out. This counseling should not be done by relatives
- To help maintain a satisfying relationship, there are four phrases that I believe married couples have to be familiar with, and also find easy to say to each other when the need arises. They are: **"I'm sorry", "Thank you", "I love you", "I forgive you".** The first and the last are the most difficult for a lot of people to say, however, practice makes perfect and using these may defuse a potential quarrel or prevent situations from turning from bad to worse
- I personally believe that if each of the partners has a personal relationship with God, then He unites them and they can each have the same point of reference – which is God
- God has given us a moral compass through the things He has said in the Bible. This Book which is the Word of God can be "a light to their path and a lamp to their feet" guiding them as they make the journey together with God
- I personally apply the power of Prayer to my married life and it works for me. Couples can pray together and also with their kids. When I counsel people, I tell them you cannot usually pray when there is unresolved conflict and so you may first be "forced to resolve" it and then pray together!
- Communication is vital in any marriage, and this is important in the good and the bad times as well. A spouse should not only be made aware of a "wrong" deed or attitude, but they should be praised for "good" ones. This affirmation is necessary and builds up the relationship
- I believe in "Leave and Cleave" which means you have left your original family and are in a new relationship with your spouse. Parents and relatives are great support systems, be in touch with them, but they should not dictate how one's relationship with one's spouse should go, nor run your marriage
- One can share unresolved problems with a trusted individual if needed, but one should use wisdom as to who to talk to. Try to resolve issues EARLY by oneself first, and then invite others if the two of you cannot resolve them
- Another important point is unresolved conflict which brews and leads to problems in the marriage. Once one is in any type of relationship with another

human being, conflicts will arise, but they have to be addressed and dealt with, utilizing the Four phrases mentioned above

- When things become difficult and there is lack of understanding of each other, and communication is breaking down, couples should resort to marriage counselors, family psychologists, or church marriage ministries, who may be able to help them sort out their differences and continue to stay married
- There is no doubt that some men are abusive and often this may not be obvious to outsiders. The abuse may be physical, emotional, sexual or verbal. If he does not change or does not seek counseling, then some women seek divorce and they cannot be blamed
- If one does not feel safe in a marriage MAKE SURE ONE GETS HELP. Go to a safe place and tell someone you trust. There are many organizations in different countries who help women facing or going through domestic or intimate partner violence or abuse
- With busy schedules and work, it is important to be communicating constantly and couples may have to make or schedule time for a "date night" or a time at home when they just sit and chat. This is even more important once kids become part of the family
- Mothers should make time to spend with husbands, and not just be attentive to the kids
- Sexual relationship is important and builds healthy marriages. There are many books etc. available teaching on how to build a great sex life with your spouse. Seek help if you are having challenges in this area. Talk to your spouse about it if he is too demanding, if you are not happy, or physical issues like back pain, arthritis, vaginal dryness, menopause symptoms or pain. You should also see your health care provider about these

Parenting

"Each day of our lives we make deposits in the memory banks of our children".

—Charles R. Swindoll
Christian Pastor and Author USA.

This will be discussed briefly with the understanding that it is a vast subject that cannot be fully dealt with here. In societies today, parenting may not necessarily be done by biological parents, and may involve adopted or foster parents, relatives or step parents of the child. There are resources on the internet, podcasts or print media (go to the library) which can assist adults in performing this difficult but rewarding responsibility.

Two Parents

Parenting is not an easy task and if the home is a two-parent one, then both parents have to be involved in raising the children. The mother should not assume that raising the children is her sole responsibility, because it should be a shared one, and the father has to be encouraged to be involved if he is present. Both parents have to send the same message to the children by being united when it comes to issues like discipline, showing affection etc. to the children. Kids may sometimes "test" the limits of parents, and they are also aware or cognizant of ambiguity when it is demonstrated by parents sending different messages to the kid(s). When this happens, they can play one parent against the other in order to get what they want, and this brings conflict.

Single Parent

Being a single parent is not easy and most times it falls on women, but there are some men who play the role as well. The single parent wears two hats as "mother" and "father" and it is important to let other significant people in your lives help you. For example, a mother can encourage a trusted male role model to be involved in the life of her son(s) and do things with him (them). Note that I mention 'TRUSTED' since there are Predators who may be potential child sex abusers, so don't let your guard down. Always talk to your kids to find out about what they did etc. if they go out with another adult. You should also make sure your kids know some adults can abuse them, teach them to recognize and feel comfortable discussing any "Red Flags" with you which may have occurred in the company of another adult. (More information is found in the chapter dealing with child sexual abuse). It is safer if a friend of your son is part of the company if possible, for safety sake. Involvement in sports, church and other social groups like Girl Scouts and Boy Scouts may help with the socialization of your children. But make sure they are safe.

There are many books and internet sites which help with parenting. Some include: https://www.focusonthefamily.com/parenting/; https://www.focusonthefamily.com/shows/focus-on-parenting-podcast/; www.nationalparenthelpline.org/find-support https://stopparentingalone.com/ops.

Kids Must Know They Are Loved

Whether the home is a single parent home, two-parent home, a blended family (each parent comes with kids from a previous relationship/marriage), or adopted family, kids must know that they are loved and appreciated. They must also know that there are rules of the house that they are expected to obey. Children often learn by the example that they see in their home and from outside the home, and so if they do not receive love from the home, then they look for it elsewhere; which may lead them to be involved with the wrong crowd or gangs. If they do not feel accepted and valued at home, they will try and find it elsewhere.

Discipline and Affirmation

Not only should there be discipline but there should also be encouragement, praise, and affirmation from parents to boost the kids' morale and confidence. Kids need to be made aware that their parent or parents are in their "corner" and cheering for them. It is important for parents to ask their school-age kids about their friends, and talk to them about issues like drugs, tobacco, alcohol abuse, and bullying in school or in the neighborhood. Many kids have been bullied and have not been able to share it with their parents for various reasons. The bullying may be verbal, physical, emotional or cyber (social media). Teaching them about safety at home, at school and in the neighborhood is important, especially how to identify and report sexual abuse to trusted individuals.

Discussion and Family Time

Parents need to spend quality time with each of their children, as this gives them the opportunity to know what is happening in their kid's life. Drugs, tobacco and alcohol use need to be discussed by the family and even the issue of sex at an appropriate age. Some parents have a "date night" with each child periodically and this can allow the child to feel comfortable in a parent's presence and open up to the parent. Maybe mothers can go with the girls and fathers with their sons to start off with. Limiting how much time they spend watching TV, or screen time on phones, tablets, computers etc. must be regulated by parent(s). Parental controls are needed on devices including TVs.

Praying for Your Kids

Lastly, with the task of parenting becoming more challenging due to the bombardment of messages (which may be good or bad), from both print and social media, I suggest that prayer is important and parents must pray for and with their children from a young age. This helps them learn how to pray and be comfortable praying by and for themselves. Due to my faith in God, I strongly recommend that kids be introduced to church early in life so that at an accountable age, they can come to personal faith in God for themselves, because I don't believe a parent's faith can automatically be transferred to a child. Faith in God is through a personal experience, this is unlike mere religion. Its religion which is transferred or handed down by parents. Personal faith requires a personal trust and decision making, not a coerced or forced one. Faith in God provides a compass that they can use to direct their lives in these challenging times.

Divorce

This is a painful development in a marriage and I have had many women come to see me in my practice as a physician who have gone through, are going through, or have already gone through divorce. When divorce results from cheating or a husband saying he does not love his wife anymore, because he has found a younger woman or another woman, it is very painful and a wife feels betrayed and abandoned. She may start having low self-esteem and blame herself, feel guilty or get depressed. It is even more painful if the couple have been together for several years and when there are younger children involved. It is a more stressful time especially if the woman would have preferred the relationship to continue. There are of course circumstances when the woman is the person who wants to get out of the relationship for a number of reasons which may include infidelity (cheating) on the part of the husband, or physical, verbal and other kinds of abuse by the man. She may also be the cheating spouse.

Mediation and or counseling

This must be tried first unless it's a case of abuse and the woman's safety is at stake. If this is the case, she has to go to a safe place first, and get counseling. Unfortunately, experience shows that men generally, do not often want to go for help through counseling with professionals. It may be so because the man may feel vulnerable and may not want his shortcomings exposed during such times, or may feel guilty admitting to faults in the presence of a marriage counselor or mediator.

Children and Divorce

Usually, separation occurs first and, in that case, one parent or spouse may move out with the children if they are young. If unfortunately, reconciliation is not possible, and divorce does occur, then if there are children involved, there may be shared custody, unless one parent signs over their rights for shared custody of the child(ren) to the other parent. In shared custody, each parent must try to be civil with each other and not play the children against the other parent. Kids can be "caught in the middle" of divorced couples and used as "pawns" by either parent: this must be avoided at all costs. It is important to communicate to the children (before the separation and or divorce occurs) that they are not the reason for the divorce and that both parents love them very much. This is important since some kids may think they are the reason for their parents' problems and desire to separate and or divorce.

Help during Divorce

If the woman has custody of the children, then for the sake of the children, she should be civil at least with the ex-husband and allow him to be in touch with the kids, unless he chooses not to, or is prevented from doing so due to violence, abuse, a restraining order etc. Most times, both a mother and her children may need counseling to go through this difficult time of their lives. Kids are most times innocent victims and should be made to go through this experience with as little pain as possible. It takes determination and resolution from both parents to let this happen, and make the kids live their lives as normal as can be, in this difficult situation. Some churches and other organizations have "Divorce Care" groups and meetings. One can check these out and go to their meetings. These can be useful, and some have separate meetings for kids involved.

Dating after Divorce

A question sometimes arises as to whether one should be dating while going through divorce or right after a divorce. It is probably not a good idea to do so at the early stage (first year), given the emotions one is going through at that time. Whether it is during or just after separation or divorce, getting into another relationship during this time may not give one sufficient time to grieve or learn new lessons which may help in the next relationship. This is a pretty vulnerable time as one is already looking for someone who has a listening ear, and will sympathize with you; and so anyone one meets who is willing to do that is attracted to you and the close attention may cloud one's judgement at that time. Waiting a while to settle down and be healed by time and counseling, will make one more objective, and then one can later get into a relationship which is not based just on sympathy from the new man. TAKE TIME TO HEAL, HOLD OFF A NEW RELATIONSHIP UNTIL LATER.

Widowhood

Losing a spouse or significant other (for those who have lived with boyfriends), is a very devastating and painful experience. It is often described as losing part of oneself. People who lose a spouse will go through grieving which is described below. It is said that time is the healer and if one is a person of Faith, accepting the Comfort and Peace from God is needed to go through these difficult times. The grief gets better with time, and one should not feel guilty if one gets back into socialization etc. by six months because it depends on the cause of death and if the death in a way freed the deceased from his suffering when death occurs; for example for someone who dies after a long fight with Cancer and pain, dying may give relief for both the deceased and the relatives, although the individual will be missed.

Remarrying After A Divorce or Death of A Spouse

Some people choose to remarry after a divorce or death of a spouse, while others feel content being single. Men tend to remarry much quicker after the death of a spouse or significant other than women do. When it does occur, it is important to go into the second marriage with a fresh start, by not always comparing the present spouse with the former one. That can lead to a lot of marriage problems. If divorce is the reason for the remarriage, it is prudent for one to take some learnt lessons from the first one to the new one. It is also a good idea to have Premarital Counseling prior to the second marriage, because this will involve a new set of "rules of engagement". There are many good books that counsel and advise people about remarriage and the blended family which may result from the new union, since each person may bring their own children into this new marriage.

Bereavement and Grieving

When one loses a loved one to death (bereaved), grieving is the normal response to this. Grieving is the multiple ways of reacting to loss, especially of a loved one. Losing a loved one is always a painful process, and the grieving process is complex and involves adapting in many areas of one's life especially if the departed one was a close relative or friend. The depth of one's grief depends on the relationship one had with the departed one, and whether the departed one was going through a lot of physical suffering, in which case, death tends to be a relief because the deceased one will not have to suffer anymore.

Kubler-Ross Model of Grief

In the field of grieving and loss, there is a model of grieving called the KUBLER-ROSS MODEL of grief. Dr. Kubler-Ross was a psychiatrist who proposed this pattern of adjustment after working with dying patients for years. Her original model was proposed for people who were sick and were facing death, however; it has been applied to grieving after a loved one dies as well. This model involves the emotional adjustments a person may go through and she proposed five stages which are:

DENIAL: No, it cannot be
ANGER: How did this happen? Who is responsible?
BARGAINING: I would do anything to have them back
DEPRESSION: I can't go on
ACCEPTANCE: There was nothing I could have done

She suggests that other emotions may be felt by some people and not others, and also that not everyone, will go through the continuum above or in the proposed order.

(Elisabeth Kubler-Ross Foundation; www.HealGrief.org)

Other Changes Associated With Grieving

Reference: loss (www.Medscape.com)

However, there are a whole lot more emotions, physical changes and even lifestyle changes that can accompany the process of grieving. These include:

Emotions: Disbelief, sadness, sorrow, guilt, confusion, resentment, loneliness, hopelessness, mood swings and shame due to sense of unfulfilled promises to the departed one

Physical: Insomnia (inability to sleep), frequent dreaming of the lost one, palpitations, lack of appetite, weight loss, overeating and weight gain, weakness, and fatigue. In severe cases, heart attack and death have resulted and recent studies have alluded to possible factors like stress hormones (Citroner, G. Grief Tied to Death – Medscape – Oct 25, 2018)

Behavior: Some individuals may have prolonged or complicated grief and may experience depression. Other behavior changes are withdrawal from social activities, conflict, and keeping busy so that one does not think about the loss. Lastly, some may adopt changes which are self-destructive like alcohol and drug abuse, and food addiction

One has the right to grieve or mourn a loved one, and this is encouraged. There may be non-professionals who initially can be of help to the individual.

Family and Friends

The presence of friends and family act as good social support for an individual who is grieving, and it is always good to be there for a friend who is going through grieving. As a friend or relative, one may not have answers to questions about why the person had to die, however; one's presence – being available as a friend or family member – is more than enough, and it is comforting for the bereaved person who is going through grieving.

Support Groups and Para-Professionals

Hospice, churches, bereavement counselors, and grief support groups may be available to help individuals who are having difficulty coping with their loss. There are also internet sites and books which help with grieving and mourning. The "Mourner's Bill of Rights" below may be a useful tool which was developed by a psychologist, Dr. Alan D. Wolfelt, Ph.D.

Treatment of Complicated Grief
Professional Help

If grief is prolonged and leads to some long-lasting emotional changes and states, then one will need professional help and or medications. One can talk with a health professional like one's family doctor, a psychologist or grief counselor/therapist. If depression is present, treatment with anti-depressants and or talk therapy may be needed.

Grieving for Other Losses

Apart from grieving after the death of a loved one, people may also grieve for other reasons like after experience of rape, sexual abuse, an abortion, loss of a job, move from a house, state or country, death of a pet, divorce, or separation etc. The emotional responses can also be intense; however, they may not be as prolonged or severe as in the loss of a loved person due to death. However, in some individuals these may also lead to Depression or Post-Traumatic Stress Disorder (PTSD), both of which were described above under mental disorders and may need treatment with counseling and medications.

Resources

There are many free online resources a grieving person can turn to, and one such is a free grief club community forum at Melody Beattie's website: https://thegriefclub. net. Several books on grieving can be found on eBay, Amazon and Christianbook. com. Some have also been written for specific cultures since the culture of a people or nation has a lot to do with how a widow griefs or is expected to mourn.

The Right to Mourn

Below are "rights" that a renowned psychologist, author, and grief counselor Dr. Alan Wolfelt has put together to help people who are mourning. In a way it gives people the choice or permission to do or not do certain things when they are mourning.

The Mourner's Bill of Rights
By Alan D. Wolfelt, Ph.D.

Though you should reach out to others as you do the work of mourning, you should not feel obligated to accept the unhelpful responses you may receive from some people. You are the one who is grieving, and as such, you have certain "rights" no one should try to take away from you.

The following list is intended both to empower you to heal and to decide how others can and cannot help. This is not to discourage you from reaching out to others for help, but rather to assist you in distinguishing useful responses from hurtful ones.

1. **You have the right to experience your own unique grief**

   No one else will grieve in exactly the same way you do. So, when you turn to others for help, don't allow them to tell what you should or should not be feeling

2. **You have the right to talk about your grief**

   Talking about your grief will help you heal. Seek out others who will allow you to talk as much as you want, as often as you want, about your grief. If at times you don't feel like talking, you also have the right to be silent

3. **You have the right to feel a multitude of emotions**

   Confusion, disorientation, fear, guilt and relief are just a few of the emotions you might feel as part of your grief journey. Others may try to tell you that feeling angry, for example, is wrong. Don't take these judgmental responses to heart. Instead, find listeners who will accept your feelings without condition

4. **You have the right to be tolerant of your physical and emotional limits**

   Your feelings of loss and sadness will probably leave you feeling fatigued. Respect what your body and mind are telling you. Get daily rest. Eat balanced meals. And don't allow others to push you into doing things you don't feel ready to do

5. **You have the right to experience "griefbursts."**

   Sometimes, out of nowhere, a powerful surge of grief may overcome you. This can be frightening but is normal and natural. Find someone who understands and will let you talk it out

6. **You have the right to make use of ritual**

   The funeral ritual does more than acknowledge the death of someone loved. It helps provide you with the support of caring people. More importantly, the funeral is a way for you to mourn. If others tell you the funeral or other healing rituals such as these are silly or unnecessary, don't listen

7. **You have the right to embrace your spirituality**

   If faith is a part of your life, express it in ways that seem appropriate to you. Allow yourself to be around people who understand and support your religious beliefs. If you feel angry at God, find someone to talk with who won't be critical of your feelings of hurt and abandonment

8. **You have the right to search for meaning**

   You may find yourself asking, "Why did he or she die? Why this way? Why now?" Some of your questions may have answers, but some may not. And watch out for the clichéd responses some people may give you. Comments like, "It was God's will" or "Think of what you have to be thankful for" are not helpful and you do not have to accept them

9. **You have the right to treasure your memories**

   Memories are one of the best legacies that exist after the death of someone loved. You will always remember. Instead of ignoring your memories, find others with whom you can share them

10. **You have the right to move toward your grief and heal**

    Reconciling your grief will not happen quickly. Remember, grief is a process, not an event. Be patient and tolerant with yourself and avoid people who are impatient with, and intolerant of you. Neither you nor those around you must forget that the death of someone loved changes your life forever

The Mourner's Bill of Rights (By Alan D. Wolfelt).

Part Five

Spiritual Health

Spiritual health will involve the following topics

Relationship with God
Living with Offense
Forgiveness
Prayer Life
Blessed to be a Blessing
Achieving Contentment
A Balanced Life and its Rewards

28

Spiritual Health

Introduction

....

The spiritual health of any individual is just as important as one's emotional and physical health. I have decided to add this section on spiritual health from my point of view, since we are discussing "Holistic Health" which for me involves health of the Body, Soul, and Spirit. I am basing it on my experience with the God of the Bible and His relationship with mankind. Even if you do not believe in the God of the Bible, I pray and trust that you will benefit from some of the principles discussed here.

"My prayer for you is that if you feel empty spiritually, you will have the experience that I had which has made me who I am today, and has enabled me to have Peace and Joy, to live a fulfilled life in relationship with God as my Father".

—Dr. Barbara Entsuah. Physician and Author.

Are You Spiritually Empty?

My prayer for you is that if you feel empty spiritually, you will have the experience that I had which has made me who I am today, and has enabled me to have Peace and Joy, to live a fulfilled life through my relationship with God as my Father, as is portrayed in the Bible. He is a good father figure who is loving, kind, and forgiving; and He has great plans for all of us compared to some earthly fathers who are wicked and abusive. You have read other parts of the book, so I trust you will read this section with an open mind, and be blessed by it.

If you choose NOT to read this section on spiritual health, that is okay, but please let your physical and mental lives be enriched by this book; and may it cause you to have knowledge and understanding because KNOWLEDGE IS POWER.

(All quotes from the Bible are from New King James Version (NKJV), copyright 1982 by Thomas Nelson, Inc.).

Spirituality

Spirituality according to the Merriam-Webster dictionary is defined among others as "sensitivity or attachment to religious values" and dictionary.com has a definition of "incorporeal or immaterial nature". Some may claim to be spiritual and have relationships with nature and inanimate things, however, personally I think there is a higher Spiritual Being – a Creator, who is God, and He is a Spirit to whom our own spirits are attracted to.

My Spiritual Experience

The discussion here is focused on relationship with God, our creator, as I have experienced and lived out. What I am giving account of here, is similar to what the Apostle John declared in his Epistle or writing found in 1 John 1v3: "that which we have seen and heard we declare to you, that you also may have fellowship with us; and truly our fellowship is with the Father and with His Son Jesus Christ. v4- and these things we write to you that your joy may be full". I am discussing this hoping and praying that you may find Joy in life, if you do not have it. Now Joy is not the same as happiness, because happiness depends on external circumstances, while joy is from within and comes from God. It is a fruit which God cultivates in us when we have a relationship with Him. It is similar to true Peace and Love, making you have Peace in the midst of a storm and loving the Unlovable. Happiness, on the other hand has to do with your environment and how external circumstances influence your emotions in a good way. So, one is happy when situations are favorable or good, and unhappy when situations are bad or unfavorable.

Having A Relationship With God

Who Is God?

"As a Christian, I look at spiritual health from the Christian perspective because of my own experience and my relationship with the God of the Christian faith".

—Dr. Barbara Entsuah

In Christianity, we believe in a Triune God (God the Father, Son and Holy Spirit. One God, but manifested, or revealed to man in three different forms). We believe God is the Omnipotent (all powerful), Omniscient (all knowing) and Omnipresent (always present) one and He created all things and holds all of His creation in place and in equilibrium.

Whereas for some, the issue of the reality of God is debatable, my aim is not to engage in such debate but to offer the Christian perspective of the Creator and His relationship to His creation – specifically with Human Beings – who are uniquely different from the other created beings. Scripture or the Bible says that "And the Lord God formed man of the dust of the ground and BREATHED INTO HIS NOSTRILS THE BREATH OF LIFE; and man became a living being" Genesis 2v7. For the creation of animals and birds in v19, we read God formed these out of the ground and brought them to Adam to see what he would call them (paraphrased). It does not mention animals having the breath of life from God. This breath of life I believe is the Spirit which every human being has, and which gives as a unique relationship with God, our creator. This mutual RELATIONSHIP of the Creator (God) to His creation (man), defines and undergirds the very essence of the existence and well-being of man. This makes for a possible and desirable personal relationship which is NOT conferred by birth nor proxy but acquired through a rational, thoughtful, individual and personal decision and commitment that is borne out by both experience and dogma. However, central to the relationship is the concept of sin.

What Is Sin?

When once asked, 'What is the definition of sin?' Billy Graham gave the following answer: "A sin is any thought or action that falls short of God's will. God is perfect, and anything we do that falls short of His perfection is sin".

(billygraham.org/story).

Sin is rebelling against God; a state of the heart which is manifested in various unrighteous acts and thoughts. As a result of sin, we as the human race are separated from God. Romans 3v23 puts it like this: "For all have sinned and fall short of the glory of God, …"

Christians believe that mankind was in relationship with his God in the beginning of creation; however, he became separated from God as a result of sin, which then affected this close spiritual relationship. Why so? Because, God is a Holy God and He hates sin, but loves the sinner. **Unlike other religions, the Christian belief is that man's attempt to get right with God or appease a Holy God, is not possible, because it falls short of God's standards. In many religions man tries to appease or get into a right standing with God through rituals, sacrifices, self-mutilation, doing good deeds, reading holy scriptures, meditations, and other practices.** All of these fall short of His requirements, because **reconciliation is on God's own terms and not man's own attempts.**

How Do We Reconcile With God?

God wants to reconcile with mankind according to His own terms or standards. The act of reconciliation – an expression of His love for man – came from God himself, and He provided a way for sinful man to be reconciled to a Holy God. The sacrifices of animals exemplified in the Old Testament Jewish religion and in many world religions today cannot pay for the price or wages of sin. God Himself set out a plan which was fulfilled by Jesus Christ who came and lived on this earth. The plan to save man, fulfills the cry of the Psalmist in Psalm 106v4: "Remember me, O Lord with the favor You have toward your people. Oh, visit me with your salvation" (NKJV). This is also the cry of many, expressed in other words, however, they have also sought to find a way back to Him through His own terms and not by human means.

God's Plan of Reconciliation

There is a simple plan of reconciliation that God has provided for mankind to get into right relationship with Him. God has indeed visited us with His salvation or Redemption plan by providing a way back to Him. This salvation plan is based on the God of the Bible – God of Abraham, Isaac and Jacob. He sent Jesus Christ to come and die in our place (He was a substitute) so that we do not have to pay for the penalty of sin. Hebrews 7v25 NKJV says "Therefore He (Jesus) is also able to save to the uttermost those who come to God through Him, since He always lives to make intercession for them".

Is the Plan that Simple?

It is so simple that men who expect God's plan for reconciling sinful man to Himself to be more complicated, reject it, and instead try to get right with God by their own good works or deeds. However, the Bible reminds us that our good works or deeds are like filthy rags before the Holy Lord. (Isaiah 64v6, paraphrased). The choice is ours, because He has given us the free will to make choices, but each choice we make, will have consequences in the present and future. A verse from 1 Corinthians 1v18 puts it like this: "For the message of the cross is foolishness to those who are perishing (getting lost – my own addition), but to us who are being saved it is the power of God" (NKJV).

Relationship with God – My personal experience

Many of us have faith in a God who is the Creator. Personally, I have had an intimate relationship with the God of the Bible for many years, and I try to live daily to please Him, because I love Him, and I am thankful He took the initiative to reach out to me, just like He has to every other human being. He is no respecter of persons but is available to anyone who calls upon Him. As a teenager, I was a church goer because my parents went to church and I considered myself a Christian and had been "born into a Christian home", but I did not really understand that one had to have a personal relationship with one's Creator. I did not understand that the Christian Faith was not one you can inherit. I had the opportunity to attend a

Christian youth camp organized by a Christian organization called the Scripture Union which has its roots from the United Kingdom. It was at an evening meeting that a British expatriate teacher explained to us what it meant to have a personal relationship with God, the Father, through His son Jesus Christ, and how to be saved from the penalty (consequences) of sin.

As I sat in that meeting, for the first time, I saw myself as God sees me – a sinner in need of a savior, and I surrendered my life and will to God. I prayed a simple prayer and asked Him, God, to forgive me for my sins, make me His child and to lead and guide me. I was no more under condemnation for my sins, my guilt was removed, and I had a new relationship with my Creator. I became "born again" in my spirit. This was what Jesus was trying to explain to Nicodemus, a Jewish religious leader, who when he heard Jesus teach, realized that something was missing in his life. Jesus told him in John's Gospel Chapter 3 verse 3-20 that he needed to be "born again", not physically but in his spirit man. (please read the verses above).

If you have never had a personal relationship with God and you feel empty and condemned, you do not have to continue that way. You can also have that experience, by following the steps below.

Steps to Salvation (Reconciliation With God).

This is what we should all recognize and understand as outlined in the Bible.

- Man is a sinner and is separated from God; Roman 3v23 "For all have sinned, and come short of the glory of God," Isaiah 59v2, "But your iniquities have separated you from your God."
- God is a Holy God. He hates sin but loves the sinner. He makes one holy and acceptable to Him by His own way, on His own terms; 1Peter 1v15-16 "Be holy for I am holy."
- There is a penalty for sinning against God. Romans 6v23; "For the wages of sin is death, but the gift of God is eternal life in Christ Jesus our Lord"
- God has made a provision to forgive sin through Jesus Christ. John 3v16-17; **"For God so loved the world that He gave His only begotten Son, that whoever believes in Him should not perish but have everlasting life. For God did not send His Son into the world to condemn the world, but that the world through Him might be saved."**
- God has thrown out an invitation to ALL to be reconciled to Him through Jesus Christ. This is what is referred to as "Grace". In one form, it demonstrates God's unmerited favor toward us. We did not deserve His gift, but He gave it to us anyway because of His love for you and me. Ephesians 2v8-9 says, "For by

grace you have been saved through faith, and that not of yourselves; it is the gift of God, not of works, lest anyone should boast"

- God's terms for reconciliation with you **does not involve your works.** They are not "righteous" enough to save you from the penalty (consequence) of sin

- The process gives us a new identity: We become Children of God; John 1v12. "But as many as received Him (Jesus – emphasis mine), to them He gave the right to become children of God, to those who believe in His name."

- Not only do you have a new relationship with God when you received Jesus Christ into your life, but God also gives us His Holy Spirit to assist us live the way God wants us to live. He is the guide who Jesus promised His disciples when He left them

- No one who has a relationship with God, needs to live under condemnation. No guilt, no sin, or deed is strong enough to separate you from the Love of God through Christ Jesus (read Romans 8v.38-39)

What Do You Have to do to Be Saved or Reconciled To God?

After recognizing and believing in the provision God has made for you to be at peace with Him based on above paragraph, you have to take the step to acknowledge your belief in, and acceptance of the gift of salvation.

Accept the Free Gift of God

You have the obligation to accept or reject God's gift. Now, whenever a gift is being given to someone, they can choose to respond in one of three ways:

1. Accept the gift, and thank the giver for it (YES TO THE GIFT)
2. Acknowledge the gift but not accept the gift by receiving it (INDECISION)
3. Refuse to accept the gift, and walk away from the giver and the gift (NO TO THE GIFT)

To get into right relationship with God, you say YES TO THE GIFT AND THE GIVER

Oswald Chambers (1874–1917) says it like this: "many a soul begins to come to God when he flings off being religious because there is only one master of the human heart, and that is not religion but Jesus Christ" (The mystery of Believing. My Utmost for His Highest. Discovery House Publishers. Michigan).

Repent of Your Sinful State

Acknowledge you are a sinner in need of salvation, and accept God's forgiveness and cleansing of your sinful nature through Christ Jesus's death and resurrection from the dead. You do so by having faith in God's plan of salvation and talk personally to God through PRAYER.

Prayer of Salvation

You can accept Him into your life right now as you read this, if you are prepared to turn from your old lifestyle, repent, and be reconciled to God. You can pray and accept the Lord Jesus Christ as your Lord and Savior without any pomp or fanfare, all by yourself even with no one around. He, Jesus Christ, has already paid the price for your salvation, and for you to get into the right relationship with God. You do this by faith or believing that this is God's plan and you are accepting and responding to God's plan.

Sample Prayer of Salvation

You can pray this sample prayer or pray your own words: God will hear you and answer.

Lord Jesus, I realize that I am a sinner and you came and died on the cross for me. Nothing else I can do can put me in a right relationship with God. Today I accept God's plan of salvation and I invite you into my life to be my Lord and Savior. Forgive me of all my sins and come and live in me. Make me a new person and help me to live for you.

Thank you for making me your child. Give me the strength to live each day for you and to let others know of my new relationship with you. Fill me with your Holy Spirit who can lead and guide me. I pray this through Jesus Christ. Thank you.

What you just prayed is summed up nicely in Romans 10v9-10 (NKJV):

"---that if you confess with your mouth the Lord Jesus and believe in your heart that God has raised Him from the dead, you will be saved. For with the heart one believes unto righteousness, and with the mouth confession is made unto salvation"

IS IT THAT SIMPLE? YES!!!. LET ME REMIND YOU ABOUT THE 2 THIEVES WHO WERE CRUCIFIED AT THE SAME TIME AS JESUS CHRIST.

One of the thieves on the cross who was also crucified the same time as Jesus was, said to Jesus in Luke 23v42-43; "Lord, remember me when You come into Your kingdom." And Jesus said to him, "Assuredly, I say to you, today you will be with Me in Paradise". The thief had previously acknowledged that his punishment was justifiable because he was a thief and was receiving his due punishment, however, Jesus was not a sinner and had not done anything wrong. So, he saw Jesus as the Son of God (Savior of Mankind) and that He was the one who will usher in the Kingdom of God. His faith in Jesus earned him salvation and a place in heaven with Jesus. One has to BELIEVE (have faith) and ACCEPT the plan of God. The other thief REJECTED Jesus and so he did not get the opportunity to be in "Paradise" with Jesus.

Is This New Relationship Real?

So, the new relationship you have with God is spiritual in nature because God is a Spirit, and we don't see Him physically, but He communicates with us through our spirits because you and I are spiritual beings in a human or fleshy body. We do not communicate with Him through objects, or sacrifices today, because that was used before Christ came as the perfect sacrifice and fulfilled all the requirements needed to get right with God the Father. Now, since we are also physical and operate mostly in the physical, we may sometimes doubt the spiritual experience we have had when we prayed to accept the Lord Jesus Christ into our lives. It is important that the basis of our salvation be hinged upon what God has said about you and not on how you feel.

What Does the Bible Say About This

In 2 Corinthians 5v17 the Bible says: "Therefore, if anyone is in Christ, he is a new creation; old things have passed away; behold, all things have become new". We have a new relationship with God. It is a love relationship. He loved us first and we love Him back because of who He is – our Lord and Savior – (which are just two of His many attributes and titles), and also because of what He has done for us (saved us and given us His Holy Spirit). To be sure of your decision (have assurance of your salvation), is very important because people or the devil will come and play tricks with your mind. Questions like "do you think just praying a simple prayer like what you did can make you right with God?", or "God cannot accept you because you are so bad" etc. It is important to believe what God says about you.

Salvation also involves you understanding with your mind what the Bible says about you and the provision of God. It also may involve some emotions. Some individuals, when they are convicted by the Holy Spirit after they hear the message of salvation, may cry, or have a lot of joy, shout, etc. while others may not show any great emotions and that is alright because we all have different personalities and different ways of expressing our emotions. The important thing is believing in your heart what God says about you and accepting His gift of salvation.

Assurance of Salvation

Everyone who has been born again by accepting the Lord Jesus as her Savior and Lord has to be assured of the step they have taken. This is referred to as "Assurance of salvation". Dr. Bill Bright who founded the Campus Crusade organization – an international Christian Organization, also called Great Commission, sums it up in this way:

Assurance of salvation is based on:

- **The Word of God**

  What the Bible says about you is what assures you of your salvation and relationship with God. We have already discussed some of the scripture passages which explain the relationship with God after one has prayed to accept Jesus into your heart. One should not depend on what one's mind, the devil or man say about the step one took. The Bible says you are reconciled with God and that settles it. The word of God is reliable and true. It is unchangeable, and we can trust that what it says about your salvation is the truth from God

  Hebrews 7v25 says about Jesus – "Therefore He is also able to save to the uttermost those who come to God through Him, since He always lives to make intercession for them."

  Mark 16v15, Jesus said "Go into all the world and preach the gospel to every creature. He who believes and is baptized will be saved; but he who does not believe will be condemned"

- **The presence of the Holy Spirit in you**

  Before Jesus died, He promised His disciples that the Father will send them another Helper, who will be with them forever, John 14v16-17. Jesus told His disciples that The Holy Spirit will dwell in a believer of Christ

  John 14v17 says "the Spirit of truth, whom the world cannot receive, because it neither sees Him nor knows Him; but you know Him, for He dwells with you and will be in you."

  He also told them that the Holy Spirit will guide them into all truth – John 16v13–14

  So, one of the things that assures us of our salvation is the presence of the Holy Spirit in us who is our Guide and our Helper. He is referred to by Jesus in John 14v16 as a Helper who will abide with us forever

  In Romans 8v16 (paraphrased) the Bible assures us that the Spirit of God bears witness with our spirits that we are the children of God

- **The changed life that has occurred in your own life**

  You will find that once you have this new exciting relationship with the Lord Jesus Christ, there are things in your life which start changing. A genuine, new relationship of love and trust in God begins to exist and it is manifested or shown in your daily life. Your desires change and certain things you did, you do them no more, because your priorities in life have changed. You live to please God and not yourself any more. This confirms what the Bible says in 2 Corinthians 5v17: "Therefore, if anyone is in Christ, he is a new creation; old things have passed away; behold, all things have become new."

  (Dr. Bill Bright Campus Crusade for Christ)

Benefits of Salvation

There are many benefits of having this personal relationship with God, your Creator, when by faith you accept Him into your life to lead and direct you.

- You are a child of God. "Behold what manner of love the Father has bestowed on us, that we should be called children of God!" 1John 3v1
- The relationship with God grants us eternal life, which is a life lived in relationship with God at the present time as He planned and intended for you, and which will continue after physical death
- We have the Holy Spirit living in us to empower us, guide and direct us. Jesus promised Him to the church when He left. (Luke 24v49)
- For the Christian we too have victory over death and the grave, because Christ's death and resurrection caused Him to have victory over death and the grave. Physical death is not the end but a continuation of life in God's presence for the Christian
- The Apostle Paul who is the writer of most of the books in the New Testament of the Bible expresses it this way. "For if the Spirit of Him who raised Jesus from the dead dwells in you, He who raised Christ from the dead will also give life to your mortal bodies through His Spirit who dwells in you". Romans 8v11
- We don't have to be in terror or fear of God, because He is a God of Love. In fact, He is Love. "– for God is love. In this the love of God was manifested toward us, that God has sent His only begotten Son into the world that we might live through Him." 1 John 4v8
- You do not have to be afraid of death or of dying, because you know what is in store for you. Some people may say they are not sure what will happen to them after dying but we have several passages in the Bible which gives us the assurance that we will be ushered into God's presence once we lay this mortal body down in death
- Remember, that because of the fall of man as a result to sin at the beginning of creation, every man or woman will either eventually die physically; or those who remain and have Jesus in their lives, will be taken up to be with Jesus when He comes back the second time for His own. Read 1 Corinthians 15v51-54 about what happens after the second coming of Jesus Christ
- You have assurance of a place with God in heaven when you die one day. When it comes to sickness or disease, they occur because of the curse upon man when he sinned against God in the beginning. Therefore, we do get sick and God sometimes chooses to heal our bodies supernaturally or miraculously. Other times He gives doctors and other health providers the wisdom to treat and make us better or heal us. However, as a Christian you should not be

afraid of death, because your spirit will not die, but will be with God in heaven when your physical body dies and returns to the dust

God is Driving But You Are Not A Robot

Your new journey with God in the "driver's seat" has started. However, remember just like He gave man free choice in the beginning of creation, you still have freedom of choice after you give Him control. Our actions and words are not automated by God, and we need to do certain things to keep in touch with Him and learn about His ways; what pleases or displeases Him, and how to learn about Him. Below we discuss your spiritual journey with God.

The Spiritual Journey With God Has Begun

The above, hopefully helps you know that the prayer you prayed to receive Him into your life was real and that God lives in you; so, you will begin this incredible journey of a relationship with your Creator. Just like a little baby who is born, you have to grow in your new found faith and relationship.

Growing the Spirit Man

As you grow in your relationship, you become like a child who matures as it is fed and nurtured by a parent. If the things listed below are lacking in your walk with God, then you do not grow and your relationship with Him does not get intimate. To grow spiritually, you need to:

- Read God's Word daily (daily Bible reading)
- Talk to God daily (Pray every day)
- Associate with others of like faith (Go to church regularly)
- Walk the talk (live your life according to the principles in the Bible)
- Don't be selfish (share with others what you have experienced)

The walk with God is very exciting, and He gives you a future and a Hope. The Bible says "Now hope does not disappoint us. . ." (Romans 5:5). God has a bright future for those, who trust in Him. 1 Corinthians 2:9 tells us that, "Eye has not seen, nor ear heard…The things which God has prepared for those who love Him". However, you need to Grow as noted above, otherwise you will find yourself drifting away from Him and your spirit man is starved.

The starved Spirit man

If you forget to daily feed your spirit man it starves and grows weak and your relationship with Christ suffers, and the joy you had as a new Christian goes away. You may be drawn back into your old way of life, where you were in the "driver's seat".

One may forsake the things that glorify God and You may stop attending church or hanging out with Christian friends. Your love for God will grow weak, as God will not be important in your life.

These old characteristics start in a subtle way and if not haltered, our new found relationship with our Father God fizzles and wanes. He on the other hand, will always be waiting for renewed walk and fellowship with us, but He will never force us to relate to Him. Remember CHOICE is a human capability God has given us, he does not force His Will upon us.

FORGIVENESS AND OFFENSE (offence – British spelling)
Forgiving others and having or carrying offense are two important topics we need to discuss.

What is Offense?

According to the Oxford Dictionary, Offense means "annoyance or resentment brought about by a perceived insult to or disregard for oneself or one's standards or principles". Synonyms include "annoyance, anger, resentment, indignation, wrath, displeasure, vexation" to name a few. Since we are all human, it is always possible to be offended by someone, or you may even be the offender at times. Sometimes the person we are offended by does not even know they have offended us.

What Should Be the Offended Person's Attitude?

Many live with offense because they have been hurt by someone (the offender); however, whether the offender is aware or not that they have displeased us, we need to forgive them. Why, because we may rob ourselves of many blessings, or be saddled with many negative consequences by holding on to the offense and having a spirit of unforgiveness. It has been described by many as "the silent killer" because of what it can do to the offended individual.

In order to get the right perspective of forgiveness, it is important for us to examine the biblical view of forgiveness.

Biblical View of Forgiveness
What is It?

"Take heed to yourselves. If your brother sins against you, rebuke him; and if he repents, forgive him. And if he sins against you seven times in a day, and seven times in a day returns to you saying, 'I repent,' you shall forgive him."
Jesus Christ—Luke 17 v 3-4. NKJV

Forgiveness is an important issue we must all deal with in order to maintain our own relationship with God and other people. God loved us so much that He forgave us and sent Jesus Christ to come down to earth and pay the penalty for our sins by dying on the cross.

As Christians (or even if you are not one), we realize that in order for us to get into a right relationship with God, we need His forgiveness, and He chose to forgive us when we deserved condemnation or punishment. He gave of His best – His son Jesus Christ so that we could receive forgiveness.

Why Forgiveness

Forgiveness is the basis of our own restored and reconciled relationship with our Creator. When we forgive others, we are extending the very act of mercy and grace to others as we have received from our Creator.

How Often Should We Forgive Others?

So, if God could forgive us while we were still sinners, we should be able to forgive our fellow human beings who hurt us or offend us.

Jesus's Example and Teaching

- Jesus talks about forgiveness and offense a great deal in the Bible and He also exemplified it. While hanging on the cross, after having been beaten, maimed, and going through suffering and pain, He said, "Father forgive them for they know not what they do" (Luke 23:34 NKJV)
- When Peter, the disciple of Jesus asked Him how many times he should forgive a brother, and whether up to seven times was enough?, Jesus's response must have blown Peter's mind. Traditionally, in that culture, it was usual to forgive someone up to three times, and Peter had increased the number to seven and must have felt very pious; but Jesus replied that up to seventy times seven!!!! (Matthew 18v21-22). In effect Jesus was saying as many times as possible, since it is virtually impossible to keep counting and recording up to 490 (70 × 7) times
- In another place, we find Jesus teaching His disciples about learning to keep forgiving an offender if they repent or are sorry. In Luke 17v3-4, He said "Take heed to yourselves. If your brother sins against you, rebuke him; and if he repents, forgive him. And if he sins against you seven times in a day, and seven times in a day returns to you saying, 'I repent,' you shall forgive him." He knew it was possible by His help, (though not easy by one's own strength) that was why He taught them to do so
- In teaching his disciples how to pray when they asked Him, Jesus told them to pray "And forgive us our trespasses as we forgive those who trespass against us" (Luke 11:4)

Apostle Paul's Teaching on Forgiveness

In the New Testament of the Bible, the Apostle Paul in his letters, encourages believers in Christ to forgive one another.

- Ephesians 4v32 says, "And be kind to one another, tenderhearted, forgiving one another, even as God in Christ forgave you"
- In Colossians 3v13, he says, "bearing with one another, and forgiving one another, if anyone has a complaint against another; even as Christ forgave you, so you also must do" (NKJV)

How Are We Able to Forgive?

It is a difficult thing to do so in your own power or strength; however, we know that it is possible to forgive someone who has hurt you with the help of God's power and grace. These two scriptures can encourage us in our quest to forgive: " I can do all things through Christ who strengthens me" Philippians 4v13 (NKJV), and "And He said to me, 'My grace is sufficient for you, for My strength is made perfect in weakness'." 2 Corinthians 12:9 (NKJV). Jesus knew we can do it, that is why He told Peter to do it as many times as necessary. For it is when we forgive that we truly begin to live in peace and freedom, and we are released from the spirit of unforgiveness. Forgiveness may be instantaneous or may take time. However, you must come to a point in your life when you can start the process of forgiving an offender. There has to be a decision day, when you make up your mind you are going to forgive an offender, because unforgiveness imprisons you and keeps you in bondage, tied up in the inside. Forgiveness on the other hand liberates you who was offended.

Steps Toward Receiving Forgiveness and Releasing an Offender

It can begin by:

- First ask God to forgive you
  Talk to God through prayer. First, we need to ask for and receive forgiveness from God whenever we have held on to unforgiveness. Someone will say what do you mean? "He or she was the one who offended me"! However, we must remember that the prayer which Jesus taught us (The Lord's Prayer) says "And forgive us our trespasses as we forgive those who trespass against us" (Luke 11:4). Holding onto unforgiveness is a sin, or offense against God, and it prevents us from getting all that God has for us. We deny ourselves of so many blessings if we hold on and do not let go of our unforgiving disposition. God will help you let go of unforgiveness and He will bring healing to your mind

and your spirit and set you free from negative emotions, like anger, hatred, bitterness and unforgiveness

If you agree that you need forgiveness from God and are prepared to receive His forgiveness, pray the sample prayer below (you can make up your own prayer):

Prayer Asking for Forgiveness for Yourself

Dear Heavenly Father, I pray that you will forgive me for holding on to unforgiveness. I confess bitterness, anger, and resentment toward _____ (insert name). I pray that you will cleanse me and forgive me for this sin. I thank you that the blood of Jesus is powerful enough to cleanse me and change my thinking. I ask this in the name of Jesus Christ. Amen.

- Forgive the Offender

  How do we forgive? In order to forgive, we must let God be the judge. We must give God (the Greatest One who forgave us), the opportunity to give us the ability to forgive

  First of all, we have to forgive by faith, because our whole Christian life is hinged on Faith. To forgive by faith means we do it because God says to do so in His Word, regardless of how we feel toward the person or what the person did. This is forgiving from your heart and not emotions

  Secondly, we do so because Jesus and men of God throughout the scriptures encourage us to do so, and Jesus Himself forgave His tormentors and those who hated Him. We lay aside anger, bitterness, and resentment and pray for God to help us forgive the person that harmed us

  The day you make that decision to forgive your offender, is the beginning of a journey of walking in forgiveness. One may not forget but one can move on and live a "liberated life", a life devoid of bitterness and revenge or desire to pay back. It is important to remember that sometimes we may hold something against someone, and they MAY NOT EVEN KNOW THAT THEY HAD OFFENDED US

- Pray for the offender

  Pray a prayer forgiving the individual who offended you. Make up your own or use the one below. You can copy it on a sheet of paper and keep close to you, so you can refer to it when you feel bitterness rising up in you

  "Lord, I choose to forgive _____ (put in their name) who has caused me great harm and sorrow. I choose to forgive him/her because you God FIRST forgave me my sins. Please forgive me for holding on to unforgiveness and offence. Jesus said I should forgive so by faith, I forgive with His help. Increase my Faith to forgive (name)_____. Help me to forgive and bury what happened and help me let go of the anger and bitterness. Let me walk in forgiveness each day by the power of your Holy Spirit and to move into the future as one who is liberated from offense. Amen

Walking in forgiveness

"Forgiveness is a funny thing. It warms the heart and cools the sting".

—William Arthur Ward, American writer (1921—1994).

This is a process and it may take some time to be completely free from thinking about the incident etc. It tends to get better with time, because not only is "Time a healer" in many ways, but God uses that to lessen the hurt or anger. Walking in forgiveness means you allow God to take control of the situation by you turning the offender over to God, because He, God, is the rewarder or judge of the offender. "Vengeance is mine, I will repay says the Lord" (Rom 12:19). God is aware of what happened and He has a record of it. Trusting in God, knowing He will fight for you, builds up your faith, giving you hope for the future, and prevents you from dwelling mainly on the past.

Meeting with the offender

There is a role in meeting with the offender if you are in a position to do so, or circumstances make this possible. Sometimes this is not possible due to the passage of time, the danger it may involve, your desire not to do so (consider the motivation – it is not right, if there is still bitterness driving this decision), or the absence of the individual/offender. In Matthew 18v15-17, Jesus outlined a process of dealing with a brother who has offended another in a fellowship or church situation. It involves confronting the individual in a loving way and the use of other individuals if necessary, to resolve the issue in a firm but loving way so that the offender admits their wrong and is reconciled to the offended individual. Sometimes a meeting will bring other issues to the surface and that may also include the fact that the offender may have seen things differently or did not even realize that he/she had offended you. You may also write a letter to the offender.

What about an unrepentant offender?

What if the offender does not admit he or she is wrong or is unrepentant? One still needs to forgive the offender even if they do not admit their fault. God will be their judge. It may mean not having the same relationship with them; however, one still has to forgive them, and move on. This is because the act of forgiving brings healing and freedom to the individual who is offended or hurt.

Missed Blessings as a Result of Not Forgiving Others

There are many blessings that one misses, if one does not forgive an offender. These missed blessings are replaced by:

Lack of God's power from working in one's life
Denying oneself healing in one's body, soul and spirit
Bitterness and anger which can literally suck the energy or life out of a person
Absence of the favor of God on one's lives
Attracting certain illnesses and diseases to your body
Lack of joy, peace or love in one's life
Unforgiveness which drains one physically, emotionally, mentally and spiritually
Prayers that are hindered or not answered (Mark 11: 25)
Anger toward friends who may still be on good terms with the offender
Unforgiveness affecting one's growth as a Christian

Medical Advantages Resulting From Forgiving Someone

Physical Healing

People who walk in unforgiveness are usually stressed or on edge. If one learns to forgive, there will be a reduction of certain illnesses which are associated with stress. The levels of certain chemicals produced in your body during times of stress (Cortisol and Adrenaline) will go down when stress goes down. Normally in times of stress or danger, these chemicals are released, used for a short time and are then supposed to disappear or decrease to the pre-stress levels. However, if one's anger or stress is constantly present or ongoing, then the body is always under the influence of these chemicals, leading to high blood pressure, heart conditions, bodily aches and pains and even death. The surge in these chemicals also causes decrease in production of cells which protect the body from sickness and diseases and can make you more likely to have cancer. You will always seem stressed and anxious, and not be relaxed or happy in life because you are always carrying anger, hurt or unforgiveness. According to a chief of surgeon with the Cancer Treatment Centers of American, Dr. Steven Standiford, negative emotions and unforgiveness hinder healing of cancer patients and so they have incorporated "Forgiveness Therapy" for cancer patients. According to him, it is important to treat emotional pain and wounds as part of the healing process (Lorie Johnson, CBN news). www1.cbn.com/cbnnews/healthscience/2015/June/The-Deadly-Consequences-of-Unforgiveness

Emotional Healing

There is healing of your negative emotions when you forgive. Emotions like anger, bitterness, and resentment will fade away and will be replaced by good emotions of forgiveness, joy, and hope by God's help (Proverbs 22:24-25). You will feel as free as a bird released from a cage.

You Become An Agent of Change

Once you let go and let God have His way in your life, the negative emotions are replaced by positive ones, you can then become an agent of change; because you become someone who can help others who may also be living with unforgiveness. You have been liberated and so can be of help and a blessing to someone else going through what you went through. You are now living at a higher level because by forgiving, you are in league with Jesus, and have chosen to live above your natural, fleshly tendency to hold on to unhealthy human feelings and behavior. You have conquered the spirit of unforgiveness.

Forgiving Yourself When You Are the Offender

There are also some individuals who need to forgive THEMSELVES because they feel like punishing themselves for something they regret doing or saying. Some people feel that they have committed certain offences against others which are so grievous or unpardonable that they are not ready to forgive themselves. However, if God is willing to forgive you, then why continue to torment yourself by living in guilt or under condemnation? Secondly, this self-torment, does not erase the wrong you did. If you have wronged someone, just sincerely ask God and the individual for forgiveness and move on. If you need to take a trusted friend or relative with you to meet your offended friend or relative, do so. If meeting face to face is difficult, one can write a letter, send an email, or send someone to intervene and bring about reconciliation on your behalf.

What Does Forgiveness Not Mean?

What does forgiveness NOT mean? First of all, remember that forgiveness does not mean that the person did not commit the offence. Neither does it mean that you are excusing his or her actions or deeds, or that you are forgetting their horrible action or words if that is the case. You can forgive and may not forget. However, when forgiveness takes place, you will find that even when you remember the deed, the negative emotions and feelings that used to come up will not be as strong, or they simply will no longer occur. That is when healing has occurred.

Walking the Journey of Forgiveness

Walking in forgiveness is a continuous process and we can only do this through God's grace or favor. One does so, one day at a time with God's help. Some of the things you can do to walk in forgiveness are:

- Praying for your offender: (Matthew 5v44)
  You may not feel like doing this but make the choice to release him or her and pray for them. As you continually do so, the personal pain you experience will gradually ease off (Matthew 5v44)
- Asking the Holy Spirit each day to help you walk in forgiveness: (John 16v13-15)
  Whenever you think about what happened, instead of getting bitter, say a quiet prayer to God on behalf of the offender. Ask God to help him/her come to know God and repent of his/her sin if that is involved
- Agreeing with God that He is the one who judges all men including your offender (John 8v16)
  Consequences for an offender's sins or actions
  Remember, although God will forgive them if they sincerely repent, they will still face the consequences or the punishment for their actions. The Bible has many examples of the consequences of sin. One important one is King David and Bathsheba. (2 Samuel 11: 1-23)

King David committed adultery (sexual sin) with Bathsheba, a married woman, and then he had her husband Uriah murdered. He later repented when God confronted him with the sin through a prophet of God. After he repented, God forgave David his sin, however, the consequence of his sin was that the child born from that unlawful union would die, and David's house or family will see great internal conflict. He prayed and fasted that his child with Bathsheba would live and not die. However, God caused the child to die, and David accepted the consequences of his sin.

Summary

"That old law about 'an eye for an eye' leaves everybody blind. The time is always right to do the right thing".

—Martin Luther King, Jr. Minister and Civil Rights Activist, USA.

In conclusion, I trust this discussion on forgiveness and letting go of offense will help anyone who is struggling with these two important issues and recognize God's viewpoint about them. If it is difficult for you, talk to a trusted friend or another child of God to help you take that step. Secondly, I hope that this will result in yielding oneself to God in order to receive freedom and live according to God's plan. Forgiveness is liberating for both the offended and the offender, so I challenge anyone carrying such a load to lay it down, by allowing God to work in their lives and free them from these. It is possible to be free from holding offense.

Offense and unforgiveness affects both the offender and the offended. God is able to help you forgive someone who has offended you and help you let go of offense. Forgiveness is a process but there must be a starting point when the offended decides to "let go and let God" have His way which is forgiveness. Jesus Christ is the greatest example of one who forgave his enemies when he was hanging on the cross. We must follow His example. "Therefore if the Son makes you free, you shall be free indeed" (John 8v36 NKJV). THE BURDEN OF CARRYING AN OFFENSE IS NOT WORTH THE DAMAGE IT CAUSES

Prayer

. . . .

This is a broad subject and a bit of discourse on it in this book is appropriate since we are addressing spiritual health as part of holistic health. We will just touch on a few aspects of prayer, and hopefully, this will help women to pray more, especially those who for whatever reason, do not pray regularly or find it difficult to do so.

"To be a Christian without prayer is no more possible than to be alive without breathing".
—Martin Luther King, German Christian Reform leader (Nov. 10, 1483—Feb. 18, 1546).

Why Do People Not Pray?

. . . .

Some women/men do not pray regularly because of:

Lack of time, or too busy
Not sure how, when or what to pray about
Having bought into some myths associated with prayer or praying
Not believing that God hears them
Fear that they may not do it right

Our reference will be the Bible, the Christian guide book for knowing God and His will for us

What Is Prayer?

Prayer is simply talking to God, your loving Creator, Savior and Father. The Bible encourages us to "Pray without ceasing" 1Thess. 5v17 (NKJV). This simply means at any time and at any place. Great men of God believed in the power of prayer. For example, John Wesley, cofounder of Methodism said "God does nothing except in response to believing prayer." Believing prayer is praying by faith that God can do something about the situation.

Come Let's Explore Prayer and Break Down Some Myths

"Prayer is the simplest form of speech That infant lips can try; Prayer the sublimest strains that reach The Majesty on high"

—Prayer is the soul's sincere desire.
James Montgomery (1771—1854) Hymn

In the Bible we have the perfect example of what to pray and how to pray. This was exemplified by Jesus, and His desire to teach us how to pray and show us how important it is to Him.

Luke 18v1 says: "Then He spoke a parable to them that men always ought to pray and not lose heart". This passage is about Jesus speaking to His disciples. Prayer was very important to Him and by example and teaching He tried to let His disciples make it a priority in their lives as well.

There is a mystery in Praying: God sends the answer to our prayers even before we pray, but if we do not pray, circumstances might prevent us from seeing or hearing His answer.

Myths about Prayer and Praying

"I have researched many of the great men and women of God over the years, and all of them had one thing in common. They were men and women of prayer"

—Pastor Duke Taber, viralbeliever.com

There are certain myths about praying which have hindered some women from being praying women who can intercede (stand in the gap) or cry on behalf of their families, their nation, other nations, and themselves to God.

The common ones include:

- Myth #1. Some people have been given the gift of prayer
  Nowhere in the Bible where gifts of the Spirit are mentioned is a gift of prayer mentioned. It is available for ALL of us to use as a means of communicating with the Lord our God
  "The greatest thing anyone can do for God and for man is pray. IT is NOT the only thing, but it is the chief thing. The great people on earth today are the people who pray. . . . I mean those people who take the time and pray" (S.D. Gordon)

- Myth #2. I am too busy or do not have the time to pray
  Time is like a currency and the LORD has given all of us 24 hours of it. Using part of it to communicate with the one who gave it to you will help you to better manage time. If you are too busy to pray, then you are too busy. YOU can choose to make the time. It is a choice one has to make
- Myth #3. Prayer is a monologue
  We give God our list and go off on our merry way. No, it should not be so. It's a two-way conversation and intimacy with God. John 10v3 says, "My sheep hear my voice" and Jeremiah 33v3 says "call to me and I will answer you and show you great and mighty things. Isaiah 30v21 says, "Your ears will hear a voice behind you saying this is the way." God speaks to us through His Word, through others and also through our minds when we are listening to Him

"Prayer is simply a two-way conversation between you and God". Billy Graham (Evangelist).

Cultivating the Habit of Hearing From God.

Hearing from God is a learnt behavior. You do not need a special gift or anointing to hear from God. You can cultivate the habit by asking Him his opinion about the smallest things as well as the large issues. He is always speaking; as you pray, expect to hear from Him. We just have to open our spiritual ears to listen AND hear Him. Ask Him to give you a listening or sensitive spiritual ear and pray for wisdom and discernment from Him. We hear from God through His Holy Spirit who lives in us. These are some of the ways He communicates with you:

- When He speaks it is not usually in an audible voice but He does so through your conscious or mind that has been "decluttered" – like during a quiet time of prayer or meditation with Him
- You may get confirmation from His Word as you read it
- Confirmation from other believers
- From a sermon, from a letter or talking to trusted individuals etc
  If you have sincerity of heart and a desire to please Him, you can act upon what you hear or see which is not contrary to His Word. If you are not sure of something, but have sincerely prayed that He guide and lead you in the right way, and you, after having done all due diligence, find a "door open" before you, walk through that door in faith, which means move, take an action. Don't be afraid of missing Him, move by faith. In everything our ultimate purpose is to please Him and bring Glory to His name, and that should be the purpose of all we do. Even when we goof or miss it, He can still work all things together for our good and for His Glory – "And we know that all things work together

for good to those who love God, to those who are the called according to His purpose" (Romans 8v28)

- Myth #4. Praying is boring

  As you cultivate the habit, you find that you come to love the discipline of praying. You can develop or use different ways of praying. For example:

- Use the ACTS model – Adoration, Confession, Thanksgiving and Supplication (This is just a guide – don't replace relationship with formula)

  ADORATION: Worship and praise God for who He is. Many examples are in the Psalms

  CONFESSION: Confess your sins to Him. Things you may have done against Him and the bad ways you may have treated or talked about other people

  THANKSGIVING: Thank Him for the things He has done for you, family, friends, health etc. Thank Him in advance for answering your prayers

  SUPPLICATION: Verbalize your requests to Him. Don't just ask for yourself, but pray for others, your church, country, and yourself

- Use the Lord's Prayer model

  This is the prayer Jesus prayed when His disciples asked Him to teach them how to pray. They also did not know how to pray initially, but learnt how, as they spent time with Him and heard Him pray. In Luke 11v1-4, He gave them the model prayer popularly known as "The Lord's Prayer". Read through it and pray some of the things He prayed about

- Pray with someone

  There is power in agreement and Jesus Himself said in Matthew 18v19 "Again I say to you that if two of you agree on earth concerning anything that they ask, it will be done for them by My Father in heaven." Have a praying buddy or friend. You can pray in person – on the phone or online with them

  There are examples of Paul and Silas in the prison, praying and praising God and the Lord sent an earthquake and caused them to be free (Acts 16v25-26), Peter and John in Acts 3v1-7 met a lame man and prayed for him and he was healed in Jesus's name

- Pray with a group

  This may be a family prayer time at home, with co-workers at work, or at a prayer meeting at church or at a fellowship meeting. Examples of groups praying together and tapping into the power of agreement is found in the early church. After Jesus's resurrection, His disciples met together and prayed. They were in one accord (united) and God released the Holy Spirit on them. This was the power that Jesus told them to wait in Jerusalem for. They were empowered and boldly proclaimed the Word of God. (Acts 2v1-4; Acts 4v23-31). I am part of several prayer groups: a prayer group at my church, with friends on an online platform, and with other group via phone conference calls. So, this gives me ample opportunities to pray either in person or online with other people

- Use a book of Prayer

Several are available in book shops, but some examples are "Rules of Engagement", by Dr. Cindy Trimm, "God's creative power will work for you" by Charles Capps, and several books by Stormie Omartian on Power of a praying wife, praying woman, praying mother etc

"Satan does not care how many people read about prayer if only he can keep them from praying" Paul E. Billheimer

- Pray the Word of God

In the gospel of John 17v9-26, Jesus prays for all believers and one can use some of the prayers He prayed. The apostle Paul also wrote down several prayers in some of the letters he wrote to the early churches which can be prayed by us today. Examples are Ephesians 1v15-21, Philippians 1v3-6, Colossians 4v2-6. The psalms also have heart felt prayers that David prayed as he talked to God when he found himself in difficult situations, as well as prayers of praise and worship of God

- Myth #5. Prayer has to be long to be effective

Many of us have bought into the myth that prayer/intercession has to be long to be effective. Short targeted prayers or Arrow Prayers ARE effective and powerful. It is the faith behind the prayers that we pray that matters. For the Bible says that without faith, it is impossible to please God. These arrow prayers give variety and expression to our prayer life. It's like daily divine conversations. E.g. you are driving and see young people gathered – shoot an arrow of prayer on their behalf. You see a mother with several young children under 6 years, pray for wisdom and strength for her

". . . True prayer is measured by weight, not by length. A single groan before God may have more fullness of prayer in it than a fine oration of great length" C. H. Spurgeon

- Myth #6. I don't know how to pray

Just like everything else, the more you practice it, the better you become at it. Remember, it's not the length of your prayers or the elaborate words we use that matter, it is talking to God in everyday language and expressing what is in your heart. God delights in sincerity of the heart and loves it when His children make time to talk to Him. One can also pray in any language

"Don't pray when you feel like it. Have an appointment with the Lord and keep it. A man is powerful on his knees" Corrie ten Boom (A Dutch Christian who helped Jews escape the Nazi Holocaust)

- Myth #7. My pray is not effective

It is important to know that our enemy the devil does not want us to pray because he knows it is one of the powerful weapons that God has given to His children to use against him. The Bible in James 5v16-18 (**NKJV**) says "**The effective, fervent prayer** of a righteous man avails much. 17 Elijah was a man with a nature like ours, and he prayed earnestly that it would not rain; and it did not rain on the land for three years and six months. 18 And he prayed again, and the heaven gave rain, and the earth produced its fruit". The prophet of God prayed and things changed; be encouraged to know that YOU, made righteous or in good standing with God through your relationship with Jesus Christ; can also pray and be heard by God, just like He heard Elijah. Do not underestimate the power of your prayers. It's a weapon God has given to you as His Child. "Satan trembles when he sees the weakest Christian on his knees" William Cowper

Praying Women in the Bible

There are many examples in the Bible of women who prayed to God and each of these women exhibited a certain character which we can learn from. Please look up the verses below to learn something about the particular woman mentioned, and the type of prayer she prayed. You can even use this as a personal Bible Study.

MIRIAM – **Praise and worship**: (Exodus 15v20-21).
The sister of Moses and Aaron praised and worshipped God. After crossing the Red Sea and seeing God destroy the Egyptians she led other women in praise and worship. Like Miriam we can come to the Lord and give Him worship and praise. Let Him know we love Him and appreciate who He is and what He has done for us. Love on Him with a song and a dance. Psalm 100v1-5.
Praise and worship is a type of prayer.

HANNAH – **Fervent intense prayer with fasting**: (See 1 Sam 1v1-18).
Hannah, who later gave birth to Samuel the Prophet, started out as a barren wife and was tormented by her rival because she had no children. In v10 she wept and poured out her soul to the Lord for a son and at the same time, made a vow to the Lord. He remembered her prayer and gave her a son, while she in turn fulfilled her vow she had made to God by giving Samuel back to God to serve in the temple.
Prayer with fasting shows our determination to see something change.

RIZPAH – **Persistence, sacrifice and determination:** (2 Sam 21v10-14).
Rizpah was a concubine of King Saul whose two sons, together with five other sons of Saul were killed to avenge what Saul had done by killing the Gibeonites during the time of his rule. The Gibeonites were supposed to have been protected by the children of Israel, but instead they were killed. To appease God and remove His judgement against Israel (a 3 year famine), David ordered Saul's sons hanged because of possible involvement in the crime. Rizpah, after her children's death

608   Part Five: Spiritual Health

camped on a rock near the area for about six months, protecting the dead bodies from the birds and animals' day and night. When King David was told about it, he intervened and in the end gave them a decent burial. Not only did it happen for them, but he also ended up giving the dead King Saul and his son Jonathan a decent burial as well, since that had not been previously done.

We have to keep on asking and not give up easily, especially if praying according to God's will.

ESTHER – **Fasting and prayer:** (Esther 4v15-17):
Queen Esther, a Jewish girl who was made queen in a foreign land by God's divine intervention, mobilized the Jews in exile by calling for fasting and praying when a plot was hatched by an evil man to annihilate the Jews. With power and boldness from God, she went before the king without being summoned (which could have resulted in her death) and petitioned him on behalf of the Jews. She was able to get the decree against the Jews reversed, and the evil man was put to death by the king. She was used by God to save the Jews in exile from destruction by wicked men. She and others did not just pray but she acted to change the situation.

We see prayer with fasting followed by ACTION.

MARY OF BETHANY – **Worship:** (Matthew 26v7-13, Mark 14v3-9, John 12v1-8)
Mary worshipped Jesus by breaking an alabaster flask filled with expensive perfume and anointed both Jesus's head and his feet. Anointing His feet showed her devotion to Him. She was grateful He had forgiven her sins and did not condemn her like others did.

Mary Worshipped her Lord.

ANNA, Aged prophetess and widow – **Thanksgiving and Prophesy:** Luke 2v36-38
Anna in spite of her old age was always in the house of the Lord serving with fasting and prayers night and day, waiting for God's anointed (Jesus Christ) to be revealed to the world as promised. When she saw Joseph and Mary bring the child Jesus into the temple, she recognized who He was, declaring prophetically to all that the Messiah had come, and she gave thanks to the Lord.

Anna gave thanks to God when she saw or received the answer to her prayer.
She persisted in prayer to see the revelation of God's Promise.

PERSISTENT WIDOW – **Tenacity and Faith:** (Luke 18v1-8)
Jesus told his disciples the parable of the persistent widow to teach them about persevering in prayer. If an evil judge, weary of a widow's continual requests, is willing to respond to her requests when she was being treated unfairly, how much more will a loving God respond to His children who continually bring a request before Him.

The widow did not give up but kept asking until her request was granted.

Tips for cultivating a consistent prayer life

- Believe and have Faith that you can be a woman who loves to pray.
- Think of prayer as a bank deposit from which you will make withdrawals later. So, keep depositing requests, and other prayers.
- The Holy Spirit is your Helper, so when you pray invite Him to lead you to pray according to God's will.
- God hears "Short and Sweet" prayers as well as long ones.
- Pray for others (Intercessory prayer) and not just for your own needs.
- Seize every prayer time opportunity that you are presented with. Attend church-sponsored prayer times and other called or scheduled prayer times, e.g. by friends, phone, etc.
- Join the prayer team of your church.
- Note that it calls for sacrifice and discipline.
- It's a fight, but the Lord is fighting for and with you so you are not alone.
- Pray with your husband or significant other daily if possible. Your children will see you modeling praying and would grow up wanting to do the same.
- Pray with your children and send them to school with prayer. This keeps prayer in schools, even if it is not officially done by the administration. Prayer at school starts in the home.
- Write down requests on recipe cards, note pads or sticky pads, and keep them at different places, e.g. In the car, Bible, bedroom, bathroom mirror etc.
- When someone shares a prayer concern with you, pray with them there and then. Don't wait until you get home, because you may forget to pray about it.
- Buy a small bottle of regular olive oil, pray over it and use it to anoint your house, work place, the sick who you pray for etc. James 5v4 talks about anointing people who are sick.
- Anyone can pray for these issues I have listed. You have been given that authority by Jesus Christ who is our High Priest and intercedes for us before God. No other mediator is necessary.
- Use visual prayer – e.g. have a globe of the world, or a world map to pray for the world or a particular country. You can also use pictures of your kids, or families you want to pray for.
- If you fear praying aloud in a group, tell this fear to God and ask Him to set you free. God delights in hearing your prayers irrespective of the words you use. When you are praying in a group, forget about the others and concentrate on God. It is between you and God. You are not there to get the approval of the other people in the room or praying to please them. Pray with humility and confidence as you focus on God and not on others.
- Pray some of the prayers that Paul prayed in his letters to the churches, e.g. Colossians 1v9-12, Ephesians 1v16-20.
- Pray other scripture – Use the psalms, the Lord's Prayer etc.

- Use prayer guides, e.g. Dr. Cindy Trim's *Rules of Engagement* prayer book.
- Use worship music to help you enter into God's presence. It can set the atmosphere for praying.
- You may need to create a "prayer closet" in your house – this is a quiet place you can retreat to.
- Remember you are in a spiritual battle. The enemy, the devil does not want you to pray, so he will use every means to prevent you from praying. In 2 Corinthians 10v4, we read: "For the weapons of our warfare are not carnal, but MIGHTY in GOD for pulling down strongholds". Prayer pulls down strong holds and barriers put up by satan. Strongholds are impediments or obstacles satan puts in our way or the ways of our loved ones.
- We are not fighting against human beings. Ephesians 6v10-13, reminds us that our fight is not with flesh and blood and so we need the whole armor of God to fight against spiritual powers (paraphrased). Evil forces fight against us, but thanks be to God who gives us the victory which Jesus won at Calvary when He died on the cross. He has given us the power to stand against the evil forces and take authority over them using the Word of God.
- Visually pray putting on the armor of God which is found in Ephesians 6v14-18. Examples are helmet of salvation, shield of faith and sword of the Spirit, etc.
- Pray the Hebrew names of God – Jehovah Jireh (Provider), Jehovah Shalom (Peace) Jehovah Raphael (Healer) etc. You can pray – "God thank you for being my Provider, Jehovah Jireh".
- Set time aside each week to fast and pray – half a day, whole day, etc. Fast by cutting out food, TV etc. Remember to drink fluids/water when fasting.
- Watch the movie "War Room" featuring Priscilla Shirer and Karen Abercrombie. It features a prayerless woman who was challenged to start praying when her marriage was under attack.

Hindrances to your prayers

These include but are not limited to:

- Harboring a Spirit of UNFORGIVENESS and OFFENCE – We discussed this under offence and unforgiveness
- Lack of Faith or unbelief – People's faith moved Jesus to work miracles for them, and on the other hand, He could not do miracles in certain places because of the people's unbelief or lack of faith in Him. Matthew 13v. 58
- Asking outside of God's Will: – for selfish reasons, and not in the will of God. The Bible gives us principles which teach us about the broad and sometimes specific will of God in different circumstances

Below is a practical way to document some of the things you can do to "up your Praying Game".

Three things I propose to do to upgrade my Prayer Life

_____

_____

_____

I commit to pray for these people who are outside my family and church circle

_____

_____

_____

I commit to pray for my country and another country in a different continent once a week

_____

_____

_____

Blessed to be a Blessing to Others

You are Blessed

'And the Scripture, foreseeing that God would justify the Gentiles by faith, preached the gospel to Abraham beforehand, saying, "In you all the nations shall be blessed."'

Gal. 3 v 8 (NKJV).

I believe we are all blessed with gifts, talents, treasures (possessions), finances, loved ones, and friends to varying degrees. Again, I derive my concept of blessings from a biblical perspective. In the Old Testament, God called Abraham from his homeland and promised him that He was taking him to a place where he will end up being the father of a great nation. God would bless him and he was going to be a blessing to others. Most importantly, God was going to bless those who blessed him. See Genesis 12:1-3. Sometimes we need to sit down and count our blessings and find joy in the little things. Each day think about the many blessings you have received from God and then have a heart of gratitude and thankfulness. As a result of this, YOU CAN BE

A BLESSING TO OTHERS as you reach out to bless them in the ways God shows you.

Anyone Can Be A Blessing to Someone Else.

We sometimes think that the only people who can be a blessing to other people are those who are well off or rich. This is a wrong perception. No matter what one's socio-economic status is, one can be a blessing to others and in turn be blessed by God and others. A clear example, I have read in the Bible is the story of Jesus feeding the five thousand people who had followed Him into a desert listening to His teaching. It was a long day and there was no food except a young boy's lunch – which was made up of two fishes and five loaves. He gave these to the disciples and Jesus blessed the meal and used it to feed the five thousand men, plus women, and children. I am sure the boy had more than enough of the left overs to take home because of his generosity (John 6:4-13), and the disciples also had some to take home. Jesus also taught that it was more blessed to give than to receive as mentioned by the Apostle Paul in Acts 20v35. He reminds us to support the weak in those same verses. So, you can be a blessing, no matter your economic status.

Being A Blessing on A Daily Basis

Every day, one should look out for ways in which one can be a blessing to another person. It may be in a small way, like saying "Good morning" or giving directions to someone, offering someone a ride, complimenting someone, having a listening ear, hugging someone, sending a word of encouragement to people through social media, to bigger things like feeding someone, offering accommodation to someone, blessing someone financially, praying for someone etc. Having the understanding that whatever we possess are blessings from God, helps one not to be proud of one's status, or to be envious of others' good fortunes or blessings. After working hard, when we reap blessings, we have to thank God and give Him praise for giving us grace to get those blessings. Jesus watches and must be very happy and proud of His children who bless others.

Achieving Contentment in A Crazy World.
What is Contentment?

'Let your conduct be without covetousness; be content with such things as you have. For He Himself has said, "I will never leave you nor forsake you."'

—Hebrews 13v5 NKJV

In the Scriptures, contentment is mentioned several times. The free dictionary defines contentment as "the state of being contented; satisfaction" (www.thefreedictionary.com). The Apostle Paul in the books of Timothy and Philippians mentions that "godliness with contentment is great gain" and "when one has food and clothing, one is content", and lastly testified that "he has learnt in whatever state he finds himself to be content (paraphrased)". Human nature tends to covet or envy what other people possess or have achieved, but is oblivious or unaware of the struggles, difficulties or hard work that has resulted in another individual's prosperity, achievements or educational level. It is not only the have-nots who may not be content and envious of the rich, but the rich may not be content with what they have and try to gain more sometimes by dubious means.

Is Your Success Too Costly?

Most people who are living well materially, have worked hard but one thing to ask is, "at what cost?" In the process, they may compromise their principles, treasured relationships, and quality family time in order to gain worldly goods. Many professionals, especially medical doctors, who in their bid to make more money and be extremely rich have had broken marriages and no meaningful relationships with their children, because they were hardly at home to spend time with them. Others have cheated and used dubious means to make more money and have lost the trust and confidence of their patients and health regulators. This kind of 'success" is too costly and not worth it, even if one is not a God fearing individual. The advice from Paul the Apostle is worth noting: 1 Timothy 6:6-9 (NKJV) "Now godliness with contentment is great gain. [7] For we brought nothing into this world, and it is certain we can carry nothing out. [8] And having food and clothing, with these we shall be content. [9] But those who desire to be rich fall into temptation and a snare, and into many foolish and harmful lusts which drown men in destruction and perdition".

A Balanced Life and Its Rewards

"Finally, brethren, whatever things are true, whatever things are noble, whatever things are just, whatever things are pure, whatever things are lovely, whatever things are of good report, if there is any virtue and if there is anything praiseworthy-meditate on these things". Philippians 4 v 8   (NKJV).

We alluded to a balanced life at the beginning of the book and will end by recap of this. A balanced life brings contentment to one's body, soul and spirit. Physically by keeping one's body healthy with exercise, healthy eating and doing things to prevent diseases. Taking one's medicines is also important. Emotionally, enjoying time with family and friends, enjoying the material things one has been blessed with, as well as being a blessing to others. In addition mental health illnesses need to be treated by counseling, medications and self-care. Spiritually, contentment is achieved by having a relationship with God and that keeps our spirits vibrate and healthy. We are not perfect in all these areas;

however, we have to pay attention to all three areas of our lives, and that involves some efforts on our part. That is one of the purposes of this book, to encourage and motivate you to work on all three areas of your being.

Your Destiny is in Your Hands

"Your attitude plus your aptitude will determine your altitude"

—Jojo Entsuah Engineer, enterpreneur, Lay Preacher, President Gateway of Hope Inc.

Remember that you have a part to play in whatever destiny God has for you. He has already planned it, but you have to find your purpose by having a right perspective or attitude. You also acquire the appropriate knowledge or abilities to rise to where God wants you to be, in order to be a blessing to your generation. My husband has a quote which sums this up beautifully (see above).

POST SCRIPT

November 2019: During the final editing of this book, my dear friend, sister in the Lord and fellow colleague Dr. Vivian Woodard who wrote the foreword of this book, went home to be with her Lord and Savior Jesus Christ on August 20th, 2019. She was a woman of little stature physically, but a Giant in her Christian walk and as a woman of Prayer and Faith. Many have also testified of her service to mankind as a Giver, and an excellent Physician. Like me, her Faith in God was an integral part of her calling as a Physician. We view the practice of Medicine as a vocation from God, and not just a job or profession. She will be sorely missed; however, we know she is at peace in the presence of her Lord and Savior Jesus Christ; and we of like faith will see her one day. We have this Assurance and Hope from the Apostle Paul in 1Thessalonians 4v13–14. "But I do not want you to be ignorant, brethren, concerning those who have fallen asleep, lest you sorrow as others who have no hope. For if we believe that Jesus died and rose again, even so God will bring with Him those who sleep in Jesus". v.16 "For the Lord Himself will descend from heaven with a shout, with the voice of an archangel, and with the trumpet of God. And the dead in Christ will rise first. Then we who are alive and remain shall be caught up together with them in the clouds to meet the Lord in the air. And thus, we shall always be with the Lord". (NKJV).

Final Word

I trust this book will be a blessing to everyone who reads it to gain knowledge and understanding of their bodies and the conditions which may affect it; as well as their emotional/mental health and spiritual health. It is meant to be a constant companion like a second Bible for everyone (laugh). I have tried to cover the three aspects of every human life or being as I see it: Body, Soul, and Spirit. I have hopefully articulated my own walk with God in a way that I hope will be helpful to anyone who is seeking or wanting to have a personal relationship with God who is a Good Loving Father. May this book help you to know your body, your mind, and your spirit, so you will be able to fulfill your purpose on earth to the fullest.

Closing Prayer For You.

I end with these two earnest prayers for you, the reader, which are found in the Bible:

- 3 John1:2 NKJV "Beloved, I pray that you may prosper in all things and be in health, just as your soul prospers", AND
- 1 Thessalonians 5v23 NKJV "Now may the God of peace Himself sanctify you completely; and may your whole spirit, soul, and body be preserved blameless at the coming of our Lord Jesus Christ"

GOD BLESS YOU

Dr. Barbara Entsuah. MD. MHSc. (Canada); Board Certified Family Medicine (USA); Fellow Ghana College of Physicians and Surgeons (Ghana).

References/Notes

Definition of CAM. National Center for Complementary and Integrative Health: https://nccih.nih.gov/health/supplements

www.WebMD.com

Geller, A. et al. Emergency Department Visits for Adverse Events Related to Dietary Supplements. N Engl J Med 2015; 373:1531–1540.

www.worldlifeexpectancy.com; and WHO-2011 data

Top 10 causes of death in developed countries WHO Fact sheet No 310. Updated May 2014

NIH study provides clarity on supplements for protection against blinding eye disease 5/5/2013. https://www.nei.nih.gov/news/pressreleases

Zosia Chustecka. Cold Cap to Prevent Hair Loss During Chemo Cleared in US. Medscape Medical News, Dec 8th, 2015

Diabetes and Dietary Supplements – nccih.nih.gov/sites/nccam.nih.gov/files/Diabetes_11-08-2015

Mean glucose level associated with various A1C values: (http://www.uptodate.com, Wolters Kluwer Health)

Thyroid diseases. www.familydoctor.org. Written by editorial staff. Updated 03/2014

Dr. Femke Rutters. Stress, Sleep and Social Jetlag: The Obesity Epidemic's Psychosocial Side. Medscape Diabetes & Endocrinology. October 19th, 2015

James PA, Oparil S, Carter BL, et al. 2014 Evidence-based guideline for the management of high blood pressure in adults: Report from the panel members appointed to the Eighth Joint National Committee (JNC 8). JAMA 2014; DOI:10.1001/jama.2013.284427. Available at: http://jama.jamanetwork.com/journal

U.S. Department of Health and Human Services. The Health Consequences of Smoking—50 Years of Progress. A Report of the Surgeon General 2014

Chomistek AK, Chiuve SE, Eliassen AH, et al. Healthy lifestyle in the primordial prevention of cardiovascular disease among young women. J Am Coll. Cardiol. 2015; 65:43–51

Drs. Slopen, Glynn et al. Job Strain, Job Insecurity, and Incident Cardiovascular Disease in the Women's Health Study: Results from a 10-Year Prospective Study. PLOS One Journal. July 2012

Yong H, et al. Efficacy of folic acid therapy in primary prevention of stroke among adults with hypertension in China. JAMA 2015; 2274

Dr. Harvey Simon, "Music as Medicine" The Am. Journal of Med., Feb. 2015, vol. 128, No. 2

Drs. Bret S. Stetka, Felipe De Brigard. (How Memory Works (and How to Preserve It). Medscape Psychiatry, Medscape.com. Feb 13, 2015.

Snitz B, O'Meara E, Carlson M, et al. Ginkgo biloba for preventing cognitive decline in older adults: a randomized trial. Journal of the American medical Association. 2009;302 (24): 2663–2670

Shelly L. Gray, Melissa L. Anderson, Sascha Dublin, et al. Cumulative Use of Strong Anticholinergics and Incident Dementia. A Prospective Cohort Study. JAMA Intern Med. 2015; 175(3):401–407.

Dr. Majid Fotuhi et al. High Impact of a Brain Fitness Program in Improving Cognitive Function and Brain Activity in Elderly with Mild Cognitive Impairment. Alzheimer's Association International Conference (AAIC) 2015. Abstract 4331

Matthew Baumgart, Heather M. Snyder et al. Summary of the evidence on modifiable risk factors for cognitive decline and dementia: A population-based perspective. June 2015 Volume 11, Issue 6, Pages 718–726

Insomnia. www.familydoctor.org. Written by familydoctor.org editorial staff. 4/2014

Dr. Entsuah, B. March was Kidney Awareness Month Article written March 2013

Pelvic muscle exercises. Health Central hospital rehabilitation handout. Ocoee Florida

National Academy Press (www.nap.edu). Dietary Reference Intakes for Water, Potassium, Sodium, Chloride, and Sulfate. 2005

National violence against women survey. November, 2000. Source: https://www.ncjrs.gov/pdffiles1/nij/183781.pdf

Entsuah, B. The dawning of a new day. 2009. A guide to help victims of sexual abuse go through the journey of recovery, hope and healing. Accra. Legacy and Legacy Publishing.

IntimatePartnerViolence.http://www.cdc.gov/ViolencePrevention/intimatepartnerviolence/index

Female cancers. American Cancer Society

Joanne Silberner. An ounce of prevention. http://www.pri.org/stories/2012-12-05/part-iii-ounce-prevention

WebMD, Breast disorders

Cleveland clinic.org, Breast disorders

American Cancer Society

National Institute of Health Breast cancer home page

Breast cancer Immunotherapy. www.cancerresearch.org/cancer-immunotherapy/impacting-all-cancers/breast-cancer

North American Menopause Society. Sexual health after breast cancer

MonaLisa touch Laser therapy (www.smilemonalisa.com)

Siteman Cancer Center at Barnes-Jewish Hospital and Washington University School of Medicine Cancer Survivors' 8ight Ways to Stay Healthy After Cancer

M. Frenkel, V. Sierpina, K. Sapire. Effects of Complementary and Integrative Medicine on Cancer Survivorship. Current Oncology Reports. May, 2015, 17:

E. H. Allott, C.-K. Tse, A. F. Olshan et al. Non-steroidal anti-inflammatory drug use, hormone receptor status, and breast cancer-specific mortality in the Carolina Breast Cancer Study. Breast Cancer Research and Treatment. September 2014, Volume 147, Issue 2, p 415–421

Fibromyalgia treatment. University of Michigan. http://fibroguide.med.umich.edu

Living well with Sickle cell disease. (www.cdc.gov/ncbddd/sicklecell/documents/livingwell-with-sickle cell

Pauline Anderson; Medscape medical news "New 'Brain Food' Scale Flags Best Nutrients for Depression," May 26, 2016).

Dr. Ramsey, Drew. Eat Complete: The 21 Nutrients That Fuel Brainpower, Boost Weight Loss, and Transform Your Health. 2016

Medscape.com: On death and dying by Elizabeth Kubler-Ross 1969

www. Healgrief.org

The Mourner's Bill of Rights. By Alan D. Wolfelt

The Bible. New King James Version, copyright 1982 by Thomas Nelson, Inc.

Dr. Bright Bill; Transferable Concept: How you can be sure you are a Christian. Campus Crusade for Christ

Index

Made in the USA
Columbia, SC
25 March 2021